ATLAS OF URODYNAMICS

Atlas of Urodynamics

Second Edition

Jerry Blaivas
Clinical Professor of Urology
Weill Medical College of Cornell University
Medical Director of UroCenter of New York
New York, NY, USA

Michael B. Chancellor
Professor of Urology and Obstetrics and Gynecology
University of Pittsburgh School of Medicine
Pittsburgh, PA, USA

Jeffrey Weiss
Clinical Associate
Professor of Urology
Weill Medical College of Cornell University
UroCenter
New York, NY, USA

Michael Verhaaren
UroCenter
New York, NY, USA

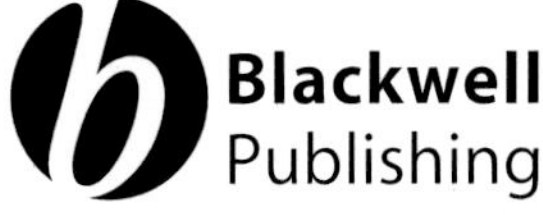
Blackwell
Publishing

Blackwell Publishing, Inc., 350 Main Street, Malden, MA 02148-5020, USA
Blackwell Publishing Ltd, 9600 Garsington Road, Oxford OX4 2DQ, UK

Blackwell Publishing Asia Pty Ltd, 550 Swanston Street, Carlton, Victoria 3053, Australia

First published 1996 (published by Lippincott Williams & Wilkins)

Second edition 2007
1 2007

Library of Congress Cataloging-in-Publication Data
Atlas of urodynamics/Jerry Blaivas, Michael Chancellor, Jeffrey Weiss, and Michael Verhaaren, 2nd edition
p.; cm.
Previous edition: Baltimore: Lippincott Williams & Wilkins, 1996.
Includes bibliographical references and index.
ISBN 978-1-4051-4625-8
1. Urodynamics–Atlases. I. Blaivas, Jerry G. II. Title: Urodynamics.
[DNLM: 1. Urodynamics–Atlases. 2. Urination Disorders–Atlases. WJ 17 A8818 2007]
RC901.9.A85 2007
16.6–dc22
2006035501
ISBN: 978-1-4051-4625-8

A catalogue record for this title is available from the British Library

Set in 10/13½pt Trump Mediaeval by Charon Tec Ltd (A Macmillan Company), Chennai, India
www.charontec.com
Printed and bound in Singapore by COS Printers Pte Ltd
Commissioning Editor: Martin Sugden
Editorial Assistant: Jennifer Seward
Development Editor: Rob Blundell
Production Controller: Debbie Wyer
For further information on Blackwell Publishing, visit our website:
http://www.blackwellpublishing.com

Contents

Preface to the First Edition

life is a journey
from childhood to maturity
and youth to age,
from innocence to awareness
and ignorance to knowing,
from foolishness to discretion
*and then perhaps to wisdom**

This book part of our journey; it is about a quest for understanding the physiology and pathophysiology of the lower urinary tract. At first glance, this seems to be a rather simple task. The lower urinary tract has but two functions, the storage and timely expulsion of urine. The bladder fills (at low pressure) with urine from the kidneys and when the urge to void is felt, micturition is postponed until a socially convenient time. During micturition, the sphincter relaxes, the bladder contracts and the bladder empties.

But there is no sphincter. For sure, the proximal urethra functions as a sphincter, but it cannot be seen with the naked eye. Nor is it apparent under the careful scrutiny of the microscope or in the gross anatomy laboratory. There is no valve, like in the heart. Nevertheless, it works perfectly until damaged by disease or the surgeon's knife or the slow pull of gravity on it's musculofascial supports.

The urodynamic laboratory is, indeed, a laboratory. It is the place where scientific observations and measurements lead to an enhanced understanding of how the lower urinary tract works. Each patient is his own experiment. The purpose of a urodynamic evaluation is reproduce the patient's symptoms or usual voiding pattern and, by making the appropriate measurements and observations, the underlying physiology becomes apparent. This approach is truly multidisciplinary and involves physicians (urologists, gynecologists, neurologists, physiatrists, geriatricians, and radiologists), nurses and enterostomal therapists, behaviorists, and physical therapists.

This book is written for all those who are interested in understanding how the lower urinary tract works and what goes wrong when it malfunctions. Urodynamics encompasses all of the diagnostic modalities used in the evaluation of bladder and urethral function. This ranges from simple diaries of micturition patterns to synchronous measurements of detrusor, urethral, and abdominal pressures, sphincter electromyography and fluoroscopic visualization of the bladder and urethra.

*Gates of Repentance The New Union Prayer Book p. 283, British edition, 1979 Central Congress of American Rabbis and Union of Liberal and Progressive synagogues, Library of Cat card # 78-3667.

The data from these measurements can be analyzed by sophisticated computer programs which quantify detrusor contractility, urethral resistance, and outlet obstruction.

We hope that this book will serve both as a comprehensive review of urodynamic technique and an atlas of normal and abnormal findings that the clinician will want to read in its entirety and keep for future reference. But most of all, we hope that the contents of the book will pique the interest of those whose future research will further enhance our understanding of this fascinating subject.

Preface

Why Urodynamics? Why an Atlas?

A man complains of difficulty voiding. He is otherwise healthy. His urinalysis is normal and his prostate is large. Without knowing any more than that you can treat him with an alpha-adrenergic blocking agent and he has about a 50% chance of clinical improvement. If that fails, you can do a transurethral prostatectomy and the chances of a successful outcome is probably about 75%. That's pretty good and it doesn't cost the health care system too much. But it's pretty bad if you happen to be the patient in the 25% who does not have a successful outcome, especially if you get worse afterwards.

A woman complains of stress incontinence. She, too, is otherwise healthy, and, without knowing any more about her, you do some kind of pubovaginal sling, She'll probably have a successful outcome too. Or maybe she'll get worse.

If you're content with these kinds of results and if you're content treating patients empirically, you don't need urodynamics. But if you want to know more about the subtle differences that distinguish one patient from another, about why one patient fails and another succeeds, why one patient does better with a medication or an operation and another with behavior modification, urodynamics usually provides the answers.

If you don't routinely use urodynamics, in our judgment, both the patient and the doctor are disadvantaged. The patient is disadvantaged because, deprived of a precise diagnosis, treatment, by definition, must be empiric. Some patients will get empiric therapy that is doomed to failures; others may undergo surgery that is doomed to failure when another treatment is more appropriate.

The doctor, too is disadvantaged because he or she is deprived of the experience and knowledge that allows one to detect the subtle differences that distinguish one patient from another. If you treat patients according to an algorithm that begins with simple, non-invasive therapies and progresses to invasive, surgical therapies, you never learn from your own experience.

These are the reasons why we consider urodynamics to be an essential component in the armamentarium of the physician who treats patients with lower urinary tract symptoms.

Why an atlas? For those with logical minds, who like to lump things together, categorize and classify, an atlas might seem redundant. Why not show a few examples of this and that and be done with it? We believe that no two people are exactly alike, that urodynamics are riddled with artifact and that human physiology is subject to the same vicissitudes that afflict every other aspect of life. Why do you have a headache one day, but not another? Why does post-void residual urine vary so much in patients with lower urinary tract symptoms? Why don't patients with overactive bladders have involuntary detrusor contractions every time the bladder fills to a certain volume? Although we can't answer these questions with any degree of certainty, we need to do the best we can. To that end, we consider urodynamics to be a snapshot that records one brief moment of time for a given patient. But if you take enough snapshots of enough people in enough clinical situations, you begin to get a picture of the whole range of pathophysiology. After all, a real time video is nothing more than a bunch of snapshots strung together. For the doctor who never gets to see the whole video, a good atlas provides enough snapshots for him to begin to appreciate the entire spectrum of voiding dysfunction.

Glossary and Abbreviations

ALPP (Abdominal leak point pressure): The lowest abdominal pressure at which leakage is observed from the urethral meatus during cough or valsalva in the absence of a detrusor contraction.

Bladder compliance is calculated by dividing the change in bladder volume by the change in detrusor pressure during that change in bladder volume. Compliance is expressed as ml/cmH_2O.

Bladder sensations: During bladder filling, the International Continence Society (ICS) recommends that the following sensory landmarks be reported: **first sensation of bladder filling (FSF), first desire to void (1st urge), strong desire to void (severe urge)**. Others have recommended that the urge or desire to void during cystometry be recorded on a four points scale [1–3]. **Increased bladder sensation** is defined as a first sensation of bladder filling and/or an early desire to void, and/or an early strong desireto void, which occurs at low bladder volume and persists. **Reduced bladder sensation** is defined as diminished sensation throughout bladder filling. In **absent bladder sensation** the patient has no bladder sensations at all. **Non-specific bladder sensations** make the individual aware of bladder filling such as abdominal fullness or pressure or vegetative symptoms.

Blaivas: Groutz Female Bladder Outlet Obstruction Nomogram. A nomogram that describes 4 categories based on detrusor pressure and uroflow (see Ch. 11, p. 123).

DESD (detrusor–external sphincter dyssynergia): DESD is characterized by involuntary contractions of the striated urethral and periurethral musculature during involuntary detrusor contractions.

DLPP (Detrusor leak point pressure): The lowest detrusor pressure at which leakage is observed from the urethral meatus during bladder filling in the absence of a detrusor contraction.

EMG: Sphincter elelctromyogram obtained with surface electrodes applied to the perineum.

FSF: The bladder volume at which the patient experiences the first sensation of bladder filling during cystometry.

IDC: Involuntary detrusor contraction.

1st urge: The bladder volume at which the patient experiences the first urge to void during cystometry.

LUTS: Lower urinary tract symptoms.

Maximum cystometric capacity is the volume at which the patient feels he/she can no longer delay micturition. In patients with impaired bladder sensation, cystometric capacity may be inferred as that volume at which the patient begins void or leak involuntarily because of detrusor overactivity, low bladder compliance or sphincteric incontinence. In patients with a sphincteric incontinence, cystometric capacity may be increased by mechanical occlusion which prevents leakage as the bladder is being filled. In those with normal bladder compliance and impaired bladder sensation, capacity may be defined as > an arbitrary volume at which bladder filling is stopped.

OAB: Overactive bladder. – "Urgency, with or without urge incontinence, usually with frequency and nocturea."

Type 1 OAB: The patient complains of urgency but there are no involuntary detrusor contractions during urodynamics.

Type 2 OAB: Involuntary detrusor contractions are present, but the patient is aware of them, can contract his or her sphincter, prevent incontenence and abort the detrusor contraction.

Type 3 OAB: Involuntary detrusor contractions are present. The patient can contract the sphincter and momentarely prevent incontinence, but once the sphincter fatigues, incontinence ensures.

Type 4 OAB: There are involuntary detrusor contractions but the patient cannot contract the sphincter on abort the detrusor contraction and is incontinent.

Pdet: Detrusor pressure is that component of Pves that is created by bladder wall forces. It is estimated by subtracting Pabd from Pves (Pdet = Pves − Pabd).

Pdet@Q_{max}: Detrusor pressure at maximum uroflow.

Pves: Intravesical pressure is the pressure within the bladder.

Pabd: abdominal pressure is the pressure surrounding the bladder. It is estimated from rectal pressure measurement.

Q: Uroflow.

Q_{max}: Maximum uroflow.

Schafer (male) Bladder Outlet Obtruction and Detrusor Contractility Nomogram: A nomogram that describes 6 categories of obstruction and detrusor contractility (See Ch. 10, p. 102).

Sensory urgency is a term, abandoned by the ICS, that refers an uncomfortable need to void that is unassociated with detrusor overactivity.

Severe urge: The bladder volume at which the patient experiences a severe urge to void during cystometry.

VH_2O: infused bladder volume at uptometry

VOID: A shorthand method of reporting uroflow and post-void residual (PVR). Q_{max}/voided volume/PVR. For example, a patient with a Q_{max} = 15 ml/s, voided volume = 250 ml and PVR = 10 ml would be reported as 15/250/10.

VLPP: Vesical leak point pressure – the lowest intravesical pressure at which leakage is observed from the urethral meatus during cough or valsalva in the absence of a detrusor contraction.

1 Pre-Urodynamic Evaluation

From a clinical standpoint, the purpose of urodynamic testing is to measure and record various physiologic variables while the patient is experiencing those symptoms which constitute his usual complaints. In this context urodynamics may be considered to be a provocative test of vesicourethral function. Thus, it is the responsibility of the examiner to insure that the patient's symptoms are, in fact, reproduced during the study. To this end, it is important that the examiner has all relevant clinical information in his or her consciousness as the urodynamic study progresses. Prior to the study, the patient should have undergone a fairly extensive evaluation as described below.

The evaluation begins with a thorough history, physical examination, and urinalysis. Urinary tract infection or bacteriuria should be treated and the urodynamic study performed about 6 weeks later. In some patients with persistent bacteriuria or recurrent infection it is advisable to perform the urodynamic evaluation while the patient is taking culture specific antibiotics. In patients who are on intermittent catheterization and have bacteriuria, we administer a culture specific antibiotic about 1/2 hour before the study begins.

We strongly advocate supplementing the history with a validated symptom and medical questionnaire. The patient should fill out these questionnaires and the physician should review them prior to taking the history so that he or she can utilize the information to help structure the history taking. A sample questionnaire is shown in Appendix 1A.

History

The history begins with a detailed account of the precise nature of the patient's symptoms. Each symptom should be characterized and quantified as accurately as possible by anamnesis, questionnaire, bladder diary, and, for incontinence, a pad test. When more than one symptom is present, the patient's assessment of the relative severity of each should be noted. The examiner should not rely on any one of these tools, but rather, use each to corroborate the other.

The patient should be asked how often he urinates during the day and night, how long he can comfortably go between urinations, and how long micturition can be postponed once he gets the urge to void. It should be determined why he voids as often as he does. Is it because of a severe urge or is it merely out of convenience or an attempt to prevent incontinence or other symptoms? If the patient is incontinent, its severity should be graded. Does stress incontinence occur during coughing, sneezing, rising from a sitting to standing position, or only during heavy physical exercise? If the incontinence is associated with stress, is urine lost only for an instant during the stress or is there uncontrollable voiding? Is the incontinence positional? Does it ever occur in the lying or sitting position? Is there a sense of urgency first? Does urge incontinence occur? Is the patient aware of the act of incontinence or does he just find himself wet? Is there continuous involuntary loss of urine? Does the patient lose a few drops or saturate the outer clothing? Is there enuresis? Are protective pads worn? Do they become saturated? How often are they changed?

Are there voiding symptoms? Is there difficulty initiating the stream requiring pushing or straining to start? Is the stream weak, dribbling, or interrupted? Is there post-void dribbling? Has the patient ever been in urinary retention?

In women, is there pelvic organ prolapse? Prolapse may present with a spectrum of lower urinary tract symptoms (LUTS) as described above and they may or not be causally related to the prolapse. In some women voiding is facilitated by applying pressure on the anterior wall of the vagina or reducing the prolapse either manually or with a pessary. In some patients, prolapse causes urethral obstruction (particularly those with grades 3 and 4). In others, it masks sphincteric incontinence that only becomes evident once the prolapse is reduced [1]. A history of prior stress incontinence that spontaneously subsided is suggestive of "occult stress incontinence."

Past medical history

The patient should be specifically queried about neurologic conditions that are known to affect bladder and sphincteric function such as multiple sclerosis, spinal cord injury, lumbar disk disease, myelodysplasia, diabetes, stroke, Parkinson's disease, or multisystem atrophy. If he does not have a previously diagnosed neurologic disease it is important to ask about double vision, muscular weakness, paralysis or poor coordination, tremor, numbness, and tingling. In women, a history of vaginal surgery or previous surgical repair of incontinence should suggest the possibility of sphincteric injury. Abdominoperineal resection of the rectum or radical hysterectomy may be associated with neurologic injury to the bladder and sphincter resulting in sphincteric incontinence, urinary retention (due to detrusor areflexia), and hydronephrosis (due to low bladder compliance). Radiation therapy may cause a small capacity, low compliance bladder, or radiation cystitis.

In men, a history of prior medical or surgical treatment for benign and malignant prostate conditions should be sought. Of particular importance is treatment for prostate cancer – radical prostatectomy, brachytherapy, external beam radiation, and cyrotherapy. Each of these may be complicated by sphincteric incontinence, or urethral or anastamotic stricture. The radiation based therapies can cause particularly difficult to treat urethral strictures and radiation cystitis.

Medications sometimes cause LUTS. Alpha-adrenergic agonists, even those contained in over-the-counter cold remedies, can cause urethral obstruction and urinary retention. Tricyclic antidepressants may also cause bladder outlet obstruction. Narcotic analgesics and antihistamines can cause impaired or absent detrusor contractility that can culminate in urinary retention. Alpha adrenergic antagonists may cause stress incontinence. Parasympathomimetics such as bethanechol may cause involuntary detrusor contractions and bladder pain.

Physical examination

The physical examination should focus on detecting anatomic and neurologic abnormalities that contribute to urinary incontinence. The neurourologic examination begins by observing the patient's gait and demeanor as he or she first enters the examination room. A slight limp or lack of coordination, an abnormal speech pattern, facial asymmetry, or other abnormalities may be subtle signs of a neurologic condition. The abdomen and flanks should be examined for masses, hernias, and a distended bladder. Rectal examination will disclose the size and consistency of the prostate. *Sacral innervation* (predominately S2, S3, S4) is evaluated by assessing anal sphincter tone and control, genital sensation, and the bulbocavernosus reflex.

In women, a vaginal examination should be performed with the bladder both full (to check for incontinence and prolapse) and empty (to examine the gynecologic organs). The degree of prolapse can be assessed by either the Baden–Walker system (grades 1–4) [2] or by the pelvic organ prolapse quantification system (POP-Q) which assesses each compartment separately [3]. With the bladder comfortably full in the lithotomy position, the patient is asked to cough or strain in an attempt to reproduce the incontinence. The degree of urethral hypermobility may be assessed by the Q-tip test [4,5]. The Q-tip test is performed by inserting a well-lubricated sterile cotton-tipped applicator gently through the urethra into the bladder. Once in the bladder, the applicator is withdrawn to the point of resistance, which is at the level of the bladder neck. The resting angle from the horizontal is recorded. The patient is then asked to strain or cough and the degree of angulation is assessed. Hypermobility is defined as a resting or straining angle of greater than 30 degrees from the horizontal. If stress incontinence is suspected, but not demonstrated with the patient in the lithotomy position, the examination is repeated in the standing position.

In men, the examination focuses on the abdomen and prostate in addition to neurologic testing of the perineum and lower extremities. As for women, if stress incontinence is suspected, but not demonstrated, the examination should be repeated in the standing position with a full bladder while the patient coughs and strains.

Bladder diary

The bladder diary records the patient's voiding patterns in his/her own environment and during normal daily activities. The diary is useful not only for diagnosis, but also insofar as the patient and physician gain insights into behavioral and environmental factors that aid in the development of a treatment plan [9]. Diary recordings have been shown to be reproducible and more accurate than patient's recall [10,11]. Although there may be great variability in the actual data accumulated by these instruments, simply asking the patient whether the diary and pad test are representative of a "good" or "bad" day can be very useful. We believe that bladder diaries are extremely useful and recommend that they be part of not only the initial evaluation, but also for follow-up. In the clinical setting, 24-hour diaries are adequate for the evaluation of LUTS.

Pad test

For patients with incontinence, a pad test allows for the detection and quantification of urine loss over a set period of time. Pad tests have been described for multiple lengths of time from <1 hour to 1 week [12–15], but we find a simple 24-hour pad test done in conjunction with the bladder diary the day prior to the next office visit to be most useful [10].

Uroflowmetry ("free flow")

We believe that uroflow and PVR should be part of the initial evaluation of all patients undergoing invasive urodynamics. The flow rate is a composite measure of the interaction between the pressure generated by the detrusor and the resistance offered by the urethra. Thus, a low uroflow may be caused by either bladder outlet obstruction or impaired detrusor contractility [16]. It should be interpreted in conjunction with the maximum voided volume (from the bladder diary) and PVR. Uroflow is discussed in detail in Chapter 4.

Post-void residual volume

Post-void residual (PVR) is the volume of urine remaining in the bladder immediately following a representative void. Unless there is another reason to catheterize the patient (for cystoscopy or urodynamic study) PVR should be estimated by ultrasound. There is considerable intra-individual variability in PVR and for that reason serial measurements are often necessary [6–8].

In summary, the pre-urodynamic assessment comprises the following information:

1 A focused history and physical examination.
2 Urinalysis with or without culture.
3 A 24-hour bladder diary.
4 A 24-hour pad test (for patients with incontinence).
5 Uroflow.
6 Estimation of PVR urine.

Further, in order to interpret urodynamic studies properly, the following information should be available to the examiner before the start of the study:

- What symptoms are you trying to reproduce?
- What is the functional bladder capacity (maximum voided volume on the voiding diary)?
- What is the PVR
- What is the uroflow?
- Is there a neurologic disorder that could cause neurogenic bladder?

When the patient does experience his or her symptoms, the resulting physiologic data provide the substrate for understanding the etiology of the patient's complaint and directing treatment. However, when the symptoms are not reproduced, the data often prove to be irrelevant and, in many instances, even misleading. For example, if a patient complains of urinary frequency, urgency, and urge incontinence, and cystometry reveals involuntary detrusor contractions which exactly reproduce the symptoms, then the diagnosis is straightforward. However, if a patient complains only of stress incontinence and the cystometrogram demonstrates low magnitude involuntary detrusor contractions of which he or she is completely unaware, which do not reproduce her symptoms, one would be misled to conclude that the etiology of the incontinence is detrusor overactivity.

Another very common source of confusion occurs when a patient is unable to void or generate a detrusor contraction during the urodynamic study. If the examiner knows beforehand that the patient has a normal uroflow, no residual urine, and complains only of stress incontinence, such urodynamic findings are little clinical value.

The widespread availability of many different urodynamic techniques and parameters may confound the practicing physician, but in principle there are only five in number – cystometry, uroflow, leak point pressure, sphincter electromyography, and radiographic visualization of the lower urinary tract. (We do not recommend urethral pressure profilometry and do not discuss it in this book.) Each may be performed alone or synchronously with one another. When done synchronously, the tests are called multichannel urodynamics and when performed with fluoroscopic visualization of the lower urinary tract, it is called videourodynamics. Each of these topics is covered in a separate chapter. The variables chosen for a particular study depend on a number of factors – the complexity of the clinical problem, the availability of electronic equipment, the ease with which the study can be performed and the interest and expertise of the urodynamicist.

Urodynamic personnel

There was a time when urodynamics consisted of nothing more than a catheter, some tubing, and a fluid reservoir. Those days are gone forever and nowadays the urodynamic staff (often only one person) must be nurse, clinician, technician, equipment repairman, software engineer, and cleaning staff. In this environment, properly trained personnel are essential to the operation of the urodynamic laboratory. In order to perform and interpret studies, the professional staff should be well acquainted with lower urinary tract anatomy, physiology, neurophysiology, and pathophysiology. They must also be well versed in interpretation of urodynamic findings and the many sources of artifact and misinterpretation of data. Further, since most urodynamic equipment is computer based, the knowledge of computer hardware, software, and troubleshooting is almost mandatory.

Suggested Reading

1 Chaikin, D, Romanzi, LJ, Rosenthal, J. Weiss, JP, Blaivas, JG, The Effect of Genital Prolapse on micturition, Neurourol Urodynam, 17: 344, 1988.

2 Baden W, Walker T. *Surgical Repair of Vaginal Defects*, Philadelphia: JB Lippincott, 1992.

3 Bump RC, Mattaisson A, Bo K, et al. The standardization of terminology of female pelvic organ prolapse and pelvic floor dysfunction, *Am J Obstet Gynecol*, 175: 10–17, 1996.

4 Bergman A, Bhatia NN. Urodynamic appraisal of the Marshall–Marchetti test in women with stress urinary incontinence, *Urology*, 29: 458–462, 1987.

5 Birch NC, Hurst G, Doyle PT. Serial residual volumes in men with prostatic hypertrophy, *Br J Urol*, 62: 571–575, 1998.

6 Griffiths DJ, Harrison G, Moore K, et al. Variability of post void residual volume in the elderly, *Urol Res*, 24: 23–26, 1996.

7 Stoller ML, Millard RJ. The accuacy of a catheterized residual volume, *J Urol*, 141: 15–16, 1989.

8 Groutz A, Blaivas JG, Chaikin DC, Resnick NM, Engleman K, Anzalone D, Bryzinski B, Wein AJ. Noninvasive outcome measures of urinary incontinence and lower urinary tract symptoms: a multicenter study of micturition diary and pad tests, *J Urol*, 164: 698–701, 2000.

9 Jorgensen L, Lose G, Andersen JT. One hour pad weighing test for objective assessment of female urinary incontinence, *Obstet Gynecol*, 69: 39–42, 1987.

10 Jakobsen H, Vedel P, Andersen JT. Objective assessment of urinary incontinence: an evaluation of three different pad-weighing tests, *Neurourol Urodyn*, 6: 325–330, 1987.

11 Chancellor MB, Blaivas JG, Kaplan SA, Axelrod S. Bladder outlet obstruction versus impaired detrusor contractility: role of uroflow, *J Urol*, 145: 810–812, 1991.

12 Burgio KL, Goode PS. Behavioral interventions for incontinence in ambulatory geriatric patients, *Am J Med Sci*, 314: 257–261, 1997.

13 Chaikin DC, Romanzi LJ, Rosenthal J, Weiss JP, Blaivas JG. The effects of genital prolapse on micturition, *Neurourol Urodyn*, 17: 426–427, 1998.

14 Kinn A, Larsson B. Pad test with fixed bladder volume in urinary stress incontinence, *Acta Obstet Gynecol Scand*, 66: 369–371, 1987.

15 Walters MD, Jackson GM. Urethral mobility and its relationship to stress incontinence in women, *J Reprod Med*, 35: 777–784, 1990.

Appendix 1A: LUTS Questionnaire

OAB & Incontinence Questionnaire

NAME: ______________________ DATE: ______________________

Instructions: Please mark only one answer for each question and do not handwrite any answers. Most symptoms vary from day to day. We understand that if you check off more than one you feel that you will be providing more information about your condition. *Please do not do this*. Just check the box that best describes you. You will have the opportunity to discuss your symptoms in more detail with your doctor.

1 How often do you usually urinate during the day?

- ______ Not more often than once in 4 hours
- ______ About every 3–4 hours
- ______ About every 2–3 hours
- ______ About every 1–2 hours
- ______ At least once an hour

2 How many times do you usually urinate during the day?

- ______ 8 or less times
- ______ 9–10 times
- ______ 11–12 times
- ______ 13–14 times
- ______ 15 or more times

3 How often do you usually urinate during the night?

- ______ Never
- ______ About every 3–4 hours
- ______ About every 2–3 hours
- ______ About every 1–2 hours
- ______ At least once an hour

4 How many times do you usually urinate at night (from the time you go to bed until the time you wake up for the day)?

- ______ 0 time
- ______ 1 time
- ______ 2 times
- ______ 3 times
- ______ 4 or more times

5 What is the reason that you usually urinate?

- ______ Out of convenience (no urge or desire)
- ______ Because I have a mild urge or desire (but can delay urination for over an hour if I have to)
- ______ Because I have a moderate urge or desire (but can delay urination for more than 10 but less than 60 minutes if I have to)

——— Because I have a severe urge or desire (but can delay urination for less than 10 minutes)
——— Because I have desperate urge or desire (must stop what I am doing and go immediately)

6 Once you get the urge or desire to urinate, how long can you usually postpone it comfortably?
——— More than 60 minutes
——— About 30–60 minutes
——— About 10–30 minutes
——— A few minutes (less than 10 minutes)
——— Must go immediately

7 How often do you get a sudden urge or desire to urinate that makes you want to stop what you are doing and rush to the bathroom?
——— Never (go to question 11)
——— Rarely (go to question 9)
——— A few times a month (go to question 9)
——— A few times a week (go to question 9)
——— At least once a day (go to question 8)

8 How often do you get a sudden urge or desire to urinate that makes you want to stop what you are doing and rush to the bathroom?
——— Once a day
——— Twice a day
——— Three times a day
——— Four times a day
——— Five or more times a day

9 How often do you get a sudden urge or desire to urinate that makes you want to stop what you are doing and rush to the bathroom but you don't get there in time (i.e. you leak urine or wet pads)?
——— Never (go to question 11)
——— Rarely (go to question 11)
——— A few times a month (go to question 11)
——— A few times a week (go to question 11)
——— At least once a day (go to question 10)

10 How often do you get a sudden urge or desire to urinate that makes you want to stop what you are doing and rush to the bathroom but you don't get there in time (i.e. you leak urine or wet pads)?
——— Once a day
——— Twice a day
——— Three times a day
——— Four times a day
——— Five or more times a day

11 How often do you experience urine leakage related to physical activity (lifting, bending, and changing positions, coughing or sneezing)?
——— Never (go to question 13)
——— Rarely (go to question 13)

- ______ A few times a month (go to question 13)
- ______ A few times a week (go to question 13)
- ______ At least once a day (go to question 12)

12 How often do you experience urine leakage related to physical activity (lifting, bending, and changing positions, coughing or sneezing)?

- ______ Once a day
- ______ Twice a day
- ______ Three times a day
- ______ Four times a day
- ______ Five or more times a day

13 How often do you wet yourself, your pads, or your clothes without any awareness of how or when it happened?

- ______ Never
- ______ Rarely
- ______ A few times a month
- ______ A few times a week
- ______ At least once a day

14 In your opinion how good is your bladder control?

- ______ Perfect control
- ______ Very good
- ______ Good
- ______ Poor
- ______ No control at all

15 How often do you have a sensation of not emptying your bladder completely after you finish urinating?

- ______ Never
- ______ Rarely
- ______ A few times a month
- ______ A few times a week
- ______ At least once a day

16 How often do you stop and start during urination?

- ______ Never
- ______ Rarely
- ______ A few times a month
- ______ A few times a week
- ______ At least once a day

17 How often do you have a weak urinary stream?

- ______ Never
- ______ Rarely
- ______ A few times a month
- ______ A few times a week
- ______ At least once a day

18 How often do you push or strain to begin urination?

——— Never
——— Rarely
——— A few times a month
——— A few times a week
——— At least once a day

19 How bothered are you by your bladder symptoms?

——— Not at all
——— A little bit
——— Pretty bothersome
——— A lot
——— I find it intolerable

Answer the next question only if you have begun treatment for your bladder condition

20 Compared to the way you were before your treatment with ————, do you consider yourself to be:

——— Cured?
——— Very much improved?
——— A little bit improved?
——— About the same?
——— Worse?

2 Normal Micturition

The micturition cycle (urine storage and voiding) is a nearly subconscious process that is under complete voluntary control. Bladder filling is accomplished without sensation and without an appreciable rise in detrusor pressure until a critical bladder volume is reached at which point one begins to feel the gradual onset of the urge to void. As bladder filling continues, the sensation of the need to void increases, but micturition can normally be delayed for an hour or more once this is felt. Voiding is normally accomplished by activation of the micturition reflex – a coordinated neuromuscular event characterized by an orderly physiologic sequence (Fig. 2.1). The first recorded event is a sudden and complete relaxation of the striated sphincteric muscles, characterized by complete electrical silence of the sphincter electromyogram (EMG). Next, there is a fall in urethral pressure followed almost immediately by a rise in detrusor pressure as the bladder and proximal urethra become isobaric. The vesical neck and urethra open and voiding ensues. The reflex is normally under voluntary control and is organized in the rostral brain stem (the pontine micturition center). It requires integration and modulation by the parasympathetic and somatic components of the sacral spinal cord (the sacral micturition center).

During urine storage, there are a number of physiologic mechanisms to maintain continence Fig. 2.2. (1) During bladder filling, there is a gradual increase in sphincter EMG activity (2) Immediately prior to cough there is a reflex contraction of the sphincter manifest as a rise in urethral pressure. (3) During straining or valsalva, there is equal transmission of pressure from the abdomen to the urethra. (4) If a person wants to stop in the midst of voiding or to prevent voiding during an involuntary detrusor contraction, he or she contracts the sphincter, interrupting the stream and then, through a reflex mechanism, the detrusor contraction abates (see Figs. 2.9–2.11).

In clinical practice, urethral pressures are no longer measured during routine urodynamic studies. The format for urodynamic studies usually includes synchronous measurement of uroflow (Q), vesical pressure (pves), abdominal pressure (pabd), detrusor pressure (pdet) sphincter EMG and infused bladder volume (Fig. 2.3). Normal micturition in a man and woman is depicted in Figs. 2.4 and 2.5, respectively. In some patients, mostly women, urethral resistance is so low that when the detrusor reflex is activated, there is either a very low or no discernible rise at all in detrusor pressure. Rather, when the detrusor contracts, because of low urethral resistance, all of the energy is converted to flow (Figs. 2.6–2.8). This is considered to be a normal variant.

Some patients are unable to urinate in their normal fashion because of the embarrassing and unfamiliar setting of the urodynamic laboratory.

In these circumstances, one can infer that the study is normal by extracting data from the study during the filling phase (sensation, capacity, continence) and voiding (detrusor pressure), and extrapolating from prior or subsequent unintubated uroflows to assess the detrusor pressure/uroflow characteristics (Fig. 2.8): Figures 10 and 11 depict normal urine storage mechanisms.

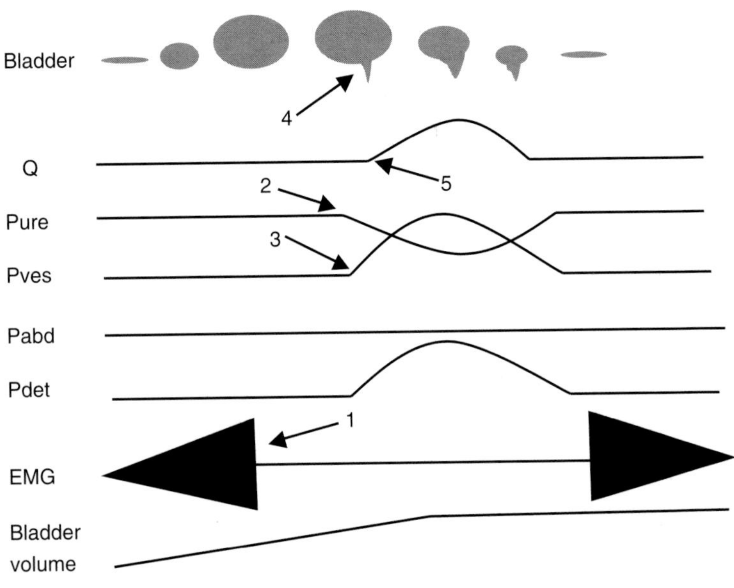

Fig. 2.1 The micturition reflex is characterized by an orderly sequence of events: (1) relaxation of the striated muscles of the sphincter (EMG silence), (2) fall in urethral pressure, (3) rise in detrusor pressure, (4) opening of the urethra, and (5) uroflow. Q = uroflow; Pure = urethral pressure; Pves = vesical pressure; Pdet = detrusor pressure; EMG = sphincter electromyogram.

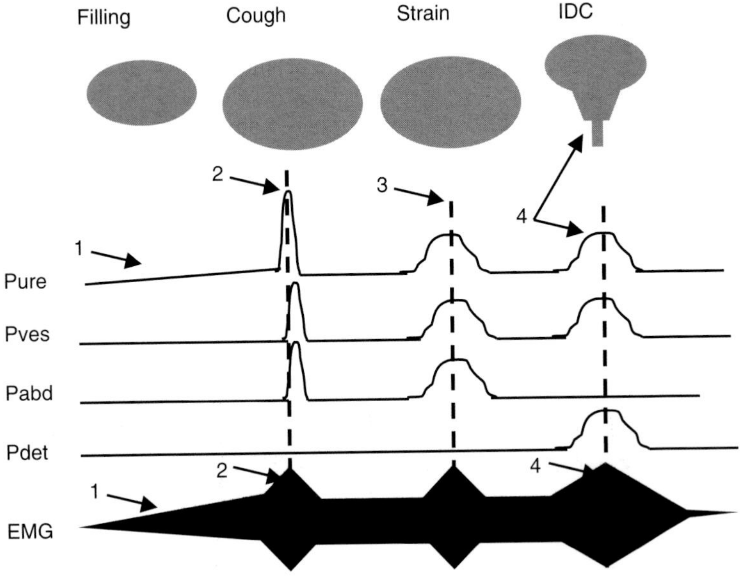

Fig. 2.2 Normal storage reflexes: (1) During bladder filling, there is a gradual increase in sphincter EMG activity that causes a gradual increase in urethral pressure. (2) Immediately prior to cough there is a reflex contraction of the sphincter manifest as a rise in urethral pressure. (3) During straining or valsalva, there is equal transmission of pressure from the abdomen to the urethra. (4) If a person wants to stop in the midst of voiding or to prevent voiding during an involuntary detrusor contraction, he or she contracts the sphincter, raising urethral pressure, interrupting the stream and then, through a reflex mechanism, the detrusor contraction abates.

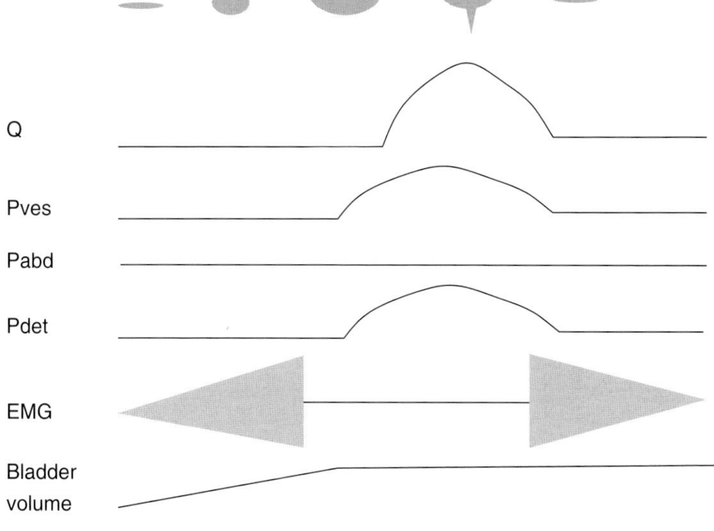

Fig. 2.3 Format for depiction of videourodynamic studies in this book. In most studies either EMG or bladder volume is displayed.

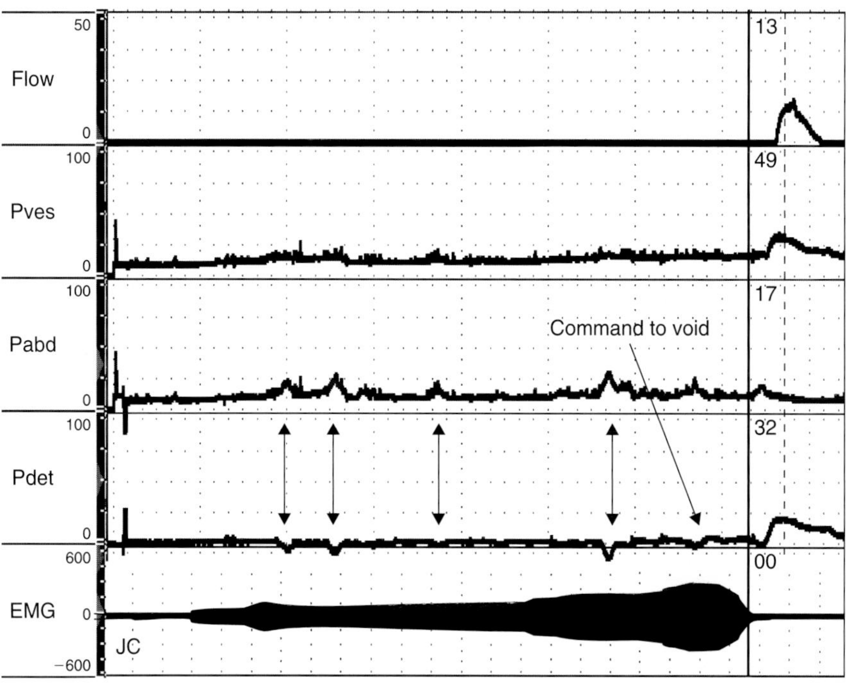

(A)

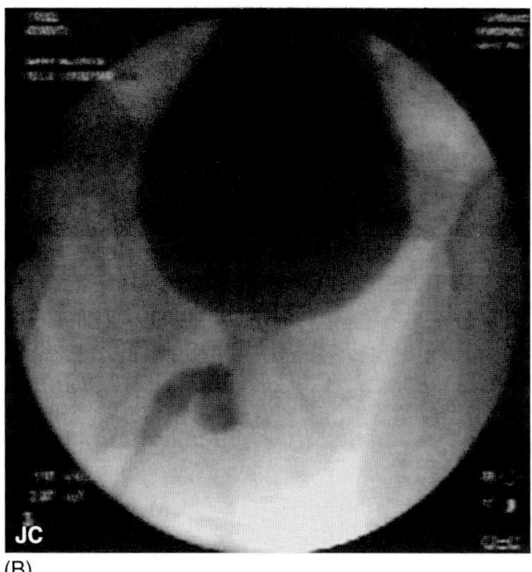

(B)

Fig. 2.4 Normal micturition in a 74-year-old man who was evaluated because of a history of urinary frequency that was determined to be caused by polyuria due to excessive fluid consumption based on his belief that "it is healthy to drink a lot of water." (A) Urodynamic tracing. FSF = 93ml; 1st urge = 210ml, severe urge = 597ml, and bladder capacity = 673ml. Note that there are several rectal contractions (arrows) that cause an artifactual fall in Pdet. When asked to void, the EMG sphincter relaxation (vertical solid line) occurred prior to the onset of the detrusor contraction. Q_{max} = 16ml/s, and Pdet@Q_{max} = 20cmH_2O (vertical dashed line). (B) X-ray obtained during the first third of voiding shows a normally funneled bladder neck and an open urethra.

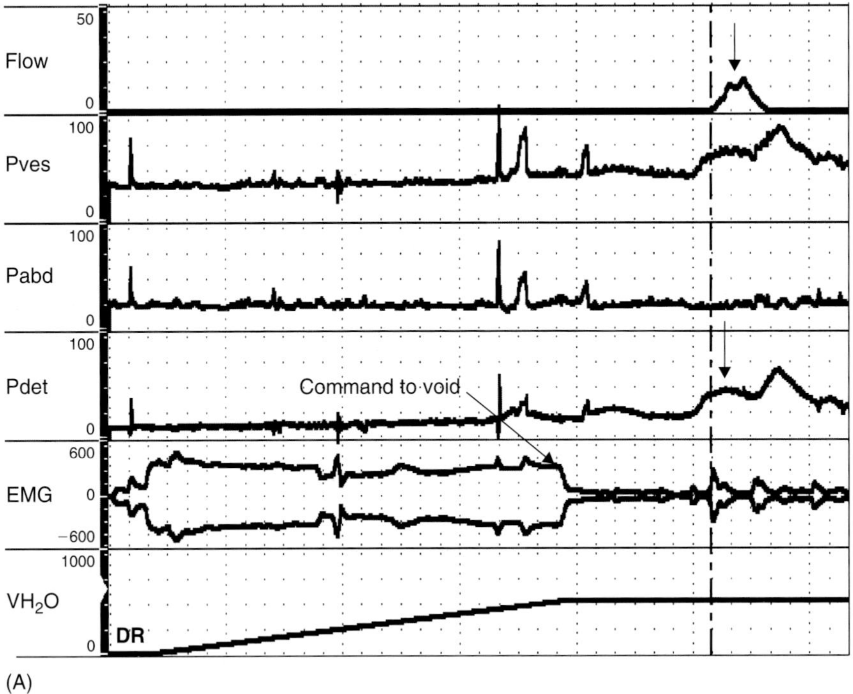

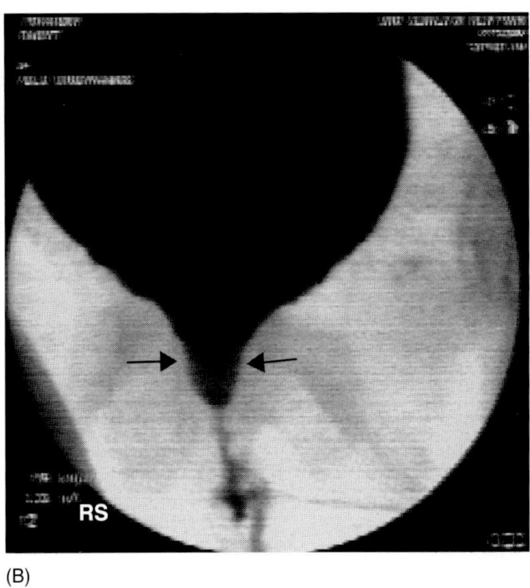

Fig. 2.5 Normal micturition in a 59-year-old woman referred for evaluation of elevated residual urine found unexpected during CAT scan done for abdominal pain. She denied any urologic symptoms. Uroflow was normal (VOID: 25/230/0). (A) Urodynamic study. FSF = 75 ml, 1st urge = 210 ml, severe urge = 523 ml, bladder capacity = 533 ml. At the command to void, the sphincter EMG tracing becomes silent and there is a slight rise in detrusor pressure followed by a sustained detrusor contraction and near normal uroflow curve. During voiding there were several small increases in EMG activity. The first one (the vertical dotted line) momentarily prevents micturition, but as she relaxes, she voids with a normal upswing in the flow curve. The second one occurs after flow has begun to decline and appears to have no effect on flow (i.e. an artifact). Once she emptied her bladder and flow ceased, there is a further rise in detrusor pressure (an aftercontraction). Aftercontractions are considered to be normal variants. Q_{max} = 16 ml, Pdet@Qmax = 43 cmH_2O, Pdetmax = 50 cmH_2O, voided volume = 533 ml, and PVR = 0 ml. (B) X-ray obtained during voiding shows a normal, funneled bladder neck (black arrows) and open urethra.

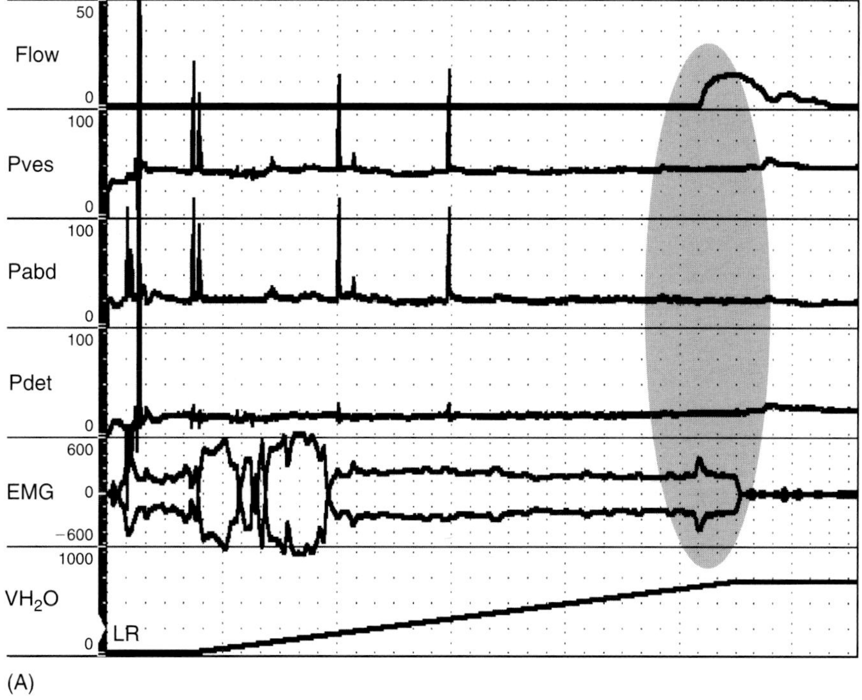

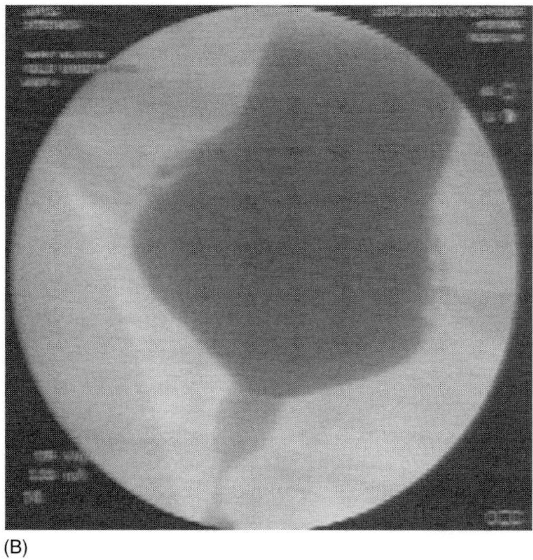
(B)

Fig. 2.6 In this 74-year-old woman, normal micturition is accomplished without an appreciable rise in Pdet. Since there is no rise in Pabd either, the only possible explanation for this is that there is a detrusor contraction, but all of the energy is converted to uroflow because urethral resistance is very low. (A) Urodynamic tracing. In this patient there is an apparent increase in sphincter EMG activity at the beginning of voiding. That it is an artifact is demonstrated by the fact that there is no rise in detrusor pressure despite a smooth rise in uroflow (shaded oval). Q_{max} = 16 ml/s, Pdet@ Q_{max} = 23 cmH_2O, Pdetmax = 28 cmH_2O, voided volume = 624 ml, and PVR = 89 ml. (B) X-ray obtained during the first part of voiding shows the proximal two-thirds of the urethra to be wide open, but there is an apparent narrowing in the distal third. However, the Pdet/Q curve excludes any possibility of urethral obstruction, so this is considered a normal variant, sometimes termed a "spinning top" urethra.

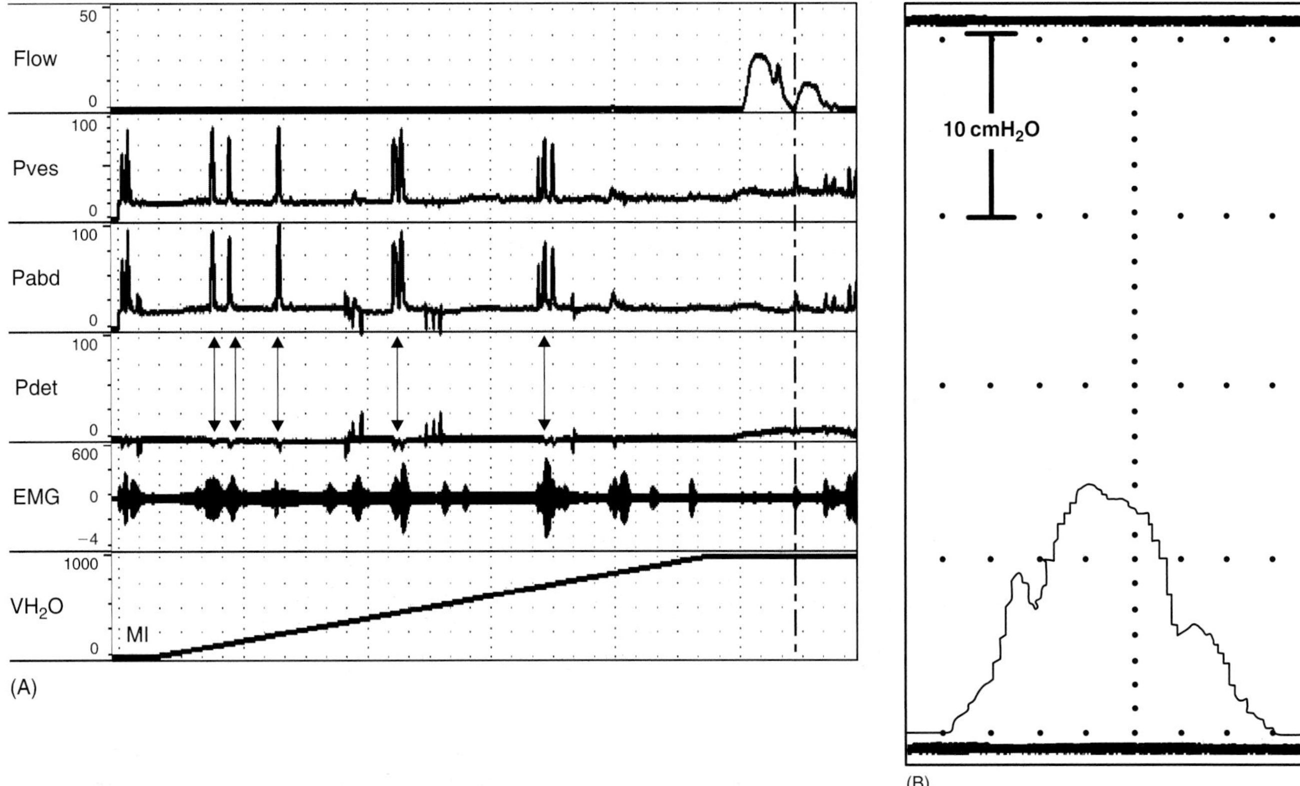

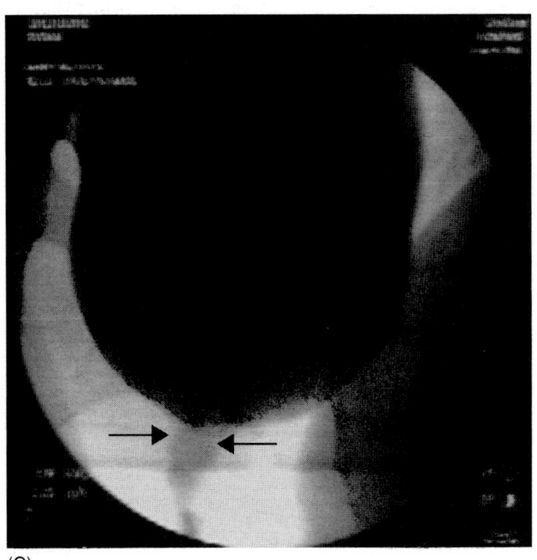

Fig. 2.7 Normal micturition in a 62-year-old woman with a low Pdetmax and a large bladder capacity. (A) Urodynamic tracing. FSF = 394 ml, 1st urge = 755 ml, severe urge occurred at 911 ml, and bladder capacity = 1001 ml. During bladder filling she was asked to cough a number of times to test for stress incontinence (arrows). The slight fall (negative deflection) in pdet is due a small subtraction error and of no significance. During the voluntary detrusor contraction, there is a single interruption of the stream caused by a momentary contraction of the striated sphincter (vertical dotted black line). Since her prior uroflow was normal (see Fig. 2.5(B)), we consider this to be a normal variant due to the unfamiliar setting of the urodynamic study. Qmax = 27 ml/s, Pdet@Qmax = 5 cmH_2O, Pdetmax = 9 cmH_2O, voided volume = 856 ml, and PVR = 141 ml. (B) Uroflow just prior to urodynamic study. Qmax = 14 ml/s, voided volume = 106 ml, and PVR = 0 ml. (C) X-ray obtained early in micturition shows a normally funneled bladder neck and open urethra (arrows).

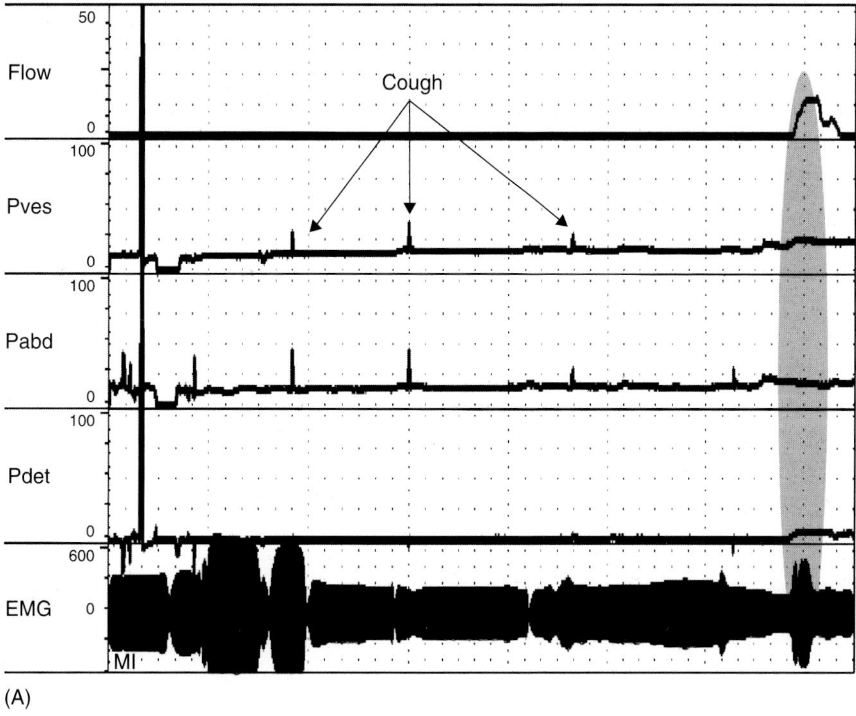

Fig. 2.8 ML is an 82-year-old woman evaluated because of recurrent episodes of bacterial cystitis. She denies lower urinary tract symptoms (LUTS). (A) Urodynamic study. FSF = 290 ml, 1st urge = 348 ml, severe urge = 382 ml, bladder capacity = 382 ml, Qmax = 15 ml/s, Pdet@Qmax = 7 cmH_2O, Pdetmax = 7 cmH_2O, voided volume = 382 ml, and PVR = 0 ml. The apparent rise in EMG activity (shaded oval) is likely an artifact since there is neither a rise in Pdet nor a fall in uroflow. Note that during each cough, pressure is transmitted equally to the bladder and abdomen (and urethra, not pictured here). This is one of the mechanisms to maintain continence.

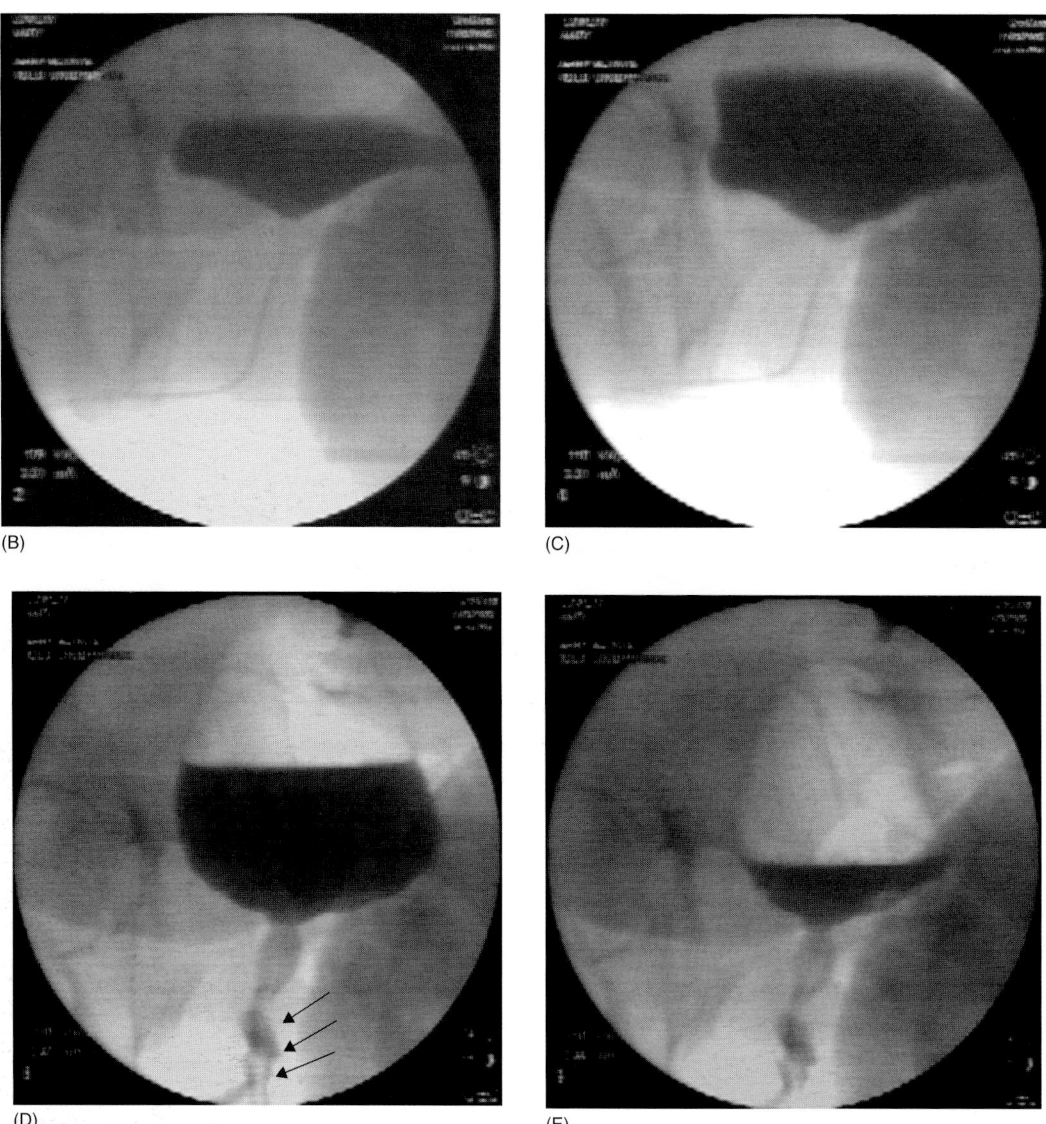

Fig. 2.8 (continued) (B+C) X-rays obtained during bladder filling showing a normal bladder contour. (D) X-ray obtained at Q_{max} shows a urethra of normal contour and some contrast in the vagina (arrows). (E) X-ray obtained near the end of micturition.

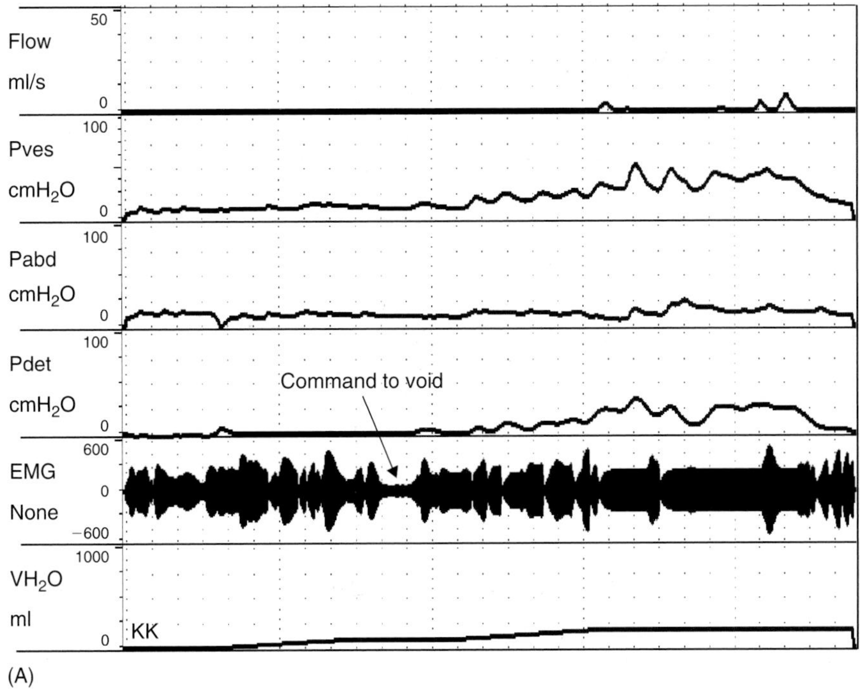

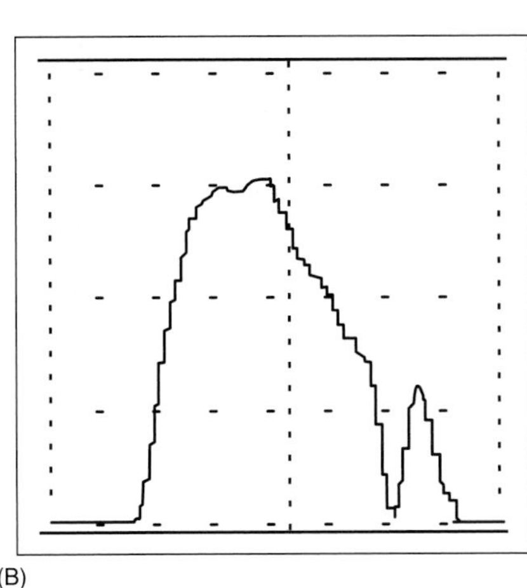
(B)

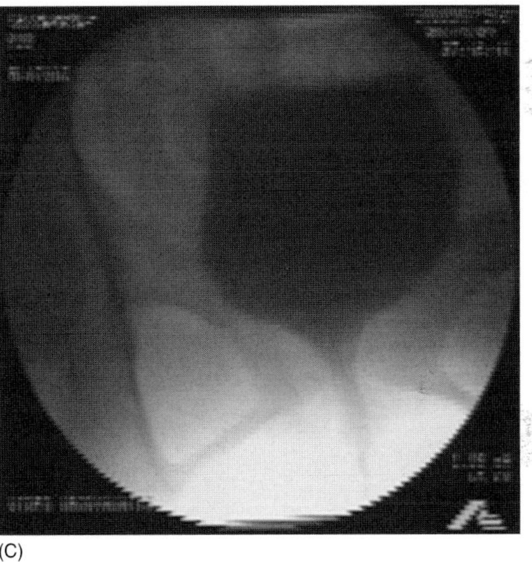
(C)

Fig. 2.9 Normal variant KK is a 23-year-old woman evaluated because of recurrent urinary tract infections associated with sexual activity. Bladder diary was normal, maximum voided volume was 360 ml and uroflow was normal. (A) Urodynamic study. FSF = 28 ml, 1st urge = 102 ml, severe urge = 124 ml, and bladder capacity = 192 ml. At the command to void, she relaxes her sphincter (EMG becomes silent) and develops a detrusor contraction, but involuntarily contracts her sphincter (increased EMG activity) and that reflexly aborts the detrusor contraction. This process is repeated over and over again during the study and she voids with a markedly interrupted stream. She stated, though, that she never voids like this and admitted that she was simply unable to relax during the study. Since her Pdetmax (43 cmH_2O) is normal and her unintubated uroflow was normal (see Fig. 2.8(B)), we concluded that she is normal. Of course, if this were representative of the way she usually voids, we would consider it to be an acquired voiding dysfunction. Q_{max} = 8 ml/s, Pdet@Q_{max} = 26 cmH_2O, Pdetmax = 43 cmH_2O, voided volume = 117 ml, and PVR = 67 ml. Normal uroflow done 1 week prior to urodynamic study. Q_{max} = 30 ml/s; Q_{ave} = 9 ml/s, voided volume = 252 ml, PVR = 0 ml, (C) X-ray obtained at Q_{max} shows a normal bladder and urethra.

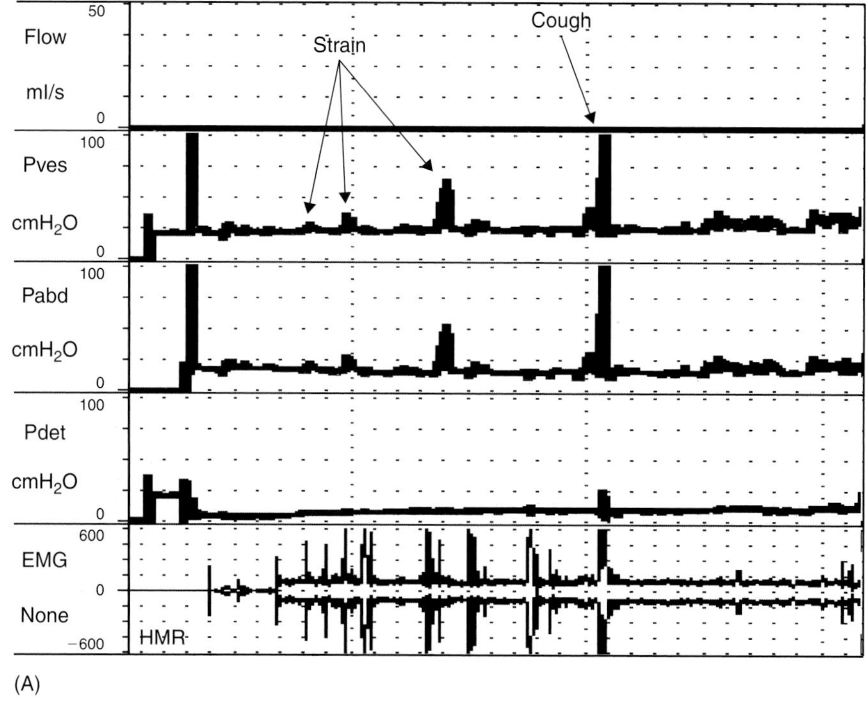

(A)

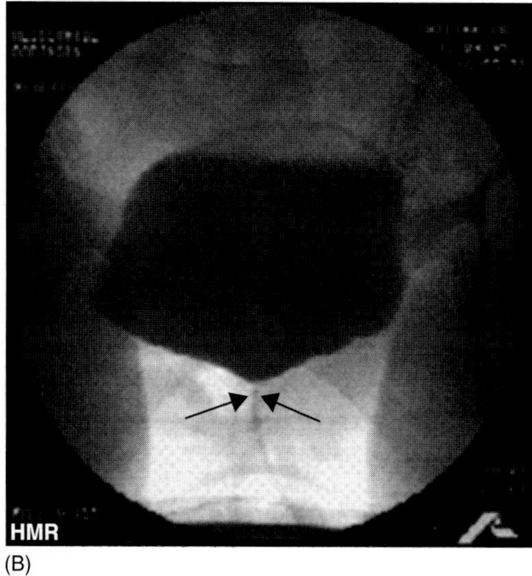

(B)

Fig. 2.10 Storage mechanisms: (A) Urodynamic tracing. During cough and strain there is equal transmission of pressure to the bladder and urethra accompanied by an increase in sphincter EMG. (B) The urethra remains closed (arrows) and continence is preserved during straining. Note that the bladder base has descended well below the pubis.

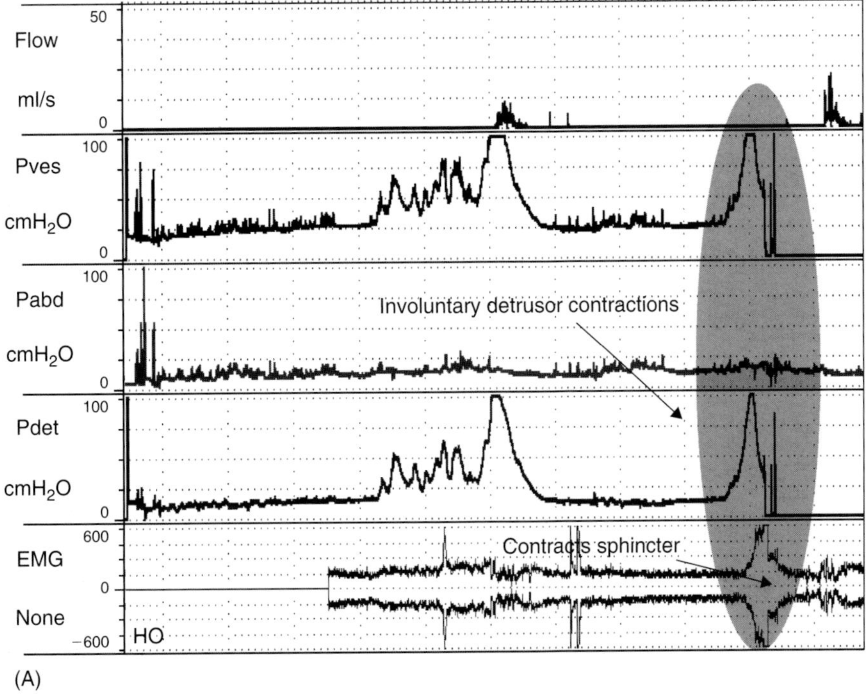

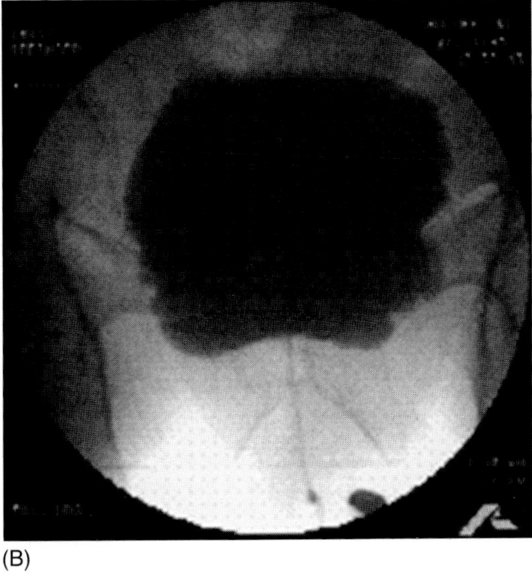

Fig. 2.11 Storage reflexes interrupting the urinary stream and aborting the detrusor contraction: The patient is a man with mostatic obstruction. (A) Urodynamic tracing. During an involuntary detrusor contraction, the patient voluntarily contracts his sphincter, obstructing the urethra. The detrusor contraction subsides and he is not incontinent (shaded oval). (B) X-ray obtained as he contracts his sphincter to prevent incontinence. One would expect the contrast to stop at the membranous urethra, but since he has prostatic obstruction the entire proximal urethra, is narrowed.

Cystometry

3

Cystometry (CMG, cystometrogram) has been described as the "reflex hammer" of the urodynamicist. It is not only the method by which the pressure/volume relationship of the bladder is measured, but it is also an interactive process which permits examination of motor and sensory function. It is used to assess detrusor activity, sensation, capacity, compliance, and control of the micturition process. Before beginning the CMG, the examiner should have access to the patient's history, bladder capacity, and post-void residual urine. After a detailed explanation to the patient, the examination is begun by passing a catheter into the bladder, measuring residual urine, and filling the bladder. Close verbal contact is maintained between patient and examiner as pre-defined motor and sensory landmarks are observed and annotated.

Terminology

The terminology presented herein is a compilation of the last two International Continence Society (ICS) reports liberally sprinkled with our own opinions about terminology [1,2]. Whenever we use a terminology different from the current ICS recommendations, we give the reasons. **Intravesical pressure (Pves)** is the pressure within the bladder. **Abdominal pressure (Pabd)** is the pressure surrounding the bladder. It is estimated from rectal pressure measurement. **Detrusor pressure (Pdet)** is that component of Pves that is created by bladder wall forces. It is estimated by subtracting Pabd from Pves (Pdet=Pves−Pabd).

Maximum cystometric capacity is the volume at which the patient feels he/she can no longer delay micturition. In patients with impaired bladder sensation, cystometric capacity may be inferred as that volume at which the patient begins void or leak involuntarily because of detrusor overactivity, low bladder compliance, or sphincteric incontinence. In patients with sphincteric incontinence, cystometric capacity may be increased by mechanical occlusion of the urethra, which prevents leakage as the bladder is being filled. In those with normal bladder compliance and impaired bladder sensation, capacity may be defined as greater than an arbitrary volume at which bladder filling is stopped. **Bladder compliance** is calculated by dividing the change in bladder volume by the change in detrusor pressure during that change in bladder volume. Compliance is expressed as ml/cmH_2O.

During bladder filling, the ICS recommends that the following sensory landmarks be reported: **first sensation of bladder filling (FSF), first desire to void (1st urge), strong desire to void (severe urge)**. The ICS recommends that the words "urge to void" not be used. We think either desire or urge to void is acceptable terminology. Others have recommended that the urge or desire to void during cystometry be recorded on a 4 point scale [3–5]. **Increased bladder sensation** is defined as a FSF and/or an early desire to void, and/or an early strong desire to void, which occurs at low bladder volume and persists. **Reduced bladder sensation** is defined as diminished sensation throughout bladder filling. In **absent bladder sensation** the patient has no bladder sensations at all. **Non-specific bladder sensations**, such as abdominal fullness or pressure or vegetative symptoms, may make the individual aware of bladder filling. **Bladder pain** during filling cystometry is an abnormal finding. **Urgency** is a sudden compelling desire to void.

Detrusor function during bladder filling is classified as normal or overactive. **Normal detrusor function** allows bladder filling with little or no change in pressure. No involuntary contractions occur despite provocation. **Detrusor overactivity** is a urodynamic observation characterized by involuntary detrusor contractions during the filling phase which may be spontaneous or provoked. **Detrusor overactivity** is a generic term that denotes involuntary detrusor contractions. There is no lower limit for the amplitude of an involuntary detrusor contraction, but when they are very low ancillary information to document their presence should be sought. These include a sudden urge to void, sudden change in sphincter electromyographic (EMG) activity, or incontinence. The ICS defines two patterns of detrusor overactivity: **Phasic detrusor overactivity** is defined by a characteristic waveform, and may or may not lead to urinary incontinence. **Terminal detrusor overactivity** is defined as a single involuntary detrusor contraction occurring at cystometric capacity, which cannot be suppressed, and results in incontinence. However, there are other instances of terminal detrusor overactivity, wherein incontinence does not result because the patient is able to contract the sphincter, prevent incontinence, and abort the detrusor contraction [6].

Filling versus voiding cystometry

From a technical standpoint, cystometry refers to the filling phase of bladder function and to the measurement of changes in vesical pressure with slow progressive increases in volume. Some urodynamicists refer to "voiding cystometry," by which they mean the pressure measurements during micturition. However, unless uroflow is simultaneously measured, little useful clinical information can be obtained. In practice, the "voiding CMG" is really part of the detrusor pressure/uroflow study.

Infusants for cystometry

Cystometry has been performed with a variety of infusants including fluid (water, saline, or radiographic contrast) and gas (air, carbon dioxide). Air should not be used because of the rare possibility of fatal air embolus. In our opinion, liquid is vastly superior to gas for several reasons: (1) when liquid is used, the bladder can be left full at the conclusion of the study, the patient checked for stress incontinence, and uroflow obtained (this is impossible with gas); (2) if incontinence occurs during the CMG it is usually obvious with liquid while gas leakage is much more difficult to detect; and (3) liquid is more physiologic and not compressible like gas. Because of the rapid filling rate that is commonly used with gas, it is often very difficult to distinguish a detrusor contraction from low bladder compliance.

Cystometric patterns

The normal adult CMG is divided into four phases (Fig. 3.1).

Phase I: The initial pressure rise represents the initial response to filling, and the level at which the bladder trace stabilizes is known as the initial filling pressure. The designation "resting pressure," though often used, is incorrect. The first phase of the curve is determined by the initial myogenic response to filling and by the elastic and viscoelastic response of the bladder wall to stretch. With more rapid rates of filling, there may be an initially higher peak, which then levels off. This peak type of initial response is relatively common with gas cystometry.

Phase II: Phase II is called the tonus limb. As the bladder fills, intravesical pressure remains low because of a property of the bladder wall known as accommodation. Compliance is normally high in phase II and uninterrupted by phasic rises in pressure.

Phase III: Phase III is reached when the elastic and viscoelastic properties of the bladder wall have reached their limit. Any further increase in volume generates a substantial increase in pressure. This increase in pressure is not the same as a detrusor contraction. If a voluntary or involuntary contraction occurs, phase III may be obscured by the rise in pressure so generated.

Phase IV: Phase IV consists of the initiation of a voluntary detrusor contraction. Some patients are unable to generate a voluntary detrusor contraction in the testing situation, especially in the supine position. This should not be called detrusor areflexia unless it is associated with a neurologic condition known to cause detrusor areflexia. Rather, it should simply be noted that the patient was unable to generate a detrusor contraction. We do not consider it to be abnormal unless other clinical or urodynamic findings are present that indicate a pathologic process.

Bladder wall compliance

Bladder compliance may be thought of as "bladder wall stiffness." It is calculated by dividing the change in bladder volume by the change in detrusor pressure during that change in bladder volume. The numeric value of compliance is dependent in large part on the volume interval over which it is measured. For example, during the tonus limb of the CMG (phase II), compliance is normally high; whereas, in phase III, it is normally much lower (see Fig. 3.1).

Technique of cystometry

Prior to beginning the cystometric examination, the examiner should plan his diagnostic approach. He should know what the patient's symptoms are, what the functional bladder is, and what the patient's lowest post-void residual urine is. The purpose of the examination is to reproduce the patient's symptoms, and by appropriate observations and measurements, the underlying pathophysiology should become apparent as the examination proceeds. Cystometry should be performed when the patient is awake and not sedated. It is generally advisable that the patient is not taking any medications that affect bladder function, but for patients being treated with medications who are not responding as expected, it is often prudent to reevaluate them while they are on their medications.

The urodynamic equipment should be calibrated and urethral and rectal catheters passed. All systems are zeroed at atmospheric pressure. For external transducers, the reference point is the level of the superior edge of the symphysis pubis. For catheter-mounted transducers the reference point is the transducer itself.

Data concerning bladder, abdominal, and urethral pressure can be obtained with microtip transducers, fiberoptic catheters, or fluid/contrast medium-filled catheters connected to external transducers. The major difference between microtip catheters and all the others is that in the former, the transducer is at the end of the catheter. The consequence of this is that there is no mechanism for achieving a standardized zero reference point; that is, the zero is the tip of the catheter itself. That means that if there is a catheter in the rectum, bladder, and urethra, they all have a different zero. Further, when the catheter is in the bladder, the weight of the urine will be recorded and added to the vesical pressure. If the tip of the catheter is at the top of a full bladder, it will record a lower pressure than if it is in the bottom of the bladder. Depending on the circumstances, these differences may or may not be clinically relevant. Although proponents of microtip technology claim that there is less dampening than with externally based transducers, artifact may be created when the catheter rests against the bladder or urethral wall.

A newly designed pressure measuring catheter utilizes microair charging of a balloon which is circumferentially placed around the catheter at appropriate locations. A miniature air-filled lumen communicates the pressure signal to an external semiconductor transducer in the cable. Its advantage is highly reproducible pressure recording measurements, particularly evident in studies of urethral pressure profilometry.

After a detailed explanation to the patient, the examination is begun by passing a catheter into the bladder, measuring residual urine, and filling the bladder. Communication between the patient and the urodynamicist is essential. Close observation of the patient is necessary because any rise in vesical pressure must be accounted for. It may reflect either a rise in the detrusor pressure, a movement artifact, or a change in abdominal pressure. To this end, synchronous measurement of Pves and Pabd is crucial; Pdet is electronically calculated by subtracting Pabd from Pves (Figs. 3.2 and 3.3). Moreover, detrusor contractions may be voluntary or involuntary. The only means of distinguishing voluntary from involuntary detrusor contractions is by talking to the patient (Fig. 3.4).

According to the ICS, "In everyday life the individual attempts to inhibit detrusor activity until he/she is in a position to void. Therefore, when the aims of the filling study have been achieved, and when the patient has a desire to void, normally the 'permission to void' is given. That moment is indicated on the urodynamic trace and all detrusor activity before this 'permission' is defined as 'involuntary detrusor activity'." We disagree with that approach (see Chapter 9 on OAB) and recommend that, during cystometry, the patient should be instructed to neither void nor inhibit micturition. Rather, the patient is instructed to simply report his/her sensations to the examiner. Periodically during the study, the patient should be asked to cough or strain, both to check the operation of the equipment and to see whether bladder activity is provoked by such maneuvers. Other techniques to provoke involuntary detrusor contractions include running water and handwashing. The volume of the FSF, 1st urge, severe urge, and desperate urge (urgency, feeling that micturition is imminent) are recorded. If an involuntary detrusor contraction occurs, the patient should be asked to try to prevent voiding (or incontinence) and his/her ability to do so is recorded (see classification of OAB in Chapter 9). It should also be noted whether or not the patient is aware of the contraction.

A normal CMG is seen in Figure 3.2(A). The pressure measured by the cystometer (vesical pressure) is the sum of detrusor pressure plus abdominal pressure. Thus, any Pves increment may be due to an increase in Pabd, Pdet, or combinations of the two. To eliminate an artifactual change in calculated detrusor pressure due to abdominal pressure changes, it is desirable to measure abdominal pressure simultaneously (Figs. 3.2 and 3.3). Once an artifactual or transmitted rise in Pdet has been excluded, there are three possibilities that can account for a rise in detrusor pressure – a voluntary or involuntary detrusor contraction or low bladder compliance. There are no characteristics of detrusor contractions that allow the examiner to distinguish voluntary from involuntary detrusor contractions (Fig. 3.4). The only way to distinguish the two is by communication with the patient during the urodynamic study. Terminal and phasic detrusor overactivity is depicted in Figures 3.5 and 3.6 respectively.

It is often difficult to distinguish low bladder compliance from a detrusor contraction and, to compound the problem further, the two conditions often coexist in the same patient. The best method for making this distinction is to start and stop bladder filling during the rise in pressure. In low bladder compliance, there is an abrupt fall in pressure when bladder filling is stopped; whereas, the pressure continues to rise or stabilizes during a detrusor contraction (Figs. 3.7 and 3.8).

Many patients strain in an attempt to initiate micturition or strain during micturition. Without multichannel studies, it is not possible to interpret the tracings properly because of abdominal straining (Fig. 3.9). In addition, rectal contractions can complicate the tracings even further (Fig. 3.10).

The ICS has made specific recommendation regarding the testing and reporting of cystometry.

The clinician should specify:

(a) Access (transurethral or percutaneous).

(b) Fluid medium (liquid or gas).

(c) Temperature of fluid.

(d) Position of patient (e.g. supine, sitting, or standing).

(e) Filling may be by diuresis or catheter. Filling by catheter may be continuous or incremental; the filling rate should be described as physiologic or non-physiologic. **Physiologic filling rate** is defined as a filling rate less than the predicted maximum (predicted maximum calculated according to the formula [7]:

$$\frac{\text{body weight (kg)}}{4}\ \text{ml/min}$$

Non-physiologic filling rate is any filling rate greater than the predicted maximum.

(f) The type (single, double, triple lumen), number of catheters (urethral, rectal), and size.

(g) Type of transducer (microtip, external, water, or air charged).

(h) Measuring equipment.

Pitfalls of cystometry

1) Calibration of electronic equipment should be done on a regular basis. Failure to do so can greatly alter the numeric values of pressure.

2) The rate of bladder filling can alter certain cyptometric findings. Non-physiologic filling rates decrease bladder compliance; the higher the filling rate, the lower the compliance [8,9] and may also proverb detrusion overactivity and bladder pain.

3) Intravesical pressure is affected by (1) the volume of fluid in the bladder, (2) the presence or absence of a detrusor contraction, (3) bladder compliance, and (4) extravesical conditions that cause compression restriction, or expansion of the bladder.

4) Vesicoureteral reflux, bladder diverticula, and leakage of water from around the catheter can lead to a decrease in recorded Pves.

5) Infections, inflammation, and radiation tend to increase the filling limb of the CMG, as do parasympathomimetic drugs.
6) Other medications, such as anticholinergics, and narcotics can increase bladder compliance and capacity.
7) Cystometric recordings are also affected by changes in the position of the patient. In the supine position patients are less likely to void or leak urine. With patients in the sitting and in the upright positions baseline vesical and abdominal pressure are higher, but detrusor pressure is unchanged.

Patient cooperation is imperative in obtaining meaningful cystometric studies. Moving, crying, extraneous muscular activity, and failure of the patient to follow directions greatly diminish the value of the study. Recordings of abnormal movement or coughing should be annotated on the tracings.

Perhaps the most important pitfall, though, is misinterpretation of the findings. Two in particular are (1) failing to fill the bladder to functional bladder capacity in patients with very large bladders and (2) ascribing pathology to patients who are unable to generate a voluntary detrusor contraction during the urodynamic study. These are discussed in more detail in the Chapter 8.

Suggested Reading

1 Abrams PH, Blaivas JG, Stanton SL, Andersen JT. Standardisation of lower urinary tract function, *Neurourol Urodynam*, 7: 403, 1988.
2 Abrams P, Cardozo L, Fall M, Griffiths D, Rosier P, Ulmsten U, van Kerrebroeck P, Victor A, Wein A. The standardisation of terminology of lower urinary tract function: report from the standardisation sub-committee of the international continence society, *Neurourol Urodynam*, 21: 167–178, 2002.
3 DeWachter S, Wyndale JJ. Frequency–volume charts: a tool to evaluate bladder sensation, *Neurourol Urodynam*, 22: 638–643, 2003.
4 Oliver S, Fowler C, Mundy A, Craggs M. Measuring the sensations of urge and bladder filling during cystometry in urge incontinence and the effects of neuromodulation, *Neurourol Urodynam*, 22: 7–16, 2003.
5 Erdem E, Akbay E, Doruk E, Cayan S, Acar D, Ulusoy E. How reliable is bladder perception during cystometry? *Neurourol Urodynam*, 23: 1–4, 2004.
6 Flisser AJ, Wamsley K, Blaivas JG. Urodynamic classification of patients with symptoms of overactive bladder, *J Urol*, 169: 529–533, 2003.
7 Klevmark B. Natural pressure–volume curves and conventional cystometry, *Scand J Urol Nephrol*, 201(Suppl): 1–4, 1999.
8 Klevmark B. Motility of the urinary bladder in cats during filling at physiologic rates. I. Intravesical pressure patterns studied by a new method of cystometry, *Acta Physiol Scand*, 90: 565–577, 1974.
9 Klevmark B. Motility of the urinary bladder in cats during filling at physiological rates. II. Effects of extrinsic bladder denervation on intramural tension and on intravesical pressure patterns, *Acta Physiol Scand*, 101: 176–184, 1977.

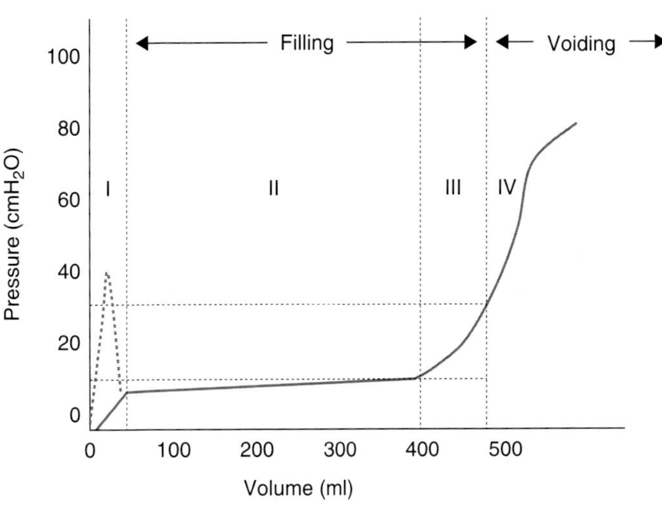

Fig. 3.1 Idealized CMG (see text for details). The dashed line in phase I is seen only with very rapid filling, such as that attained when carbon dioxide is used. It is attributed to the viscoelastic properties of the bladder wall. Note that bladder compliance changes at different bladder volumes. Bladder compliance during the tonus limb (phase II) = 400 ml/10 cmH_2O = 40 ml/cmH_2O; bladder compliance at the end of phase III of the CMG (500 ml) = 100 ml/20 cmH_2O = 5 ml/cmH_2O.

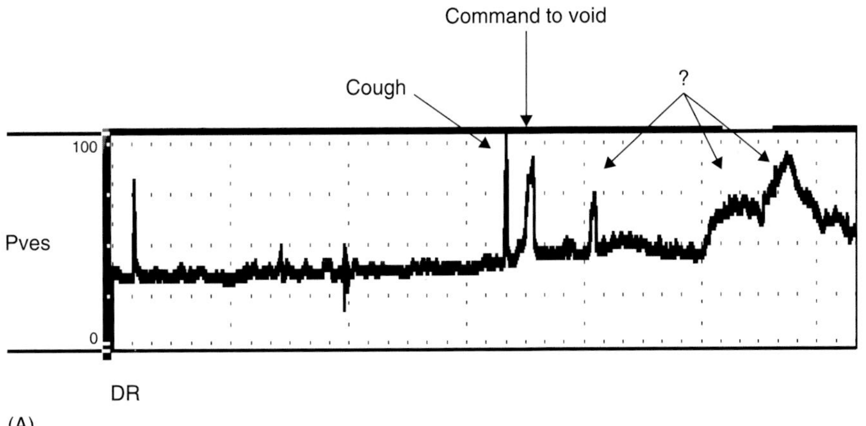

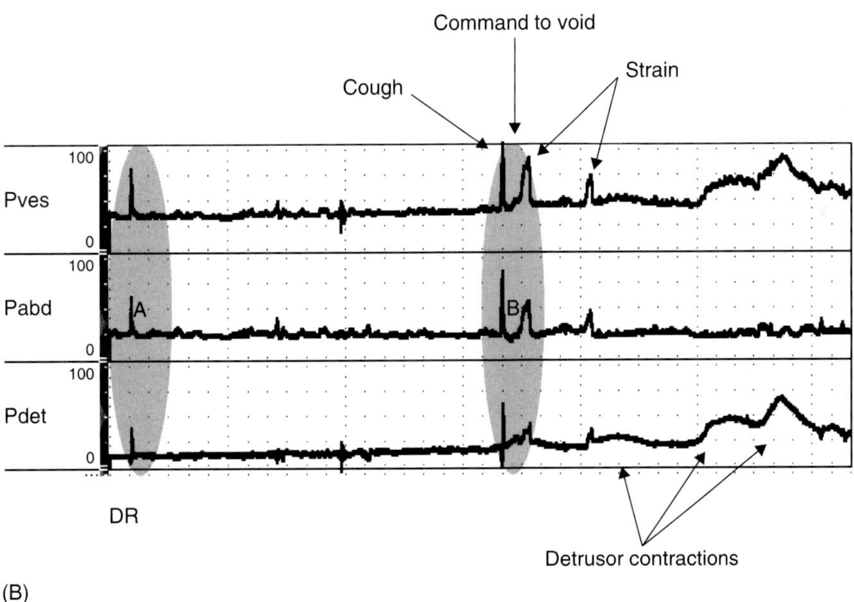

Fig. 3.2 Normal CMG in a 59-year-old woman referred for evaluation of elevated residual urine found unexpectedly during CAT scan done for abdominal pain. She denied any urologic symptoms. Uroflow was normal (voided volume = 230 ml, pattern = normal, Q_{max} = 25 ml/s, and post-void residual = 0 ml). (A) CMG. FSF (first sensation of bladder filling) = 75 ml, 1st urge = 210 ml, severe urge = 523 ml, and bladder capacity = 533 ml. At the command to void, there is a rise in detrusor pressure, but there is no way, by looking at this tracing, to determine whether this is a detrusor contraction or abdominal straining. Further, there is no way to account for the other rises in Pves (arrows). (B) When Pdet is displayed (by subtracting Pabd from Pves) it is possible to account for each rise in pressure. Note that there is an artifactual rise in detrusor pressure due to unequal pressure registration in the vesical and abdominal tracings (shaded oval B) because of a calibration error seen during a cough at the far left of the tracing (shaded oval A).

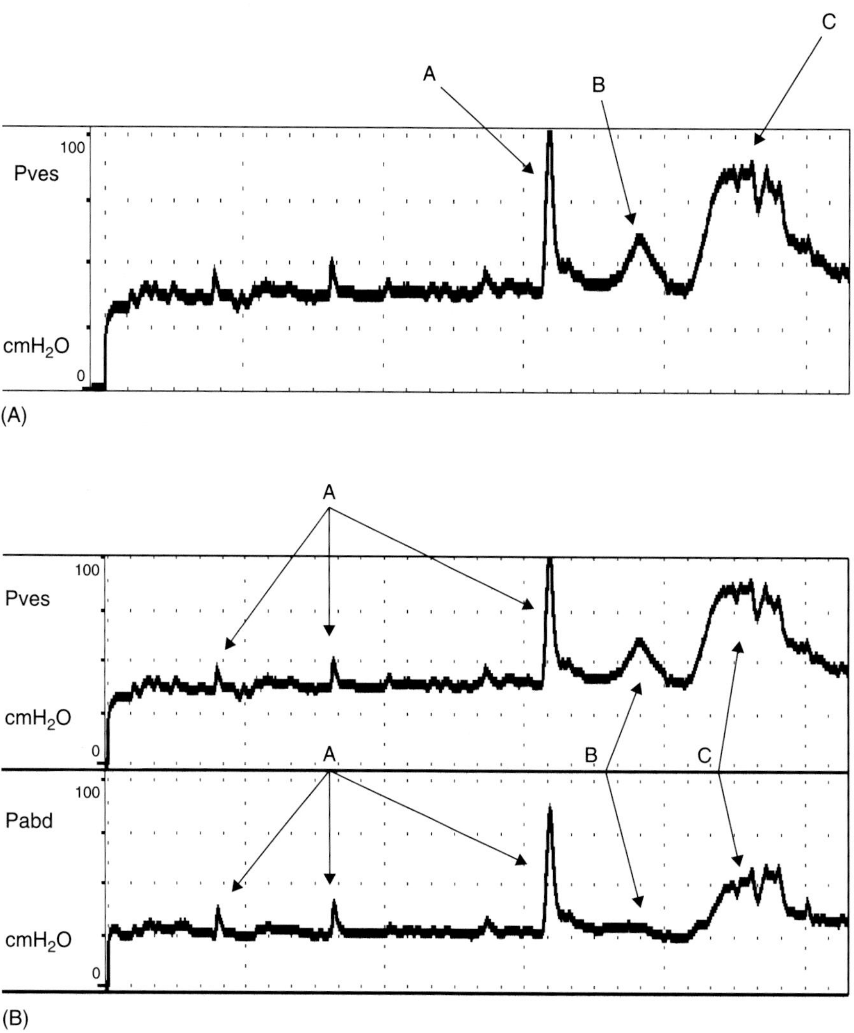

Fig.3.3 (A) With just the Pves tracing you have very limited or no information about what is happening. Arrow A – is this an artifact, straining, cough, etc.? Arrow B – this looks like straining, but it could be a short-lived detrusor contraction. Arrow C – Is the patient straining or is this a detrusor contraction? (B) More information is attained by displaying Pabd. The arrows marked "A" confirm that there is an equal rise in both vesical and abdominal pressure. This means that the rise in Pves was due to a rise in Pabd. The narrow spike in pressure suggests that these are coughs, but the only way of knowing for sure is by watching and talking to the patient. At arrow B there is a rise in Pves with no corresponding rise in abdominal pressure. The only explanation for this is that the patient is having a detrusor contraction. At arrow C, there is a nearly equal rise in Pves and Pabd. There are two possibilities to account for this. The patient may be straining during a detrusor contraction or there is a calibration error. The fact that the pressures at the black arrows were transmitted equally prove that this is a detrusor contraction accompanied by straining.

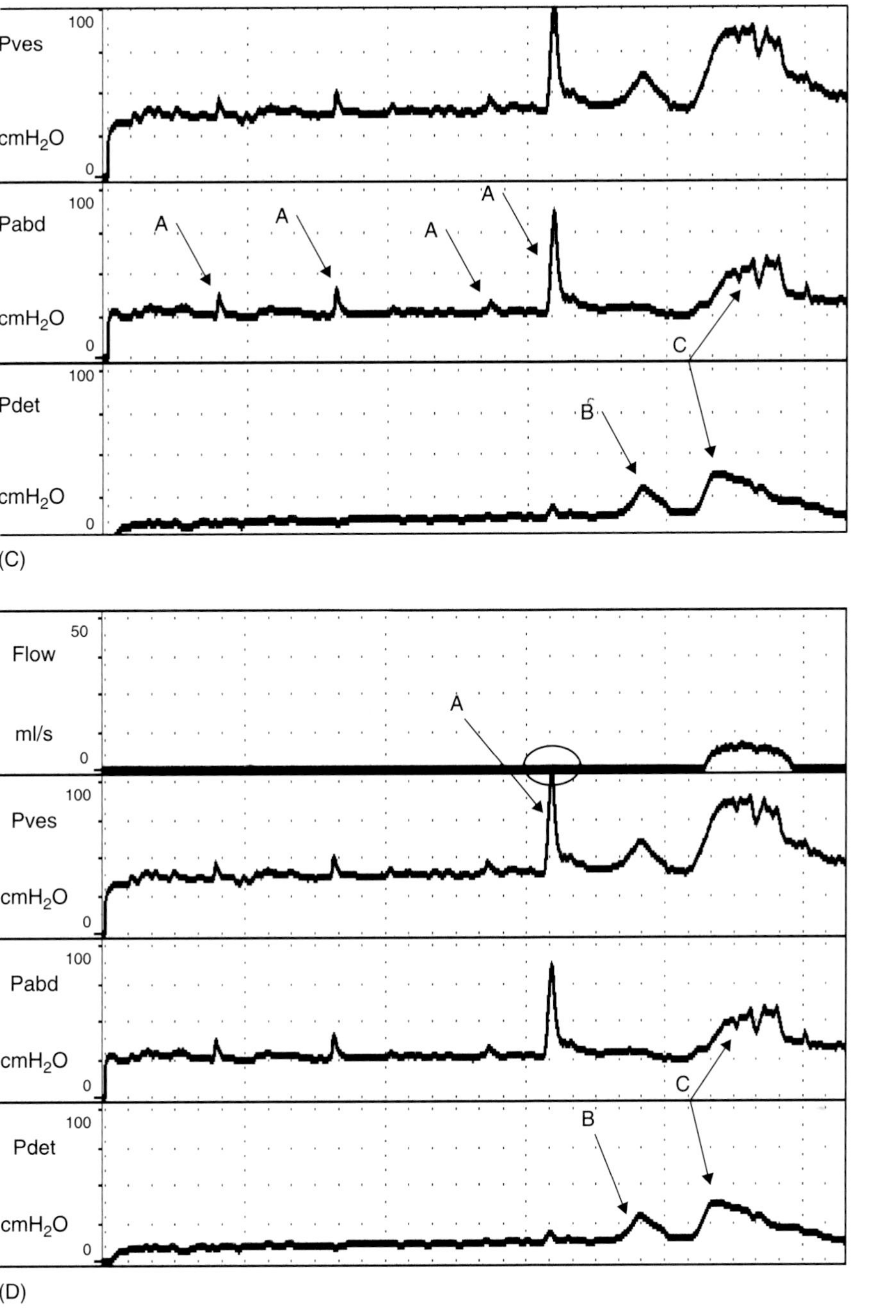

Fig.3.3 (continued) (C) Visualizing all three pressures simultaneously permits a definitive diagnosis. Arrows marked "A" point to coughs (Pves and Pabd rise equally). Arrow B shows a detrusor contraction. Arrow "C" also points to a detrusor contraction, but when you also look at Pabd it is apparent that the patient is straining. The result is that the detrusor contraction appears on the Pves tracing to be much higher than it really is. (D) When the uroflow channel is displayed an even more accurate picture is obtained. Arrow A points to a strong cough (Pves = 112 cmH_2O with no leak (black circle). Arrow B is a detrusor contraction that does not result in flow. It is not possible from this tracing to determine why. In this case though, it was an involuntary detrusor contraction that the patient voluntarily suppressed. The only way to know this is by communicating with the patient during the study. At arrow C, the patient is asked to void. She strains in an attempt to initiate micturition and almost immediately thereafter, the detrusor contracts and flow begins.

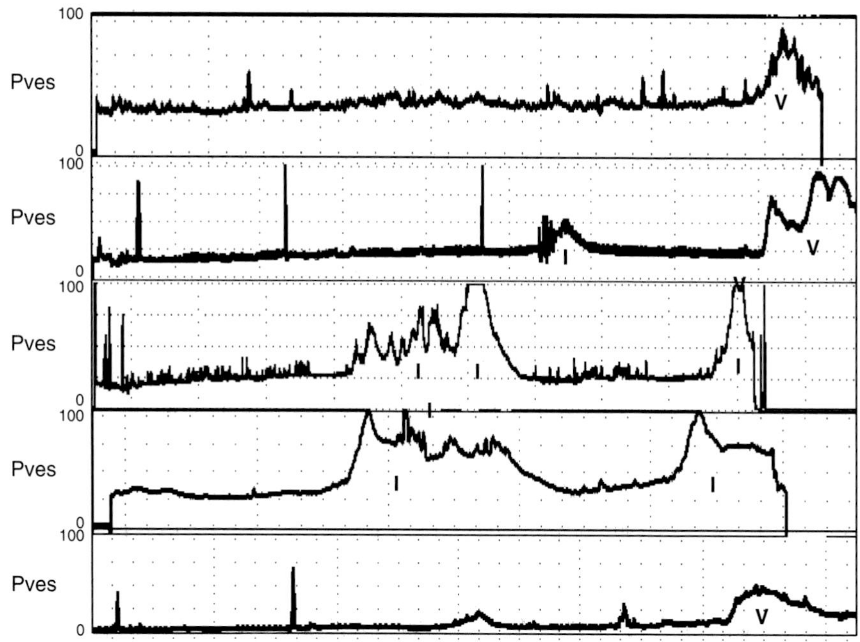

Fig. 3.4 A sampling of voluntary and involuntary detrusor contractions in men. It is not possible to determine whether a contraction is voluntary or involuntary from the tracing alone. It can only be done at the time of the urodynamic study by speaking to the patient. I = involuntary detrusor contraction and V = voluntary detrusor contraction.

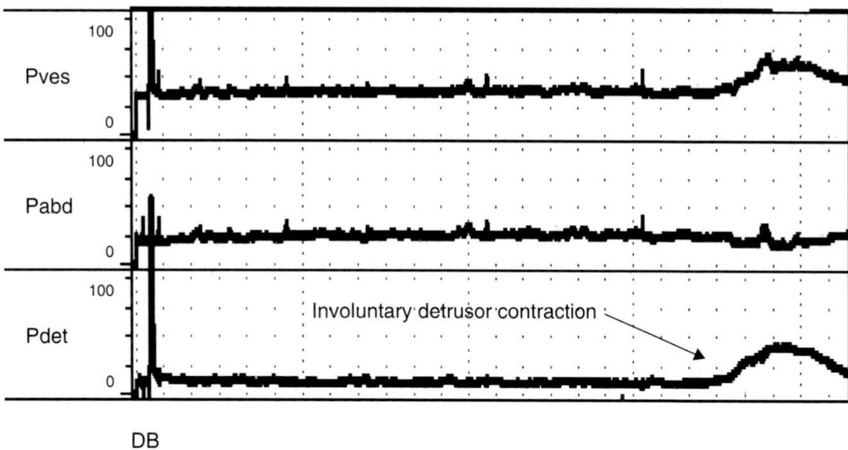

Fig. 3.5 Terminal detrusor overactivity (See text for details, p. 23).

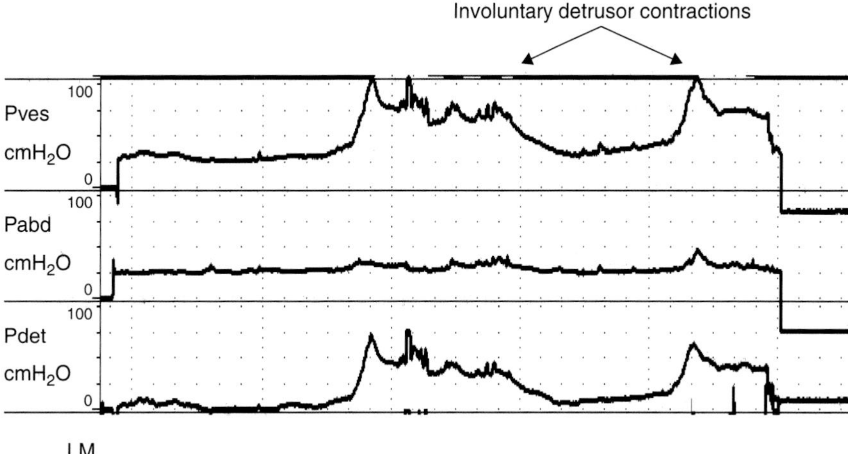

Fig. 3.6 Phasic detrusor overactivity (See text for details, p. 23).

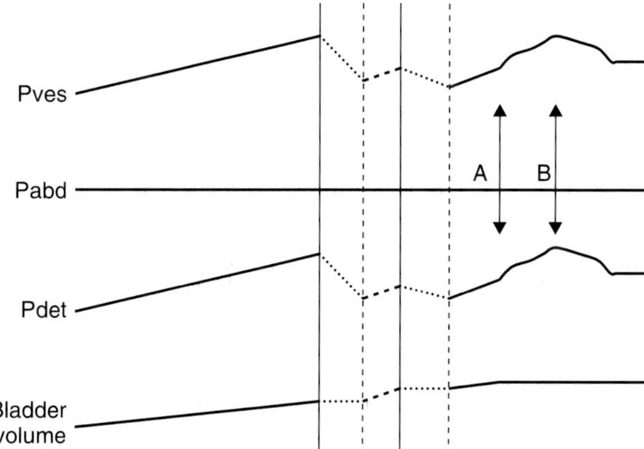

Fig. 3.7 Low bladder compliance versus involuntary detrusor contraction. During bladder filling there is a steep rise in detrusor pressure. Is this a detrusor contraction or low bladder compliance? The principal means by which this distinction is made is to stop the bladder infusion. Each time it is stopped (vertical solid lines), detrusor pressure falls (dotted lines) and when bladder infusion is started again (vertical dashed lines), detrusor pressure rises (dashed lines). At the end of bladder filling, there is another rise in detrusor pressure (arrow A) and the infusion is stopped. This time, Pves and Pdet continue to rise, proving that this is a detrusor contraction (arrow B).

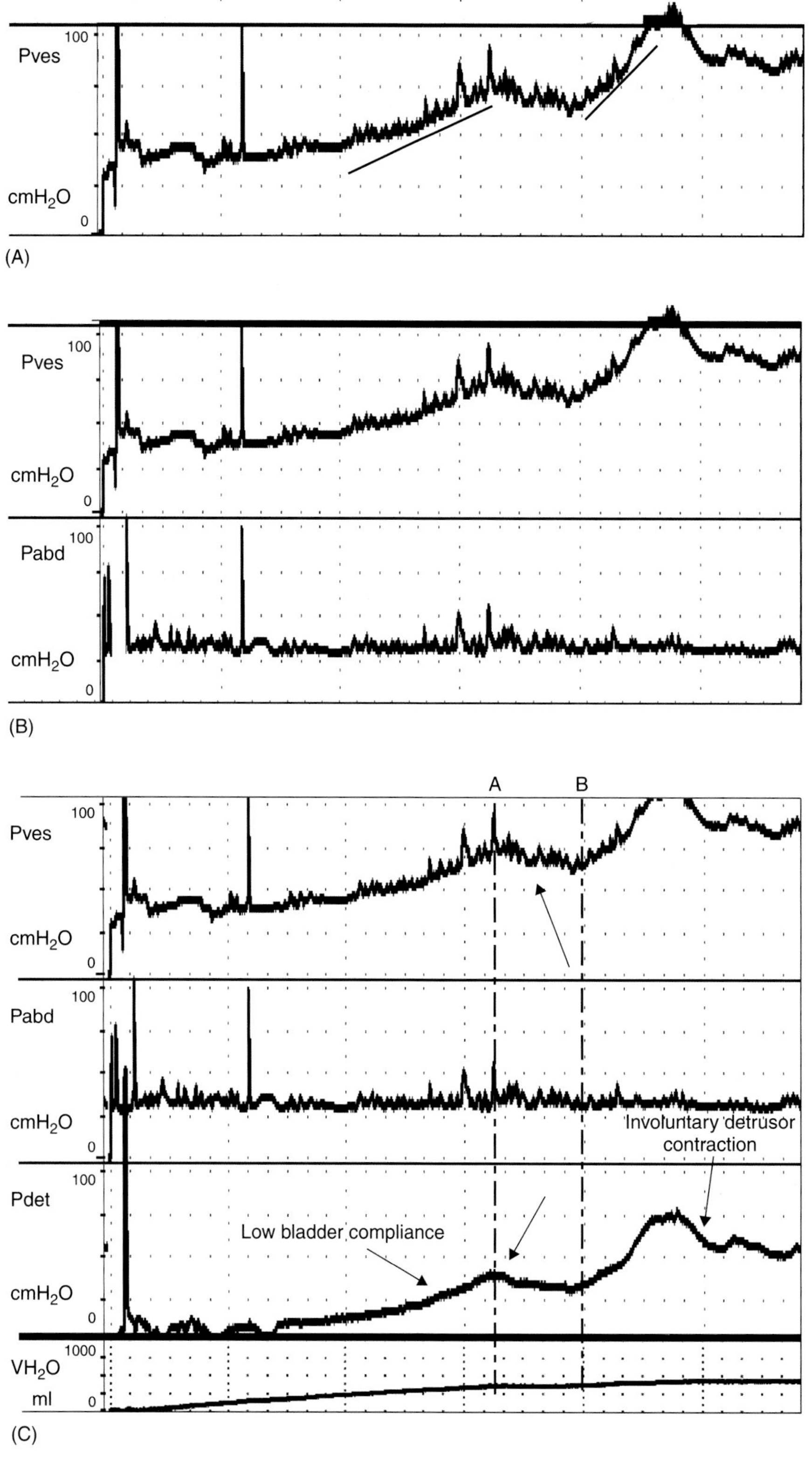

Fig. 3.8 (A) This CMG demonstrates two steep rises in Pves. The black lines parallel the pressure rises. Without further information, it is not possible to determine whether these are due to straining, detrusor contractions, or low bladder compliance. (B) When Pabd is displayed, it is apparent that the rise in Pves is not due to abdominal straining, but the distinction between low bladder compliance and detrusor contraction can still not be made. (C) The bladder infusant channel is displayed at the bottom of the graph. At the vertical dashed line A, the infusant is stopped and Pves and Pdet fall (arrows). At the vertical dashed line B, there is another steep rise in pressure and the infusion is again stopped, but this time pressure continues to rise, showing that this is a detrusor contraction, in this case an involuntary one.

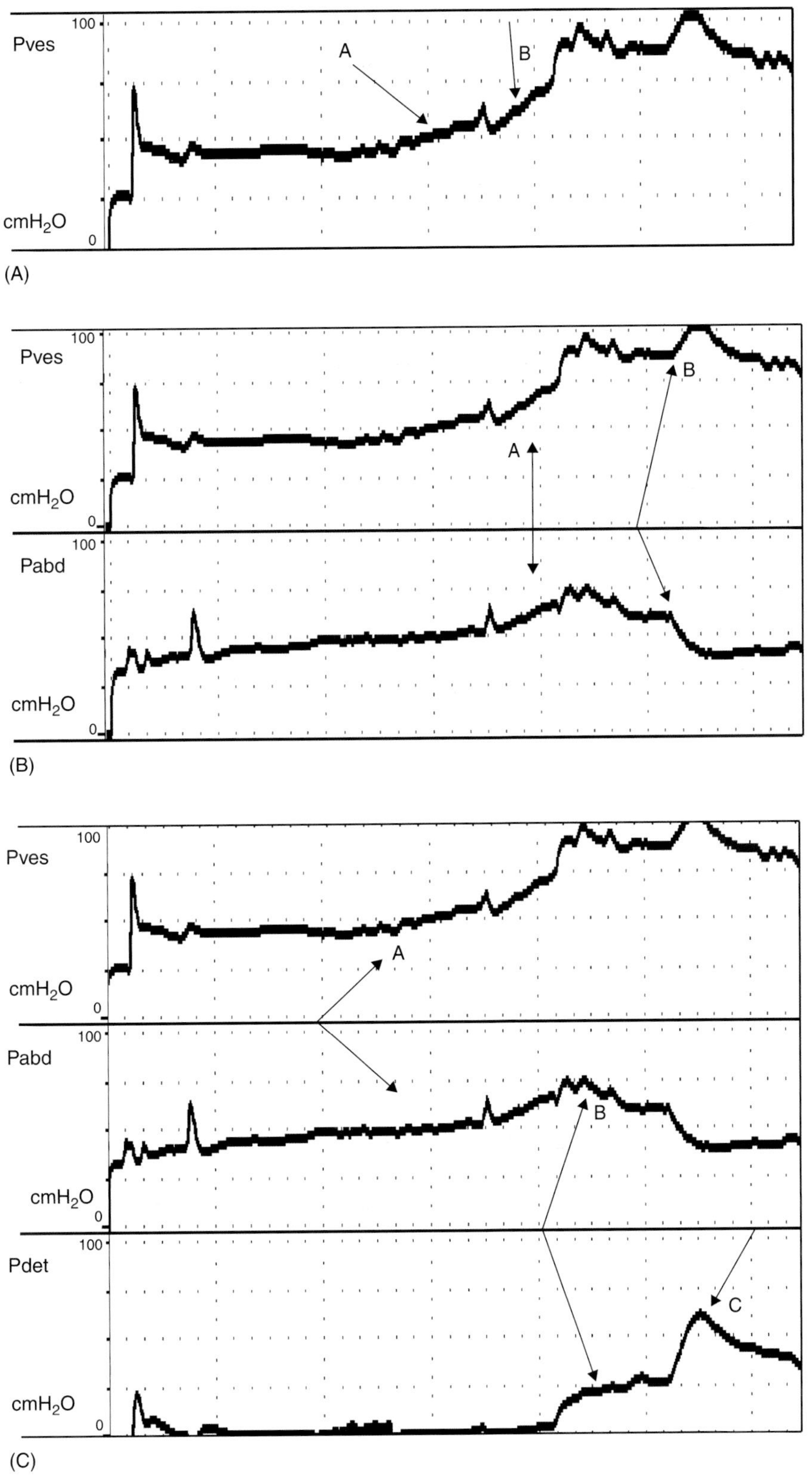

Fig. 3.9 (A) This is another Pves tracing showing a steady rise in pressure (arrow A) with a steep rise at the end (arrow B). (B) Adding Pabd to the figure we see a corresponding rise in Pabd (arrows A) and a drop in Pabd at the end without a drop in Pves pressure (arrows B). (C) Again with three tracings showing we see a lot more. There is a steady and equal rise in Pabd and Pves (arrows A) indicative of straining. The patient continues to strain and also develops a detrusor contraction (arrows B), but when straining stops, Pdet rises further (arrow C). One explanation for this is that while straining, the patient subconsciously contracted the sphincter, inhibiting the detrusor contraction, and relaxed the sphincter once straining stopped. Alternatively, the patient may have relaxed the sphincter during straining and contracted the sphincter when straining stopped. The only way to make the distinction is by measuring synchronous sphincter EMG and uroflow.

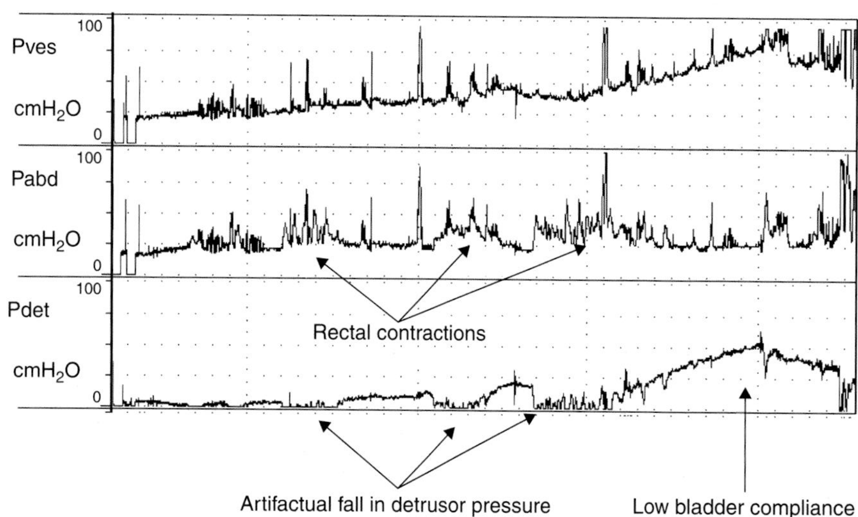

Fig. 3.10 In this patient with low bladder compliance, after radical hysterectomy, spontaneous rectal contractions artifactually lower Pdet.

4 Uroflowmetry

Uroflowmetry is a simple, non-invasive diagnostic procedure that calculates the rate of urine expulsion as a function of time. It is performed by having a person urinate into a funnel connected to an electronic measuring instrument. The measuring device calculates the mass of urine produced during the interval from initiation until completion of the void. This information is converted into an *x–y* plot with flow rate (ml/s) on the ordinate and time on the abscissa.

As originally described, uroflow was thought to be most useful as a test to diagnose urethral obstruction, especially in men with lower urinary tract symptoms (LUTS). With the evolution of detrusor pressure-uroflow studies and the recognition that uroflow reflects the net interaction of detrusor contractility and outlet resistance, the limitations of uroflow became evident. It subsequently has been shown that a diminished uroflow may be due, not only to outlet obstruction, but also to impaired detrusor contractility and low voided volumes; and, it is not possible by examining the uroflow curve to make the distinction between urethral obstruction and impaired detrusor contractility [1]. Furthermore, bladder outlet obstruction and impaired detrusor contractility can co-exist in the same patient and; finally, there is an entity called high flow urethral obstruction wherein the diagnosis is based on a very high detrusor pressure and normal uroflow [2]. Nevertheless, uroflowmetry remains an extremely useful modality in the armamentarium of the urodynamicist. Provided that an adequate volume is voided (>150ml), it is an excellent screening procedure for pathology. In men with LUTS, for example, a low flow is caused by urethral obstruction in about 65% and impaired detrusor contractility in 35% [3]. Once an accurate diagnosis has been attained by detrusor pressure/uroflow studies, uroflow is used to document and follow the progress of therapeutic interventions.

Terminology

Urinary flow rate is defined as the volume of fluid expelled via the urethra per unit time. It is expressed in ml/s. Uroflow is described in terms of its pattern and rate. The pattern may be continuous or intermittent. The **continuous flow curve** is one in which the entire micturition is completed when the flow rate drops to zero for the first time after the onset of flow. The pattern is further described as a smooth arc shaped curve (Fig. 4.1) or fluctuating when there are multiple peaks during a period of continuous urine flow (Fig. 4.2). An **interrupted flow** is one in which two or more curves fall to zero flow before the end of micturition (Fig. 4.3). The flow pattern can be further described as normal, plateau, or straining.

Maximum flow rate (Q_{max}) is the maximum measured value of the flow rate after correction for artifacts. **Average flow rate (Q_{ave})** is voided volume divided by flow time. **Voided volume** is the total volume expelled via the urethra. **Flow time (TQ)** is the time over which measurable flow actually occurs. When flow is intermittent, the time intervals between flow episodes are disregarded. **Voiding time** is the total duration of micturition, including the interruptions. When voiding is completed without interruption, voiding time is equal to flow time. **Time to maximum flow (TQ_{max})** is the elapsed time from the onset of flow to maximum flow. For patients with continuous flow, TQ_{max} is approximately one-third of voiding time in both normal and obstructed patients because the prolongation of voiding time in obstruction is primarily due to a prolongation of the descending limb of the flow curve. A uroflow report should include at the least Q_{max}, voided volume, and pattern. In addition, it should be noted whether the flow was obtained with a transurethral catheter in place (intubated) or without a catheter in place (unintubated or free flow). It should be further noted whether or not the recorded uroflow was typical of the patient's usual micturition pattern.

The equipment

Two differing technologies are used to measure urinary flow rate: **load cell systems**, employed by most manufacturers, rely on urine falling onto a pressure transducer and **spinning disk systems** rely on the change in velocity of a spinning disk as flowing urine strikes it. The latter is reported to be more accurate over a wide spectrum of flow rates and is often referred to as the "gold standard". Load cell systems, on the other hand, offer high accuracy and are more durable because they lack moving parts that may need repair or replacement. Another important factor to consider is the frequent cleaning the spinning disk system requires.

Modern electronic uroflowmeters are designed to provide high sensitivity and reproducibility of data. The technical attributes that provide high sensitivity to a uroflowmeter is the time constant parameter. From a practical viewpoint, a time constant of 0.25 seconds means that the flowmeter will register any change in flow rate lasting 0.25 seconds or more. In the case of maximum urinary flow rate, however, such high sensitivity may not be desirable, since it allows the flowmeter to capture even a brief artifactual change in flow rate. This can occur if the urinary stream directly contacts a rotating disk flowmeter or if there is mechanical movement with the weight and electronic dipstick uroflowmeters.

All uroflowmeters are equipped with an auto start capability. Data acquisition, triggered by the flow of a predetermined velocity or volume of urine, begins automatically once voiding starts. This allows the equipment to remain in operation while the patient prepares to void, prevents the waste of memory and/or paper, and provides some measure of privacy for the patient.

Before the procedure

The patient is instructed to arrive at the office with a comfortably full bladder and wait until his/her usual urge to void is felt before voiding for the uroflow. Often, patients do not do this, so after they arrive (and void in the bathroom because they couldn't hold it any longer), they are asked to drink water until they experience the sensation that they experience as their usual urge to void.

Interpretation of uroflow tracings

Uroflowmetry integrates the activity of the bladder and the outlet during the emptying phase of micturition. Flow rate and pattern are the recorded variables; if these are both normal, it is unlikely that there is any significant disorder of emptying. A normal flow, however, does not entirely exclude obstruction, which is defined on the basis of the relationship between detrusor pressure and simultaneous flow [2]. There is considerable overlap in uroflow parameters between normal and abnormal patients. This variability is more pronounced for Q_{ave} than for Q_{max}, and for this reason, most experts regard Q_{max} as the single most useful parameter.

A number of factors can influence the flow rate including age, sex, voided volume, psychic inhibition, bladder outlet obstruction, and impaired detrusor contractility [1,3–9]. For any given patient, though, the most critical factor affecting uroflow is the voided volume. Uroflow obtained at the extremes of voided volumes (too high or too low) are less reliable than those obtained with a comfortably full bladder (see Fig. 4.7). In comparing flow rates in a given individual from one time to another, whether for the purpose of evaluating treatment or following a given condition, it has been proposed that the rates should be standardized for volume. Volume–flow rate nomograms have been constructed in this regard and a number have been published. The Siroky and Liverpool nomograms are most commonly utilized [6,8,9]. The primary caveat in interpreting uroflow is to make sure that the flow event closely approximates the usual voiding event for that patient (based on bladder diaries).

Normal, continuous flow patterns are seen in Figure 4.4(A–D). A fluctuating pattern may be due to abdominal straining, fluctuations in the force of detrusor contraction, and/or fluctuations in sphincter activity (Fig. 4.4(E)). In women with sphincteric incontinence, urethral resistance may be sometimes lower during voiding resulting in a very high flow rate that has been called "superflow" (Fig. 4.4(F)). Interrupted flow patterns may be associated with a normal Q_{max} (Fig. 4.5). Computer generated reports of maximum flow rates should always be correlated with actual tracings and corrected for artifacts [5]. Transient spiky increases in flow due to accidentally jarring the flowmeter may be erroneously reported as Q_{max} in computer generated reports (Fig. 4.6). It is well documented that Q_{max} is dependent, in part, on bladder volume. In general Q_{max} increases with voided volume, but at high bladder volumes, Q_{max} tends to fall and at bladder volumes less than 150ml uroflow is inaccurate. The dependency of Q_{max} on voided volumes is seen in Figure 4.7(A–D).

Urethral obstruction and impaired detrusor contractility both result in a diminished flow rate and flattened curve, but there are no characteristics of the uroflow curve that allows one to make the distinction between the two (Fig. 4.8) [1]. Figure 4.9 shows two uroflow tracings with approximately the same numerical values and flow patterns, one due to urethral obstruction and the other due to impaired detrusor contractility. Patients with either fixed infravesical obstruction or impaired detrusor contractility may strain to void yielding characteristic spikes in flow patterns despite overall diminished flow rate (Figs. 4.10(A) and (B)). Figure 4.11 shows an unusual cause of urethral obstruction in a man after transurethral resection of the prostate (TURP). In the case of patients having undergone augmentation cystoplasty or neobladder formation, voiding may occur with straining and simultaneous pelvic floor relaxation yielding a pattern of alternating peaks and troughs in urinary flow rate (Fig. 4.12).

Pitfalls of uroflow

Certain factors or conditions may interfere with the accuracy or consistency of uroflowmetry. The most common pitfall in evaluating uroflow is not to take voided volume into account (see Fig. 4.7). Another is relying on a single flow parameter, such as Q_{max}, as it is possible for a patient to generate very high Q_{max}, which is only momentarily sustained (see Fig. 4.11). Yet another is relying on a computer generated readout that cannot distinguish artifacts (see Fig. 4.6) or that record tiny surges as Q_{max} (see Fig. 4.4(E)). Finally, one must remember that automated reports of Q_{ave} require that flow be continuous and that there is a clearly definable end point of micturition. In a patient with intermittent flow or significant terminal dribbling, a misleadingly low average flow rate may result. To guard against all these artifacts, it is important that every flow curve be manually inspected.

The uroflow machine itself can be checked periodically for accuracy. A simple technique involves applying a known volume of fluid over a fixed time interval. Q_{ave} and volume voided can be easily calculated and checked against the flowmeter. Q_{ave} = voided volume/time.

Suggested Reading

1 Chancellor MB, Kaplan SA, Axelrod D, Blaivas JG. Bladder outlet obstruction versus impaired detrusor contractility: role of uroflow, *J Urol*, 145: 810–812, 1991.

2 Gerstenberg TC, Andersen JT, Klarskov P, Raminez D, Hald T. High flow infravesical obstruction, *J Urol*, 127: 943, 1982.

3 Fusco F, Groutz A, Blaivas JG, Chaikin DC, Weiss JP. Videourodynamic studies in men with lower urinary tract symptoms: a comparison of community based versus referral urological practices, *J Urol*, 166: 910–913, 2001.

4 Drach GW, Layton TN, Binard WJ. Male peak urinary flow rate: relationships to volume voided and age, *J Urol*, 122: 210, 1979.

5 Grino PB, Bruskewitz R, Blaivas JG, Siroky MB, Andersern JT, Cook T, Stoner E. Maximum urinary flow rate by uroflowmetry: automatic or visual interpretation, *J Urol*, 149: 339–341, 1993.

6 Haylen BT, Ashby D, Sutherest JR, et al. Maximum and average urine flow rate in normal male and female populations – the Liverpool nomogram, *Br J Urol*, 64: 30–38, 1989.

7 Jorgensen JB, Jensen KME, Bille-Brahe NE, Mogensen P. Uroflowmetry in asymptomatic elderly males, *Br J Urol*, 58: 390–395, 1986.

8 Siroky MB, Olsson CA, Krane RJ. The flow rate nomogram. I. Development, *J Urol*, 122: 665–668, 1979.

9 Siroky MB, Olsson CA, Krane RJ. The flow rate nomogram. II. Clinical correlation, *J Urol*, 123: 208, 1980.

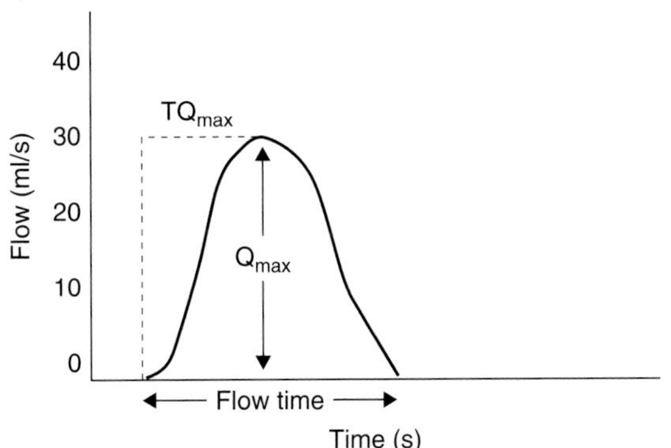

Fig. 4.1 Continuous smooth uroflow.

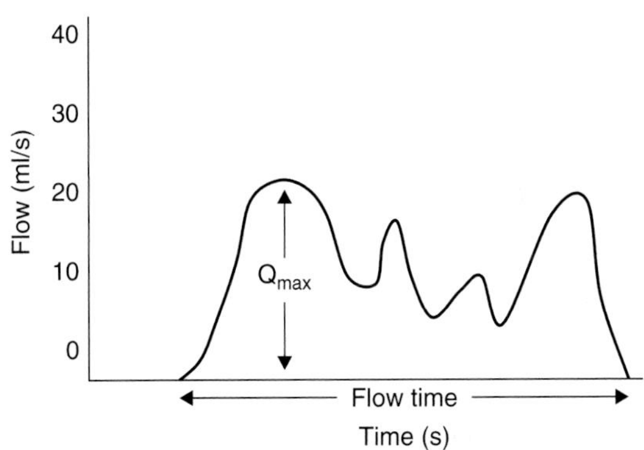

Fig. 4.2 Continuous, fluctuating uroflow.

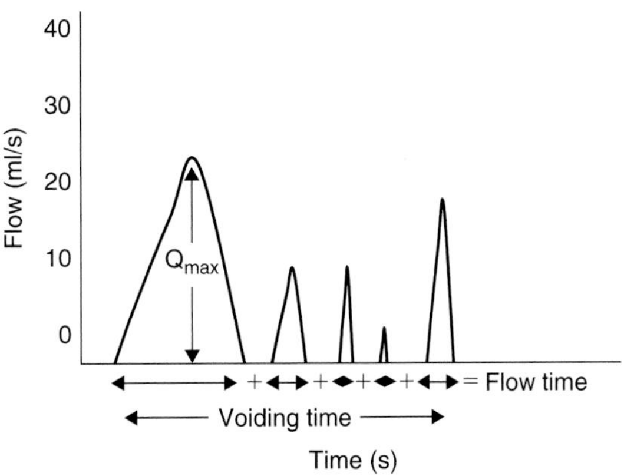

Fig. 4.3 Interrupted flow pattern.

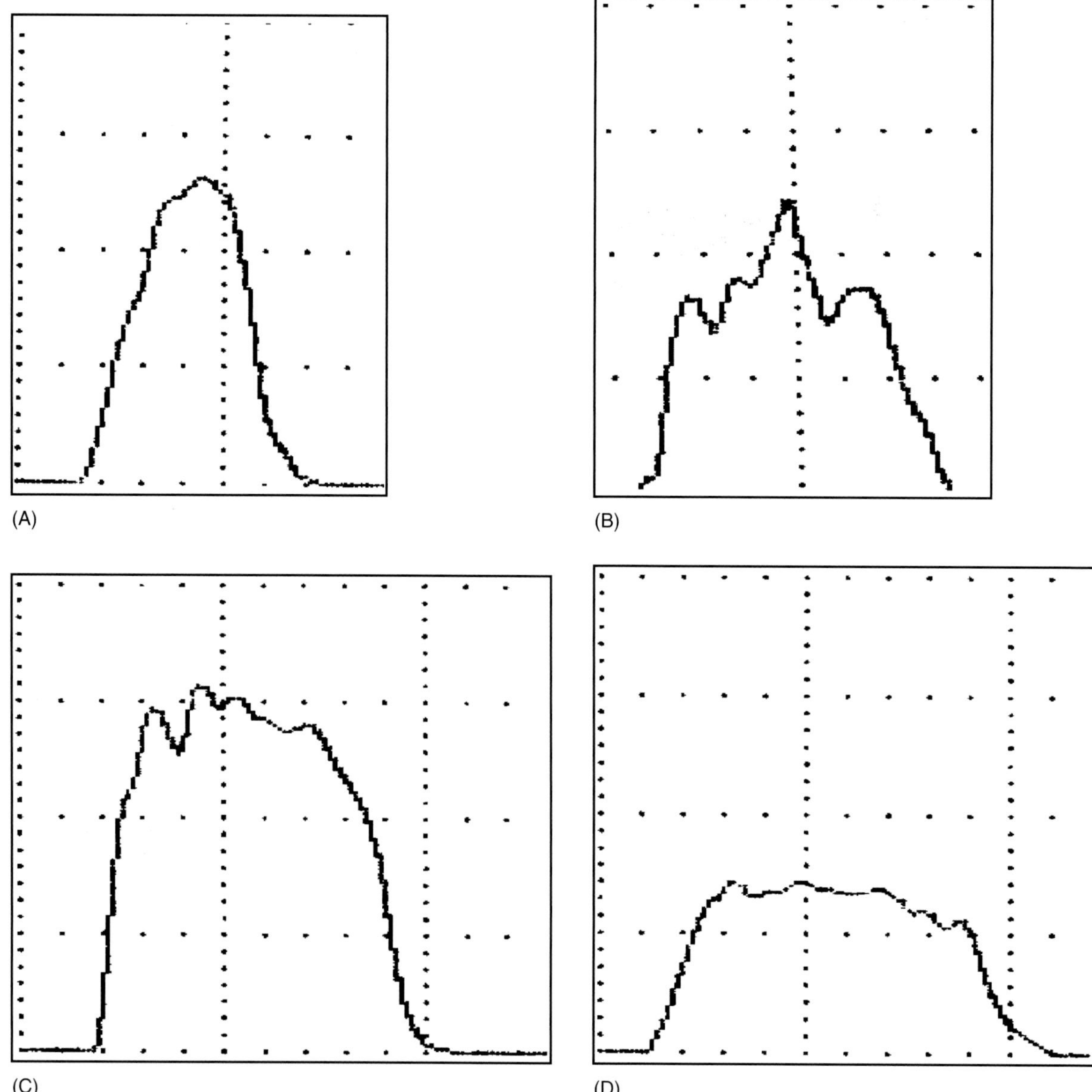

Fig. 4.4 Normal, continuous uroflows: (A) Normal uroflow in a 49-year-old woman. Q_{max} = 26 ml/s, mean flow = 15 ml/s, voided volume = 162 ml, and PVR (post-void residual) = 10 ml. (B) Normal uroflow in a 53-year-old man. The pattern is continuous and the curve is fluctuating. Q_{max} = 24 ml/s, mean flow = 13 ml/s, voided volume = 190 ml, and PVR = 0 ml. (C) Normal uroflow in a 52-year-old man. The pattern is continuous and the curve is very slightly fluctuating. Q_{max} = 31 ml/s, Q_{ave} = 22 ml/s, voided volume = 269 ml, and PVR = 0 ml. (D) Normal uroflow in a 59-year-old man. The pattern is continuous and the curve is slightly fluctuating. Q_{max} = 15 ml/s, mean flow = 10 ml/s, voided volume = 200 ml, and PVR = 10 ml.

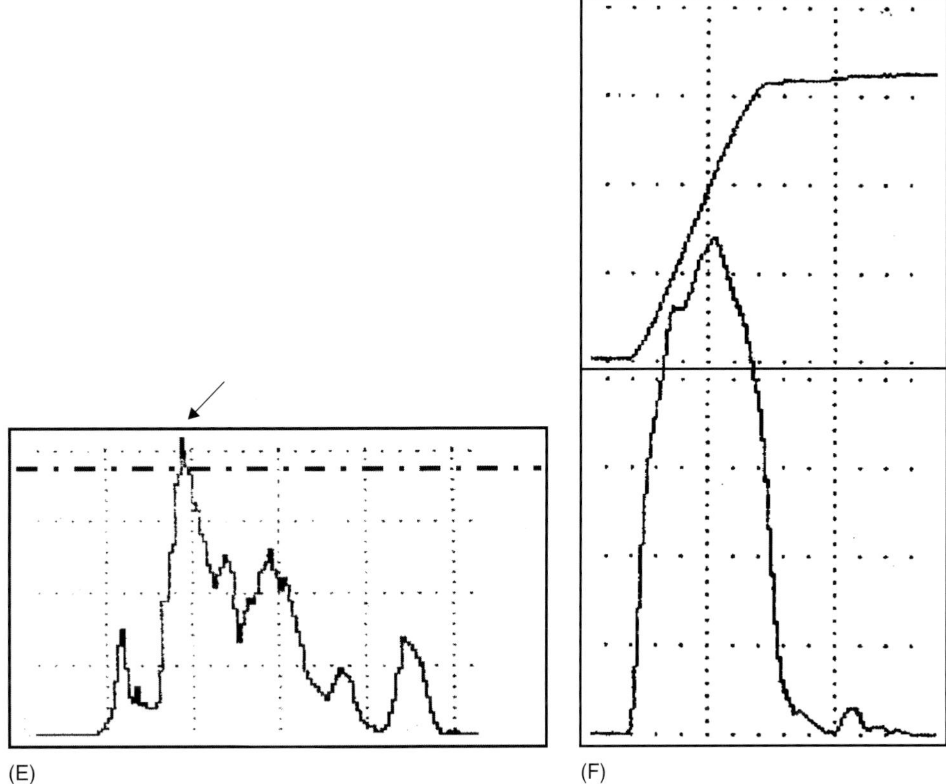

Fig. 4.4 (continued) (E) Marked fluctuations within a single continuous flow curve are usually due to dynamic changes in sphincter resistance or abdominal straining. In this young woman, it is due to pelvic floor dysfunction (subconscious contractions and relaxations of the striated pelvic floor during voiding). This results in a staccato uroflow pattern. In this instance, the computer generated readout of Q_{max} was = 42 ml/s (arrow), but it can be seen that this was due to a momentary surge that did not last long enough to be considered Q_{max}. Visual inspection of the curve gave a reading of 38 ml/s for Q_{max} (dotted line). Q_{max} = 38 ml/s, mean flow = 14 ml/s, voided volume = 273 ml, and PVR = 40 ml. (F) "Superflow" in a woman with sphincteric incontinence. Q_{max} = 56 ml/s, mean flow = 27 ml/s, voided volume = 482 ml, and PVR = 0 ml.

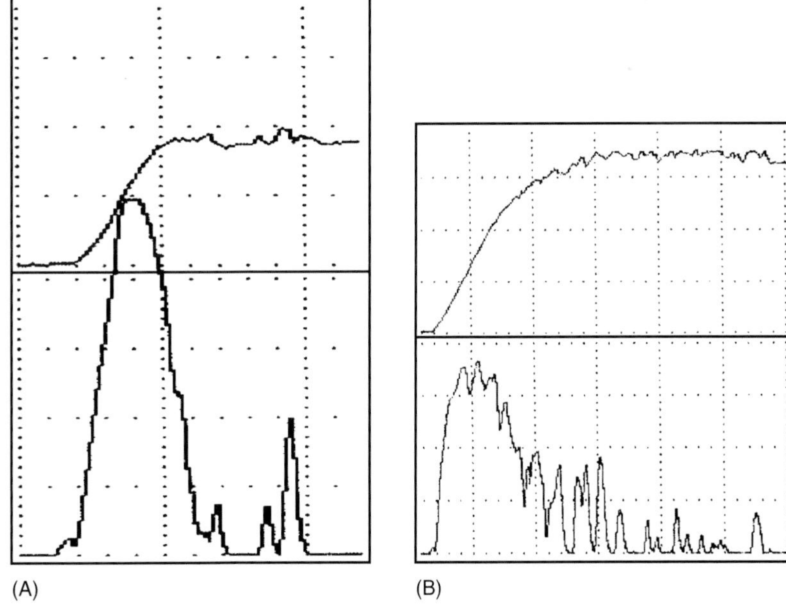

Fig. 4.5 Normal, interrupted flow patterns. (A) Normal, interrupted uroflow in a 55-year-old woman. Q_{max} = 51 ml/s, mean flow = 19 ml/s, voided volume = 273 ml, and PVR = 0 ml. (B) Normal, interrupted uroflow in an 81-year-old woman who complains of urinary frequency and nocturia. What starts off as a normal flow rate ends with straining, and a large PVR. Q_{max} = 36 ml/s, mean flow = 14 ml/s, voided volume = 510 ml, and PVR = 400 ml.

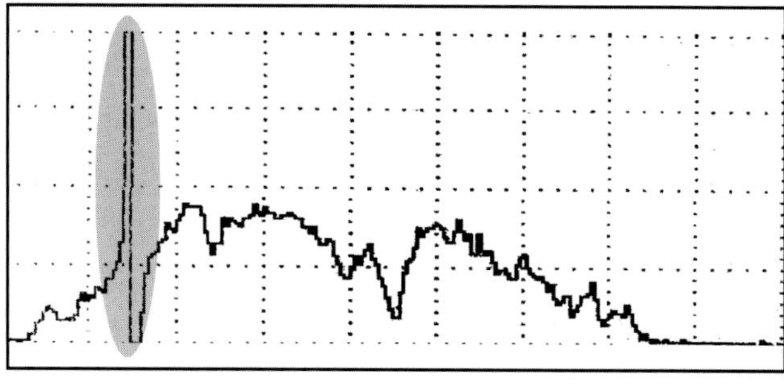

Fig. 4.6 The computer generated report read Q_{max} = 40 ml/s. On visual inspection of the flow curve, it is obvious that this is an artifact (shaded oval), likely due to mechanical jostling of the flowmeter. The real Q_{max} = 18 ml/s, mean flow = 11 ml/s, voided volume = 366 ml, and PVR = 0 ml.

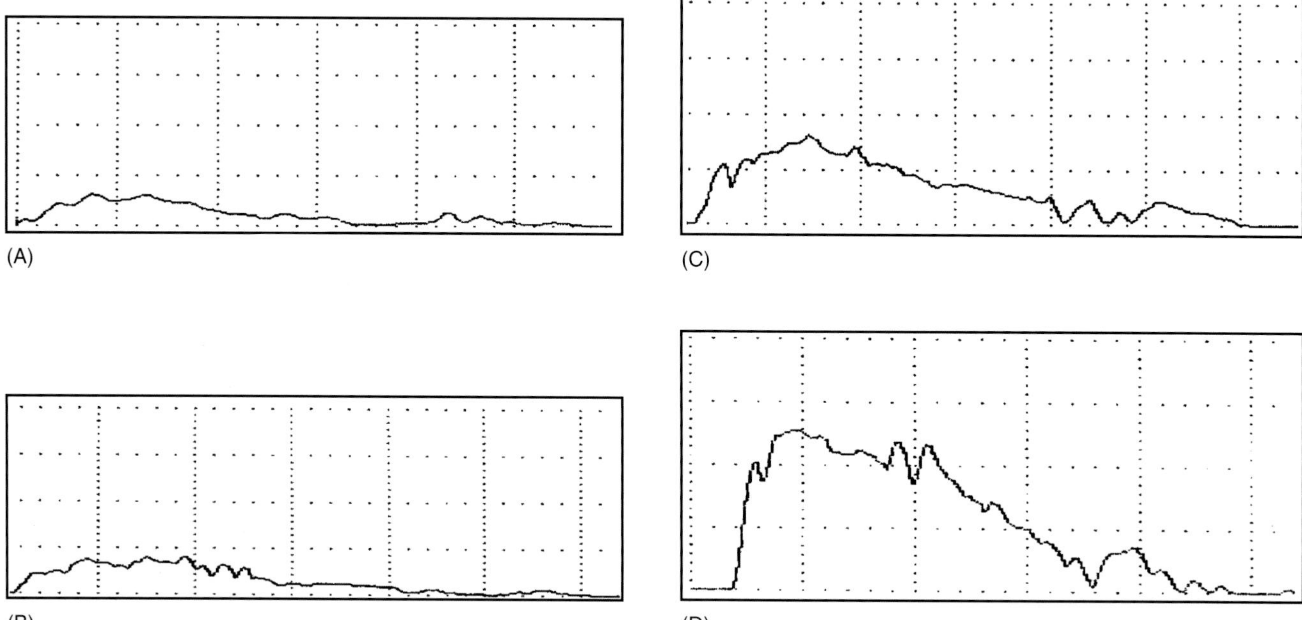

Fig. 4.7 Dependency of uroflow on voided volume. Serial uroflows in a 50-year-old man with increasing voided volumes. (A) Uroflow at 140 ml voided volume. Q_{max} = 6 ml/s and mean flow = 3 ml/s. (B) A uroflow at 200 ml voided volume. Q_{max} = 8 ml/s and mean flow = 4 ml/s. (C) A uroflow at 416 ml voided volume. Q_{max} = 16 ml/s and mean flow = 7 ml/s. (D) A uroflow at 580 ml voided volume. Q_{max} = 25 ml/s and mean flow = 13 ml/s.

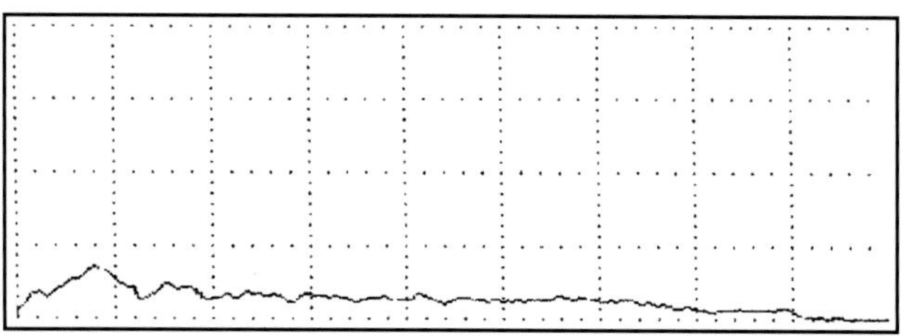

Fig. 4.8 In patients with urethral obstruction or impaired detrusor contractility, the rate and pattern of flow is usually altered resulting in a prolonged, flattened tracing. Q_{max} = 7 ml/s, Q_{ave} = 2 ml/s, voided volume = 215 ml, and PVR = 600 ml.

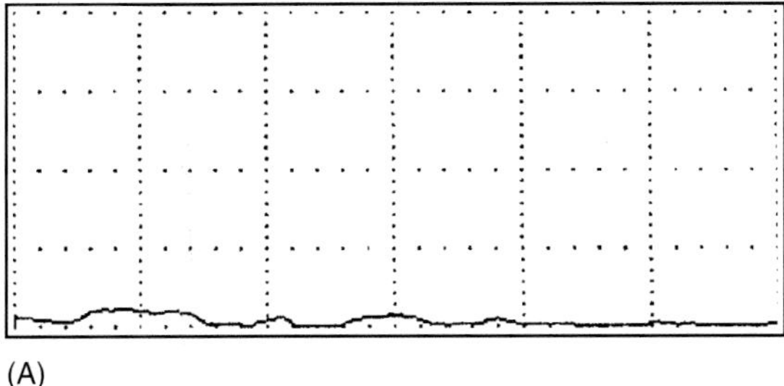

(A)

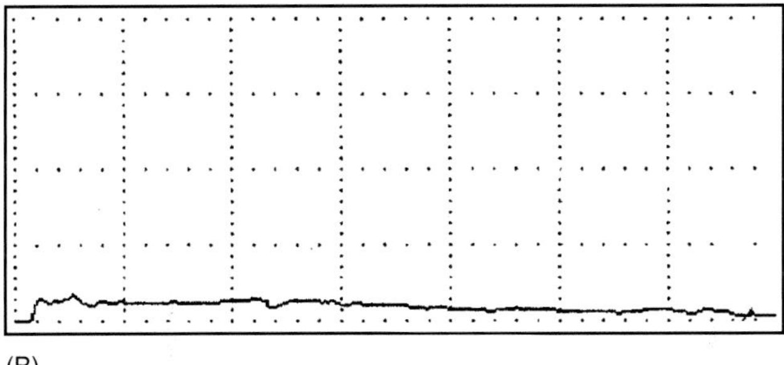

(B)

Fig. 4.9 Low uroflow due to (A) impaired detrusor contractility and (B) urethral obstruction. (A) Impaired detrusor contractility: Q_{max} = 2 ml/s, Q_{ave} = 2 ml/s, voided volume = 58 ml, and PVR (post-void residual) = 120 ml. (B) Urethral obstruction: Q_{max} = 3 ml/s, Q_{ave} = 2 ml/s, voided volume = 149 ml, and PVR = 212 ml.

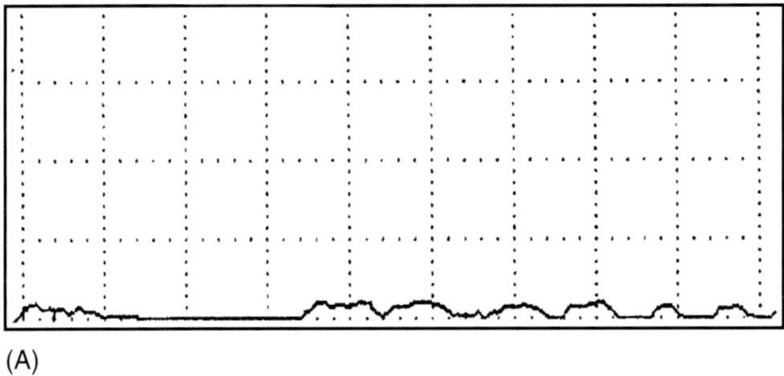

(A)

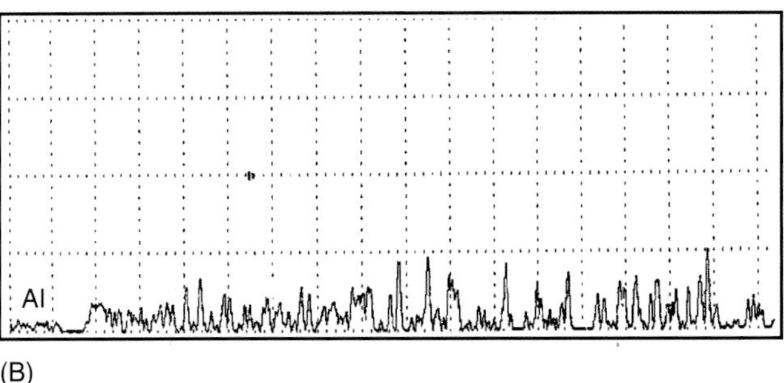

(B)

Fig. 4.10 (A) Uroflow in a 76-year-old man with prostatic obstruction and impaired detrusor contractility who strained during voiding. Q_{max} = 2 ml/s, Q_{ave} = 2 ml/s, voided volume = 97 ml, and PVR = 48 ml. (B) This 81-year-old man had a severe distal prostatic and membranous urethral stricture. He also voided with marked abdominal straining and had markedly impaired detrusor contractility. Q_{max} = 10 ml/s, Q_{ave} = 2 ml/s, voided volume = 269 ml, and PVR = 500 ml.

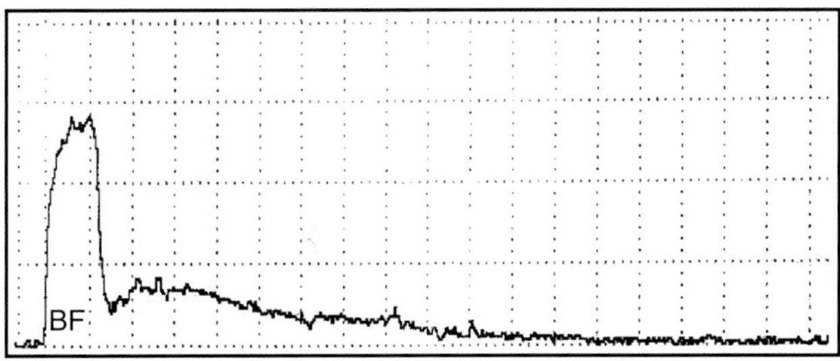

Fig. 4.11 This flow is from a 55-year-old who complained that his flow "cuts off in the middle" one month after TURP for prostatic obstruction. It shows a normal initial flow, which diminishes to a descending slope. The cause was a "ball valve" mechanical obstruction due to a retained prostate chip. Q_{max} = 28 ml/s, Q_{ave} = 7 ml/s, voided volume = 347 ml, and PVR = 50 ml.

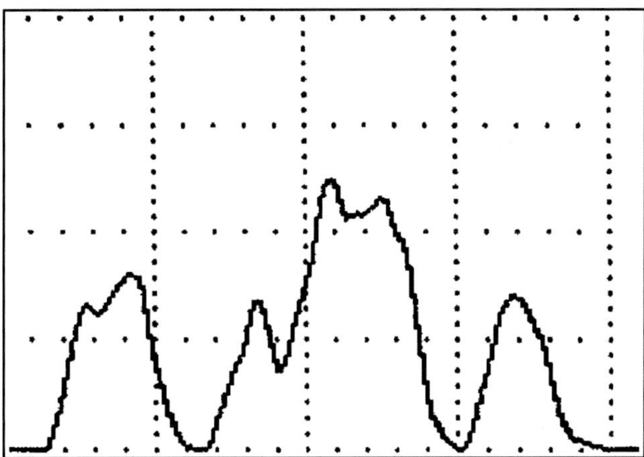

Fig. 4.12 This interrupted uroflow was seen in a man who underwent cystectomy and neobladder because of invasive bladder cancer. He voids with abdominal straining and sphincter relaxation. Q_{max} = 25 ml/s, Q_{ave} = 11 ml/s, voided volume = 366 ml, and PVR = 0 ml.

Leak Point Pressure

5

The leak point pressure (LPP) is widely considered to be the best measure of urethral sphincter strength, and we concur. This notwithstanding the fact that there is little consensus on terminology or numerical cutoffs. In a generic sense, the LPP is the lowest recorded pressure that results in urinary leakage and, as such, it is a direct measure of sphincter strength. The lower the leak point, the weaker the sphincter and vice versa. Much credit is due to Dr. Edward J. McGuire for developing the concept of LPP, how it relates to sphincteric incontinence, and pointing out the deleterious effects that elevated detrusor LPP (DLPP) has on the upper urinary tract [1,2].

The original technique described by Dr. McGuire is as follows. The bladder is filled with radiographic contrast to a volume of 150ml and the patient is asked to cough and valsalva, increasing the intravesical pressure until urinary leakage is seen by X-ray. Vesicle pressure is measured and the valsalva (vesical) leak point pressure (VLPP) is defined as the lowest vesical pressure, which causes leakage. If leakage does not occur at 150ml, the bladder is filled and the stress maneuvers repeated until leakage occurs or bladder capacity is reached.

The clinical methodology for performing the LPP has not yet been standardized and the terms abdominal LPP (ALPP), VLPP, and DLPP are used by different authors to mean different things.

The terminology used herein is defined below. There are three different pressures that are used to characterize the leak point – vesical pressure, abdominal pressure, and detrusor pressure. For all three measurements, the lowest corresponding pressure that results in visible leakage from the urethral meatus or at X-ray is considered the respective LPP. The **VLPP** is the lowest vesical pressure that causes leakage in the absence of a detrusor contraction and **ALPP** is the lowest abdominal pressure that causes leakage in the absence of a detrusor contraction. They are used to evaluate sphincteric incontinence. The **DLPP** is the lowest detrusor pressure that causes leakage. The DLPP relates bladder compliance and sphincter strength.

The examination can be performed in the lithotomy, sitting or standing position and each results in a different numeric value. Accordingly, it is important to specify the position when reporting results. We usually perform the test in the sitting position and record synchronous abdominal, vesical, and detrusor pressure and monitor the patient fluoroscopically. The bladder is filled at medium fill with radiographic contrast and the patient is asked to cough and bear down periodically during filling, usually at 100 or 150ml increments. The lowest pressure at the lowest volume that causes visible leakage is the respective LPP (Fig. 5.1). If the patient does not leak with the urethral catheter in place, it is removed and the lowest abdominal pressure is recorded as the ALPP (Figs. 5.2 and 5.3).

Despite the original presumption that urethral hypermobility and LPP were related, it has been demonstrated repeatedly that there is no correlation between the two [4,5]. Further, our experience and unpublished data from others have shown that there are a number of pitfalls with this technique. Firstly, the numeric value of LPP usually decreases with increasing bladder volume and many patients who do not leak at a volume of 150ml will leak at higher bladder volumes (Fig. 5.4). Secondly, the presence of the catheter, particularly in patients with low urethral compliance (after prostate, incontinence surgery, or radiation), may cause a false elevation in LPP. Some patients do not leak at all with the catheter in place and have obvious sphincteric incontinence and a low ALPP once the catheter is removed (Figs. 5.2 and 5.3). In these patients, the catheter size also affects LPP; the larger the catheter, the higher the LPP. Thirdly, radiologic visualization of leakage is much less sensitive than direct visualization of the urethral meatus. Accordingly, direct visualization will result in a lower LPP than radiologic detection in many patients (Fig. 5.5). Further, it should be recognized that it is the vesical and not the abdominal pressure which actually provides the energy to drive urine across the sphincter and cause incontinence. Thus, when one is using ALPP clinically it is important to (mentally) add back the estimated detrusor pressure to the ALPP to attain a true estimate of VLPP.

DLPP is useful in evaluating patients with suspected low bladder compliance; it is not relevant to patients with stress incontinence. In essence, it is a measure of the interaction between detrusor pressure and urethral resistance. The DLPP is performed by filling the bladder until either leakage from the urethra is observed or bladder capacity is reached in the absence of a detrusor contraction (Figs. 5.6 and 5.7).

The lower the urethral resistance for any given level of bladder compliance, the lower the DLPP and vice versa. In these circumstances, the sphincteric incontinence can be considered a "pop off valve" to protect the upper urinary tract at the expense of causing sphincteric incontinence. DLPPs $>40\,cmH_2O$ have been shown to cause hydronephrosis or vesicoureteral reflux [1,6].

Suggested Reading

1 McGuire EJ, Woodside JR, Borden TA, Weiss RM. Prognostic value of urodynamic testing in myelodysplastic patients, *J Urol*, 126: 205–209, 1981.

2 McGuire EJ, Fitzpatrick CC, Wan J, et al. Clinical assessment of urethral sphincter function, *J Urol*, 150: 1452–1454, 1993.

3 Abrams P, Cardozo L, Fall M, Griffiths D, Rosier P, Ulmsten U, van Kerrebroeck P, Victor A, Wein A. The standardisation of terminology of lower urinary tract function: report from the standardisation sub-committee of the international continence society, *Neurourol Urodyn*, 21: 167–178, 2002.

4 Fleischman N, Flisser AJ, Blaivas JG, Panagopoulos G. Sphincteric urinary incontinence: relationship of vesical leak point pressure, urethral mobility and severity of incontinence, *J Urol*, 169: 999–1002, 2003.

5 Nitti VW, Combs AJ. Correlation of Valsalva leak point pressure with subjective degree of stress urinary incontinence in women, *J Urol*, 155: 281–285, 1996.

6 Weld KJ, Graney MJ, Dmochowski RR. Differences in bladder compliance with time and associations of bladder management with compliance in spinal cord injured patients, *J Urol*, 163 (4): 1228–1233, 2000.

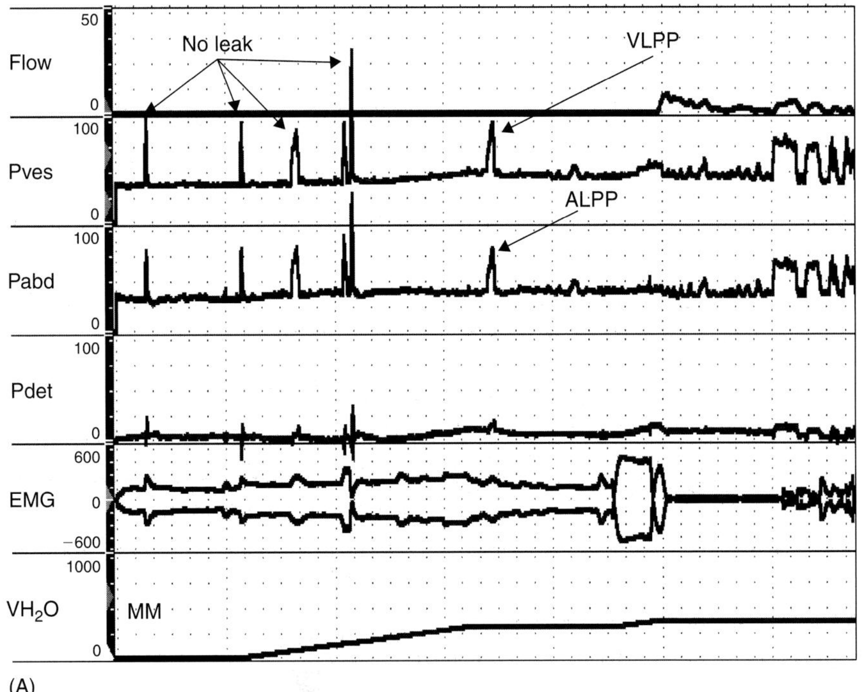

(A)

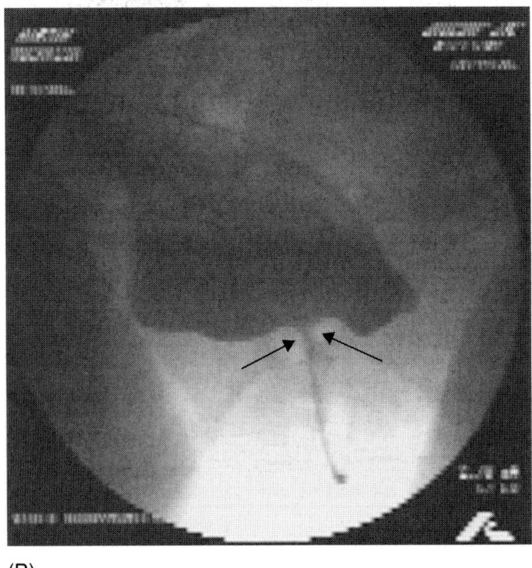

(B)

Fig. 5.1 VLPP: (A) Urodynamic tracing. During bladder filling, the patient is asked to cough and strain. There is no leakage during cough and valsalva to vesical pressures as high as 150 cmH_2O (small arrows), but at a bladder volume of 260 ml there is leakage apparent at X-ray. (B) X-ray exposed at VLPP. Note the beaked vesical neck (arrows) and contrast in the urethra.

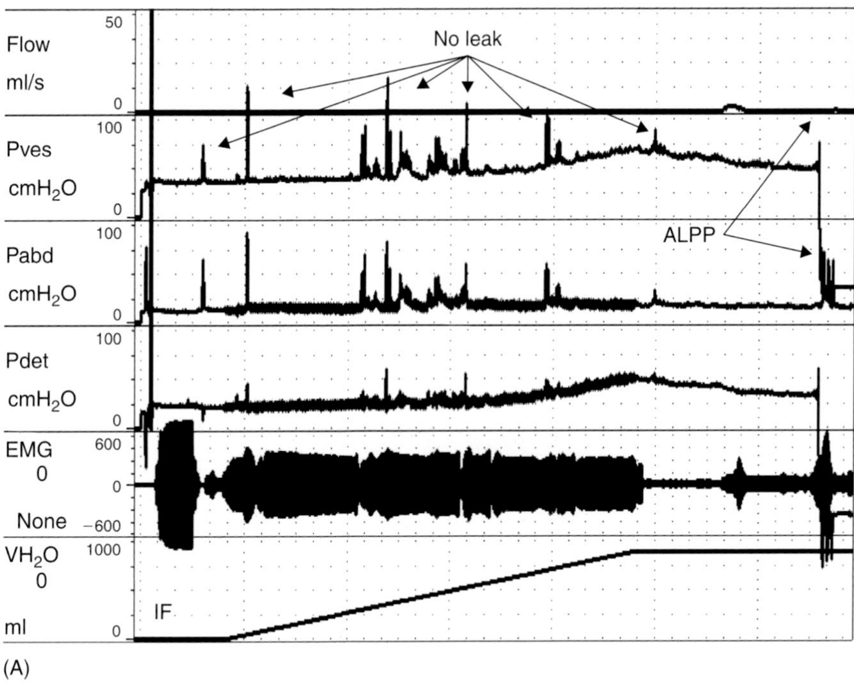

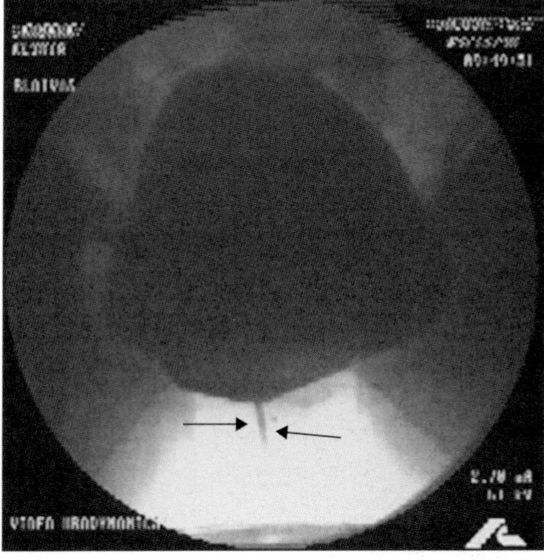

Fig. 5.2 ALPP obtained in a 78-year-old widowed woman evaluated because of stress incontinence (coughing, sneezing, walking, etc.). She has some urgency as well, but only rare urge incontinence. She ordinarily voids every hour during the day and has nocturia about every 3–4 hours at night. She has 3–4 incontinent episodes daily. She wears large pads and changes them 3–4 times a day. (A) Urodynamic tracing. Despite bladder filling to over 900 ml and multiple coughs over 100 cmH_2O, there was no leakage at all. Once the urethral catheter was removed she had an ALPP = 68 ml/s. (B) X-ray obtained at ALPP shows contrast in the urethra (arrows).

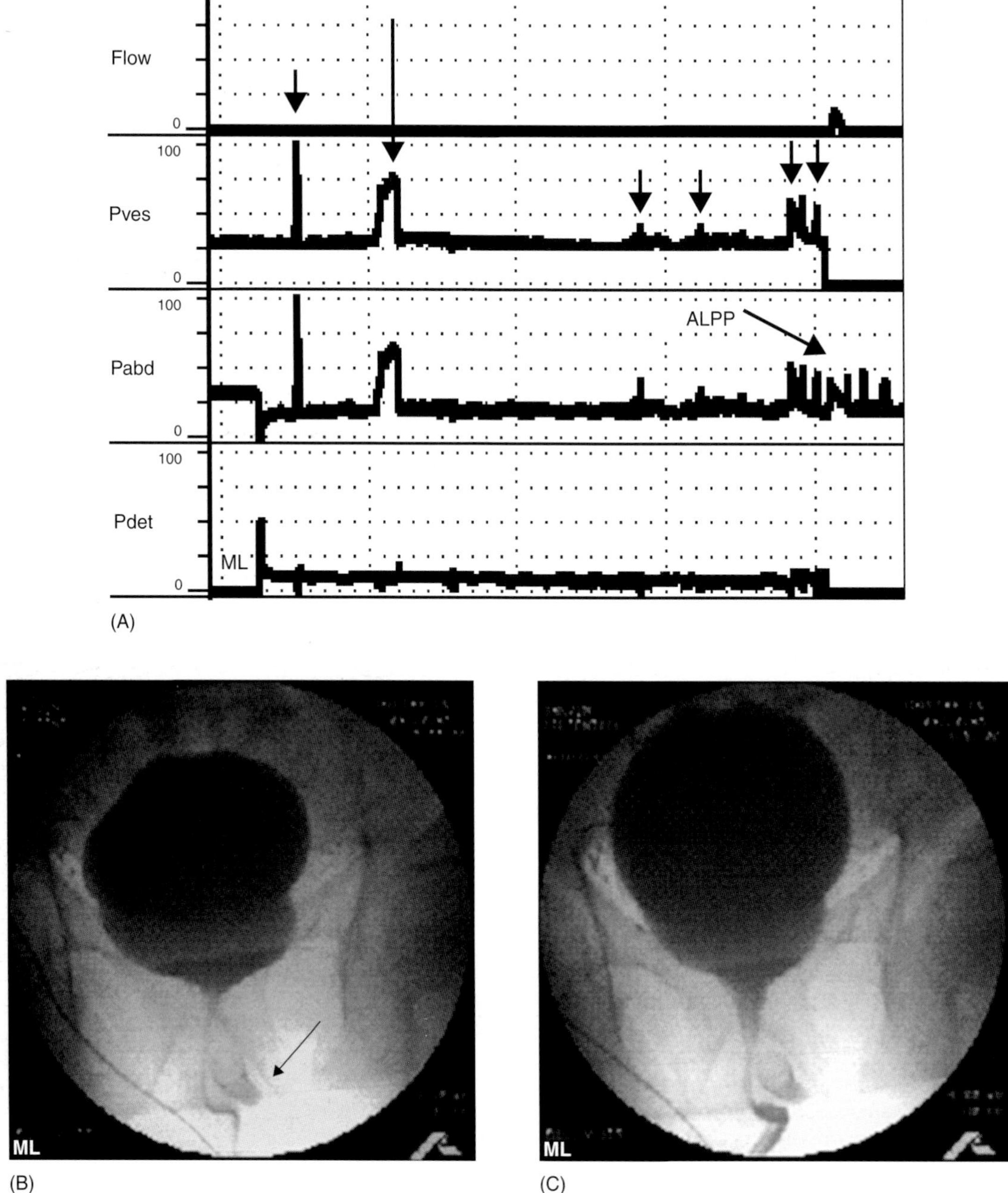

Fig. 5.3 (A) Urodynamic tracing. This is a man with post-radical prostatectomy sphincteric incontinence. During bladder filling he was asked to valsalva (large arrow) and cough (small arrows), but there was no leakage. At bladder capacity the urethral catheter was removed and he was incontinent with an ALPP = 48 cmH_2O. (B) X-ray obtained at maximum cough with 7F urethral urodynamic catheter in place shows no leakage. Incidental note is made of the cylinder of a penile prosthesis (arrow). (C) X-ray obtained at the ALPP after removal of the urodynamic catheter. Shows the unifora filled with contrast.

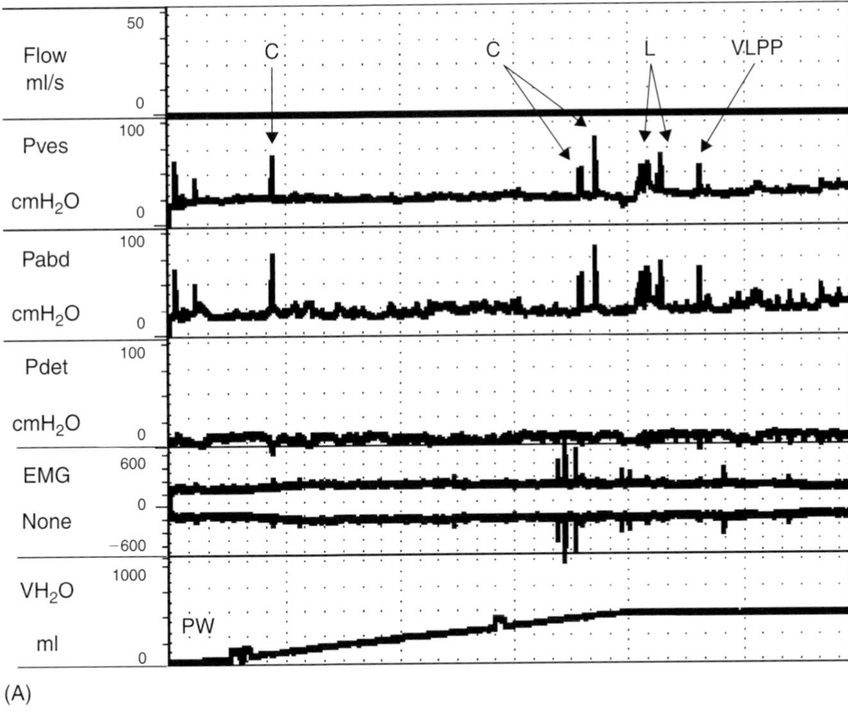

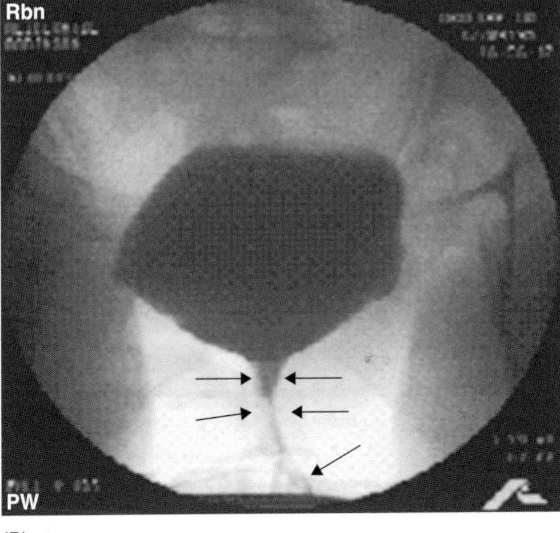

Fig. 5.4 Decreasing VLPP with increasing bladder volumes. (A) Urodynamic tracing. The bladder is filled to 150 ml with radiographic contrast and the patient is asked to cough (C), but there is no leakage. Filling is continued and there is no leakage to several more coughs (C) at a bladder volume of 240 ml. At 250 ml there is leakage visible on X-ray at Pves = 67 and 70 cmH_2O (L). The lowest pressure at which leakage occurs is 54 cmH_2O (VLPP). (B) X-ray obtained at the VLPP. Note contrast in the entire urethra and leakage into the vagina (arrows).

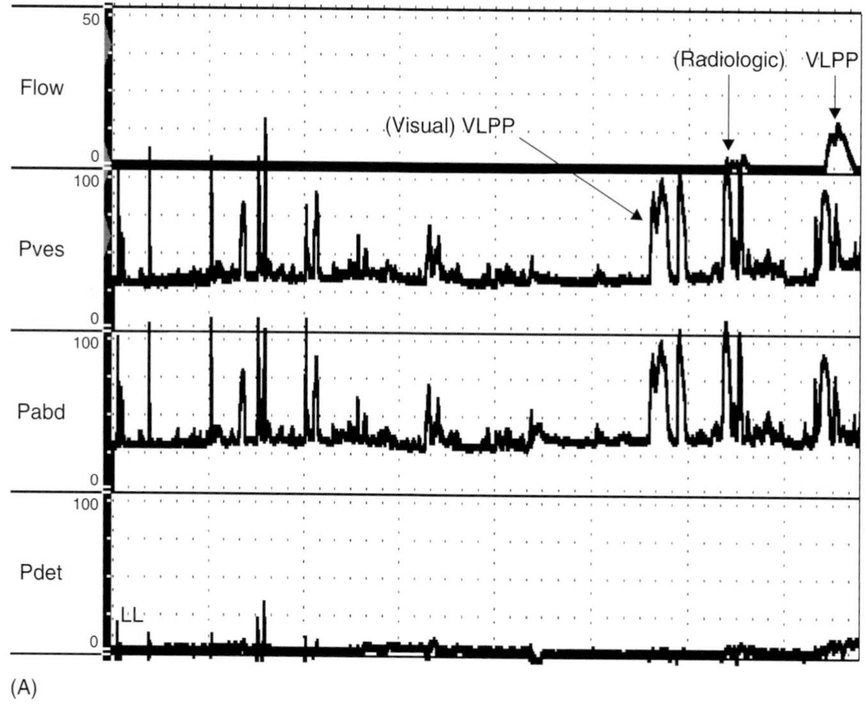

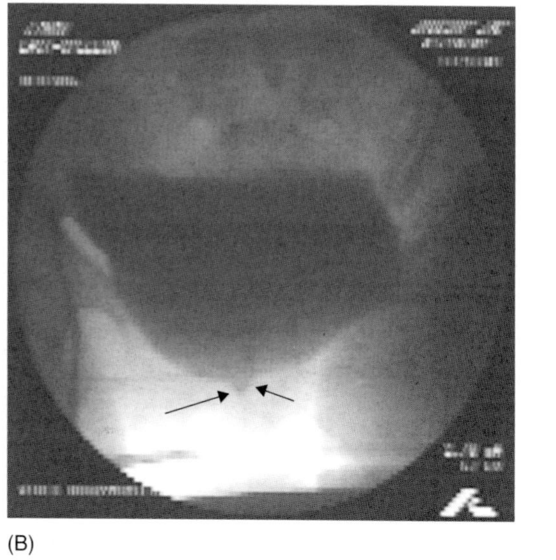

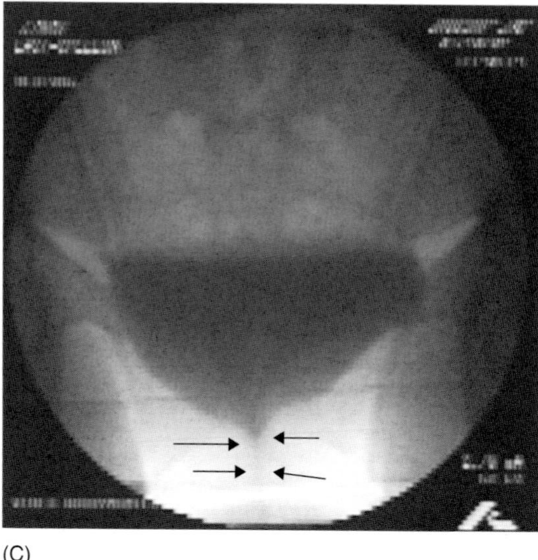

Fig. 5.5 Disparity between radiologic and visual VLPP. This is a 63-year-old woman. Her chief complaint is urinary incontinence "it's gotten worse. . .if I play tennis and hit a ball, I leak. . .I'm constantly looking for a bathroom. . .I'm constantly getting an urge. Some days I'm running to the bathroom every hour from 9 AM to 12 PM and less often afterwards." She always has stress incontinence (cough, sneeze, exercise, etc.). (A) Urodynamic tracing. During bladder filling she was repeatedly asked to cough and valsalva, but there was no visual leakage from the meatus until a bladder volume of 200 ml and a VLPP = 75 cmH_2O. Radiologic visualization of leakage did not occur until a bladder volume of 275 ml and a VLPP = 103 cmH_2O. (B) X-ray exposed with 175 ml in the bladder shows an open vesical neck at rest (arrows), but no leakage. (C) X-ray exposed at the (visual) VLPP showing descent and opening of the bladder base and urethra, but no leakage is observed radiologically. There was obvious leakage from the urethral meatus on direct inspection.

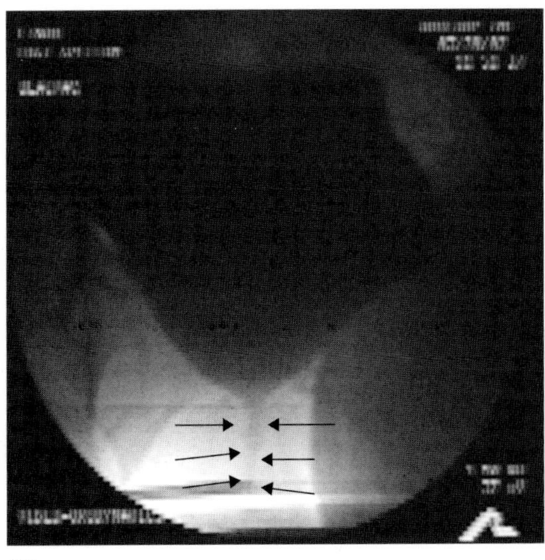

Fig. 5.5 (continued) (D) X-ray exposed at the radiographic VLPP shows the entire urethra filled with contrast (arrows).

(D)

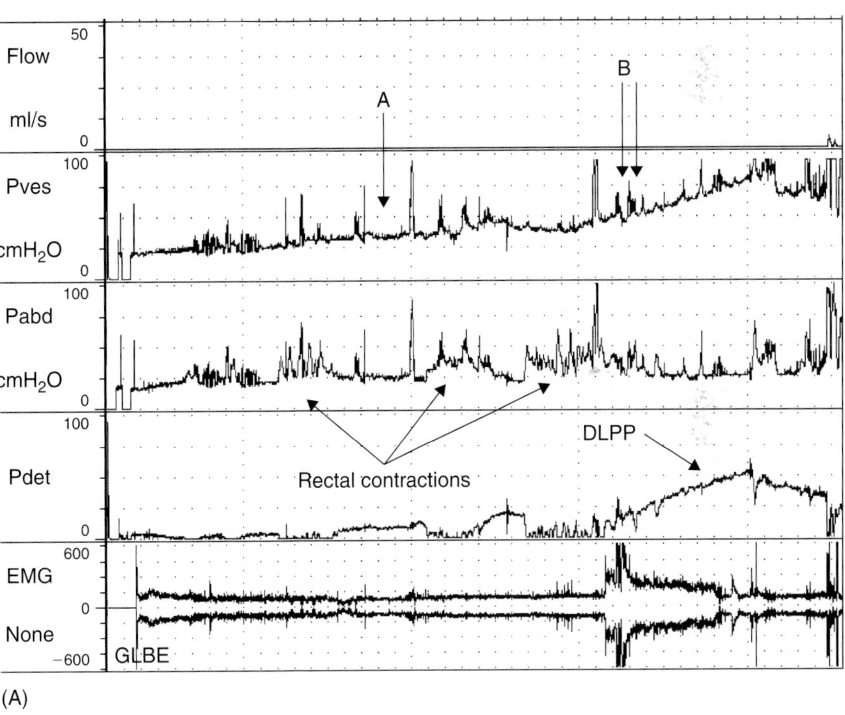

(A)

Fig. 5.6 DLPP in a 50-year-old woman two years status post radical hysterectomy, chemotherapy, and external beam radiotherapy for cervical carcinoma. She complained of a severe dribbling incontinence. (A) Urodynamic tracing. Low bladder compliance is evident by the steep rise in vesical pressure during bladder filling. Spontaneous rectal contractions cause an artifactual fall in detrusor pressure because detrusor pressure is calculated by subtracting abdominal pressure from vesical pressure. Leakage was observed from the urethral meatus at the DLPP.

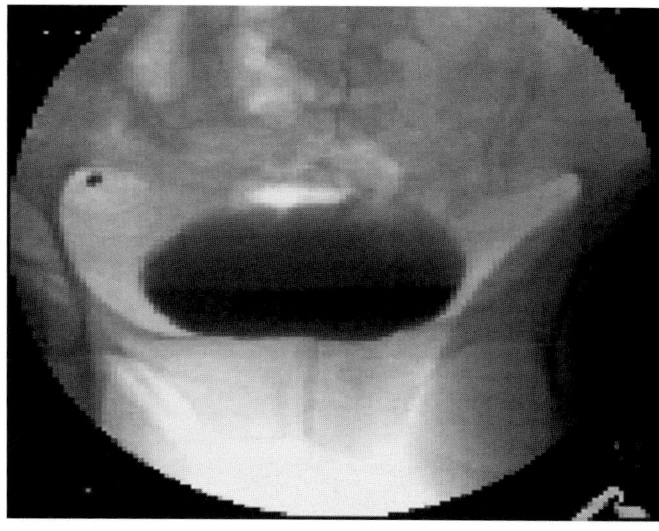

(B)

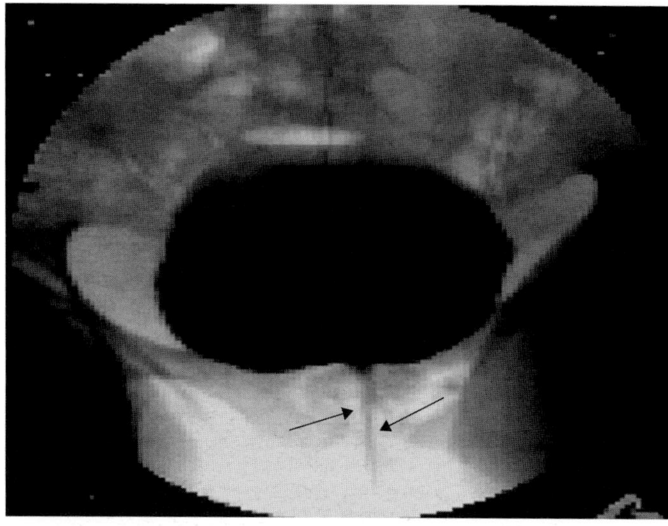

(C)

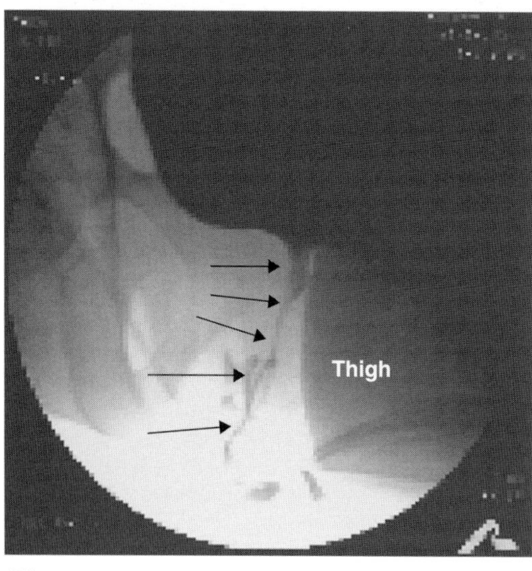

(D)

Fig. 5.6 (continued) (B) X-ray exposed during bladder filling to 75 ml (point A) shows the bladder neck to be closed. (C) X-ray exposed during bladder filling to 150 ml (point B) shows contrast in the urethra (arrows), but she has not yet been incontinent. (D) X-ray exposed at the DLPP showing contrast filling the urethra and obvious incontinence (arrows).

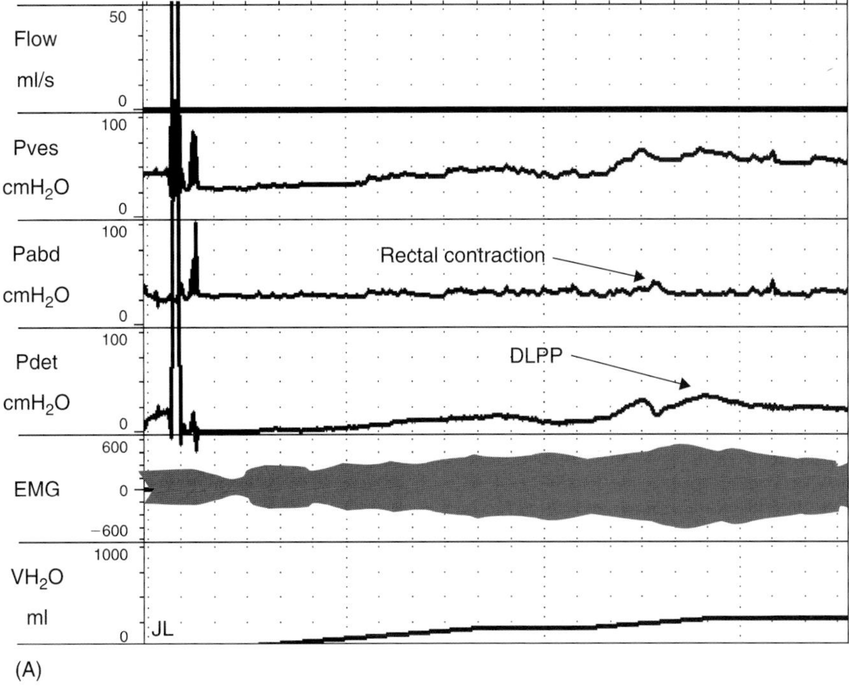

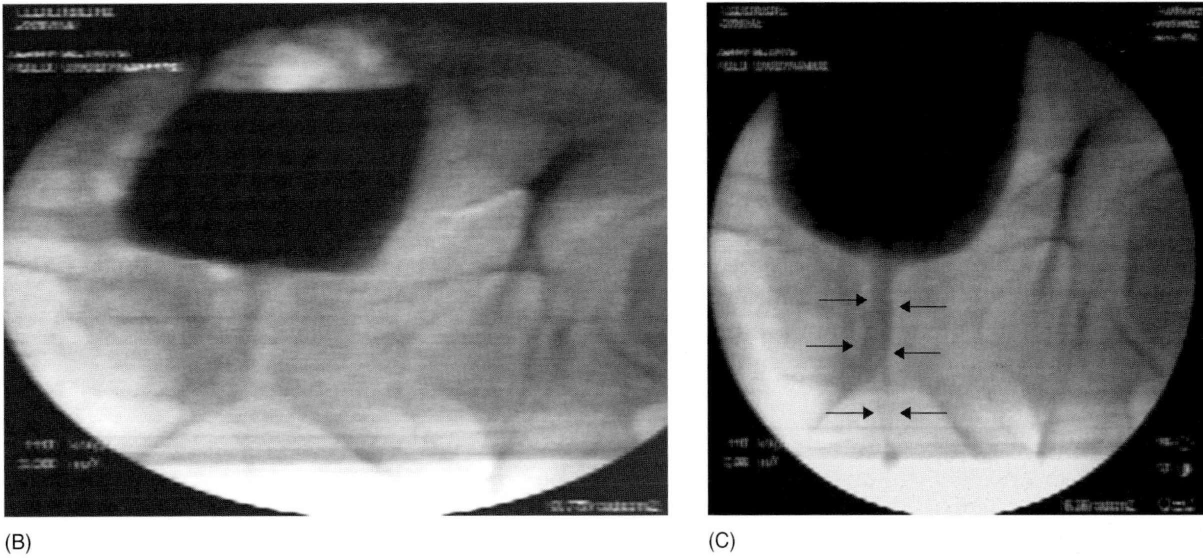

Fig. 5.7 DLPP in a 77-year-old man who developed urinary retention and incontinence after external beam radiation to the prostate for prostate cancer and subsequent unilateral S1–S4 neurologic injury during disk surgery. (A) Urodynamic tracing shows a DLPP = 37 cmH_2O. Note the artifactual fall in detrusor pressure due to a spontaneous rectal contraction. (B) X-ray exposed during bladder filling shows the bladder neck is closed and no contrast is seen in the urethra. (C) X-ray exposed at the DLPP shows contrast throughout the urethra (arrows).

Low Bladder Compliance

6

Normally during bladder filling at physiologic rates, detrusor pressure remains nearly constant because of a special property of the bladder known as accommodation. Accommodation is due to the vesicoelastic properties of the bladder, based on its composition of smooth muscle, collagen, and elastin. When accommodation is impaired, low bladder compliance ensues. In experimental animals, accommodation (and compliance) is unaffected by acute neurologic impairment or by administration of cholinergic agonists or antagonists.

Low bladder compliance is manifest as a steep rise in detrusor pressure during bladder filling. It is calculated by dividing the change in bladder volume by the change in detrusor pressure during that change in bladder volume. The numeric value of compliance is dependent, in part, on the volume interval over which it is measured (Figs. 6.1 and 6.2). In a sense, bladder compliance may be thought of as "bladder wall stiffness." Normal values of bladder compliance have not been well defined. Harris et al. suggested that the lower limit of normal in women was 40 ml/cmH_2O in women. In patients with neurogenic bladder, values of 13–40 ml/cmH_2O have been associated with a high risk of upper urinary tract complications.

Incontinence due to low bladder compliance occurs when vesical pressure exceeds outlet resistance (Fig. 6.3). Clinically, low bladder compliance is most commonly seen in a variety of neurologic conditions, especially lower motor neuron lesions (Figs. 6.1 and 6.3). It is also seen in patients with fibrosis of the bladder wall such as after multiple bladder surgeries (Fig. 6.4) and radiation cystitis (see Fig. 5.6). Bladder outlet obstruction, because of its effect on bladder ultrastructure, is known to cause low bladder compliance. Approximately 9% of men with lower urinary tract symptoms (LUTS) have low bladder compliance (Fig. 6.5).

Low bladder compliance has long been known as a risk factor for the development of hydronephrosis. It has recently been showed that relief of obstruction by transurethral incision or resection of the prostate can improve compliance. The clinical causes of low bladder compliance are listed in Table 6.1.

Table. 6.1 Causes of low bladder compliance.

I. Neurogenic
   - Myelodysplasia
   - Shy–Drager syndrome
   - Suprasacral spinal cord injury/lesion
   - Radical hysterectomy
   - Abdominoperineal (AP) resection of the rectum

II. Non-Neurogenic
   - Bladder outlet obstruction
   - Multiple bladder surgeries
   - Chronic cystitis (interstitial, radiation, tuberculous)
   - Chronic indwelling catheter

Suggested Reading

1 Klevmark B. Motility of the urinary bladder in cats during filling at physiologic rates. I. Intravesical pressure patterns studied by a new method of cystometry, *Acta Physiol Scand*, 90: 565, 1974.

2 Ruch TC, Tang PC. The higher control of the bladder, Chapter 13. In Boyarsky S (ed) *The Neurogenic Bladder*, Baltimore: Williams & Wilkins, 1967.

3 Klevmark B. II. Effects of extrinsic bladder denervation on intramural tension and on intravesical pressure patterns, *Acta Physiol Scand*, 101: 176, 1977.
4 Harris RL, Cundiff GW, Theofrastous JP, Bump RC. Bladder compliance in neurologically intact women, *Neurourol Urodyn*, 15 (5): 483–488, 1996.
5 McGuire EJ, Woodside JR, Borden TA, Weiss RM. Prognostic value of urodynamic testing in myelodysplastic patients, *J Urol*, 126: 205–209, 1981.
6 Ghoniem GM, Bloom DA, McGuire EJ, Stewart KL. Bladder compliance in meningomyelocele children, *J Urol*, 141: 1404–1406, 1989.
7 Weld KJ, Graney MJ, Dmochowski RR. Differences in bladder compliance with time and associations of bladder management with compliance in spinal cord injured patients. *J Urol*, 163 (4): 1228–1233, 2000.
8 Shin JC, Park CI, Kim HJ, Lee I. Significance of low compliance bladder in cauda equina injury, *Spinal Cord*, 40 (12): 650–655, 2002.
9 Fusco F, Groutz A, Blaivas JG, Chaikin DC, Weiss JP. Videourodynamic studies in men with lower urinary tract symptoms: a comparison of community based versus referral urological practices, *J Urol*, 166: 910, 2001.
10 Coolsaet, B.R.L.A., Bladder compliance and detrusor activity during the collection phase, *Neurourol Urodyn*, 4: 263, 1985.
11 Klevmark B. Motility of the urinary bladder in cats during filling at physiologic rates. III. Spontaneous rhythmic contractions in the conscious and anaesthetized animal, *Scand J Urol*, 14: 219, 1980.
12 Toppercer A, Tetreault JP. Compliance of the bladder: an attempt to establish normal values, *Urology*, 14: 204, 1979.

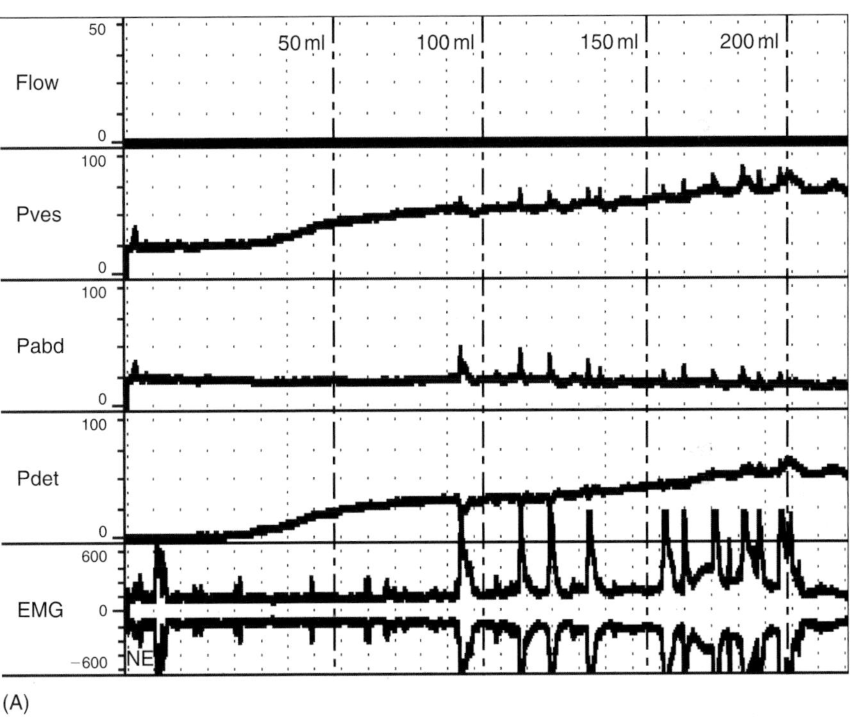

Fig. 6.1 Low bladder compliance in a 43-year-old paraplegic (T10–11) 11 years after injury. He has been managed by a condom catheter and intermittent catheterization BID (He was advised to catheterize himself at least 4 times a day, but refused because of social reasons). He has bilateral hydronephrosis and chronic pyelonephritis. (A) Urodynamic tracing. Note the small changes in bladder compliance that occurs during bladder filling. Each of the vertical dotted lines denotes the point at which bladder compliance was measured. Bladder compliance at: 50 ml = 50/23 = 2.17, 100 ml = 100/32 = 3.1, 150 ml = 150/40 = 3.75, 200 ml = 200/60 = 3.3, and 200 ml (after stopping infusion) = 200/50 = 4.

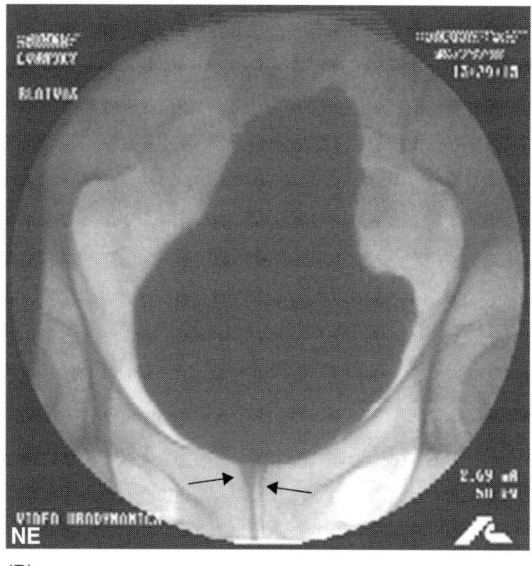

(B)

Fig. 6.1 (continued) (B) X-ray obtained during bladder filling shows an open vesical neck (arrows). Note the "Christmas tree" shaped bladder and the irregular bladder wall characteristic of a trabeculated bladder.

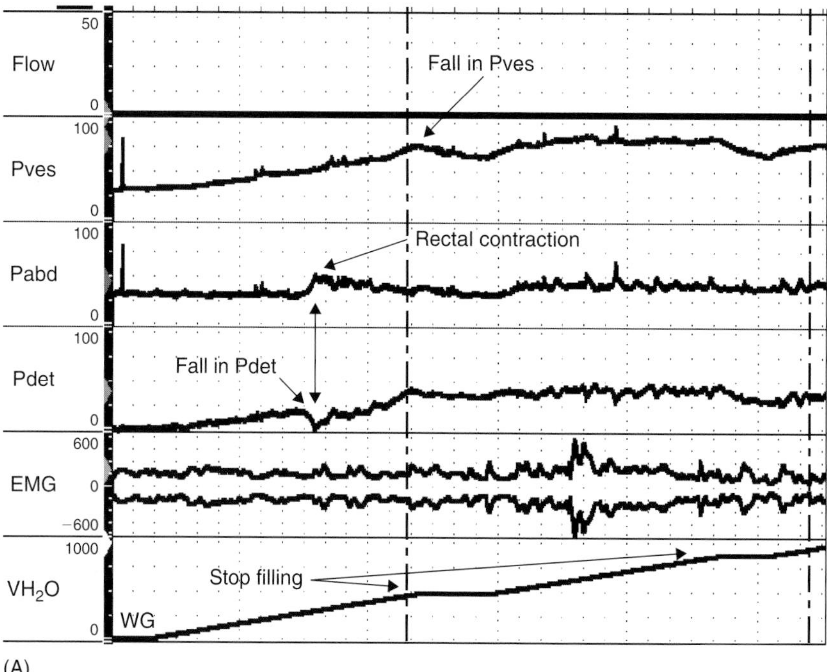

(A)

Fig. 6.2 Effect of bladder volume on bladder compliance. Low bladder compliance in an 86-year-old man with a long history of lower urinary tract symptoms (LUTS) (urinary frequency Q2H, daily urgency, and urge incontinence). Upon referral, he had a palpable bladder and was catheterized for over 2.5 l and taught intermittent self-catheterization. Renal and bladder ultrasound showed bilateral hydronephrosis and a huge bladder. He had been treated empirically for years with doxazocin for "prostatism." (A) Urodynamic study. FSF = 275ml, 1st urge = 476 ml, and severe urge = 975 ml. During bladder filling there was a steep rise in detrusor and vesical pressure, but a rectal contraction caused an artifactual fall in detrusor pressure (arrow). At the first vertical line on the left, bladder filling was discontinued because it looked like the patient might be experiencing a detrusor contraction. There was an immediate fall in vesical and detrusor pressure proving that the rise in pressure was due to low compliance and not a detrusor contraction. Bladder compliance = 500/45 = 11 ml/cmH_2O at the vertical line, but 975/40 = 24 ml/cmH_2O at bladder capacity (second vertical line on the right).

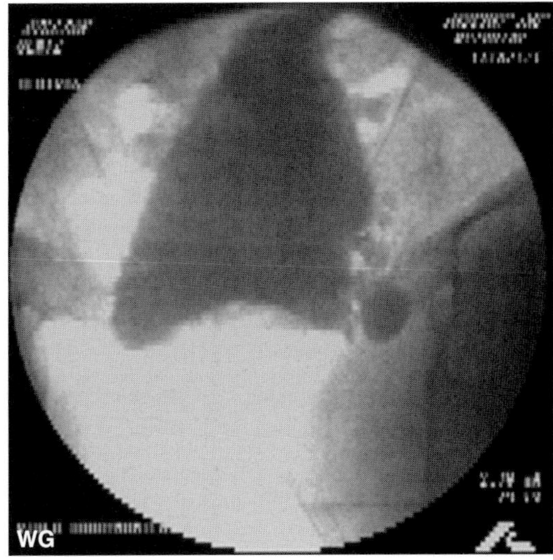

(B)

Fig. 6.2 (continued) (B) X-ray obtained during filling shows a prostatic impression on the bladder base, multiple medium and small sized bladder diverticula, and a heavily trabeculated bladder. He was treated with intermittent catheterization and his hydronephrosis completely resolved within one month.

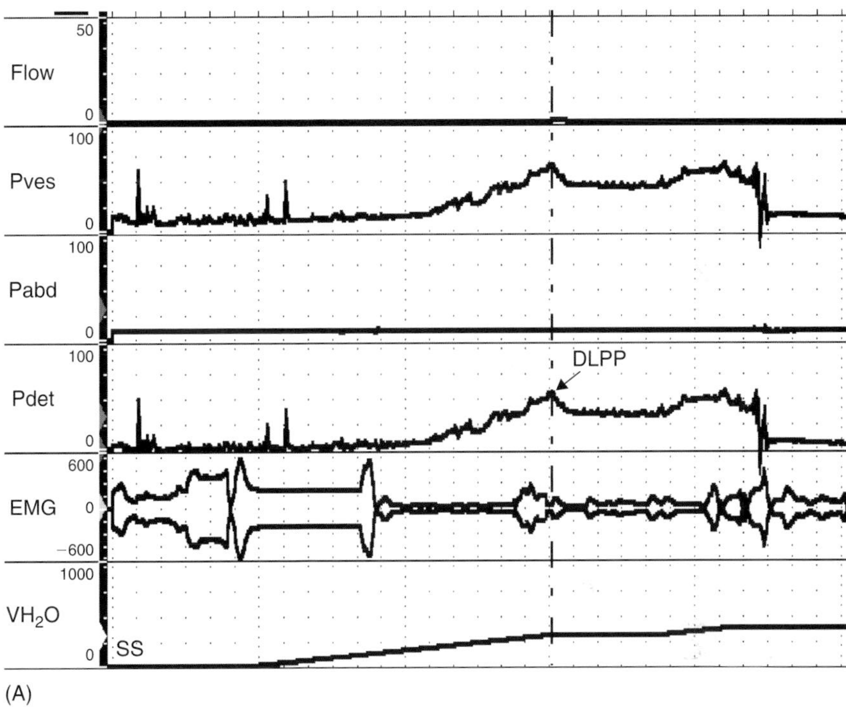

(A)

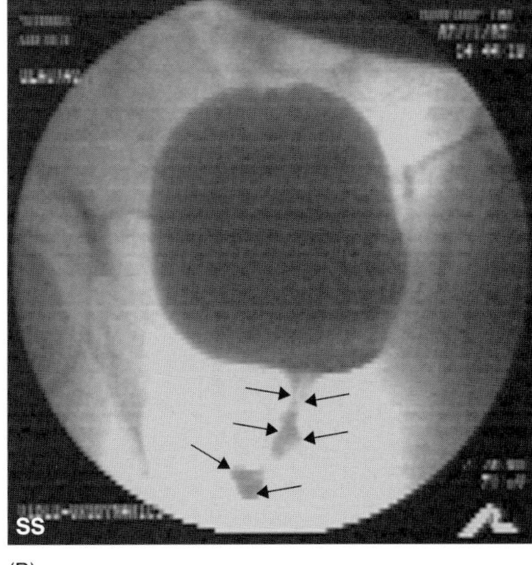

(B)

Fig. 6.3 Low bladder compliance and sphincteric incontinence in a 60-year-old man 3 months after AP resection of the rectum. He'd been treated with a Foley catheter ever since failing multiple voiding trials. (A) Urodynamic study. 1st sensation = 321 ml, severe urge = 386 ml coincident with bladder capacity, and bladder compliance = 385/58 = 6. 7 ml/cmH_2O. Urinary incontinence occurs at a detrusor leak point pressure (DLPP) = 50 cmH_2O (vertical dotted line). As soon as incontinence occurred, bladder filling was stopped and detrusor pressure immediately fell, proving that the rise in detrusor pressure (and incontinence) was due to low bladder compliance and not a detrusor contraction. (B) X-ray obtained at Pdetmax shows leakage of contrast into the urethra (arrows).

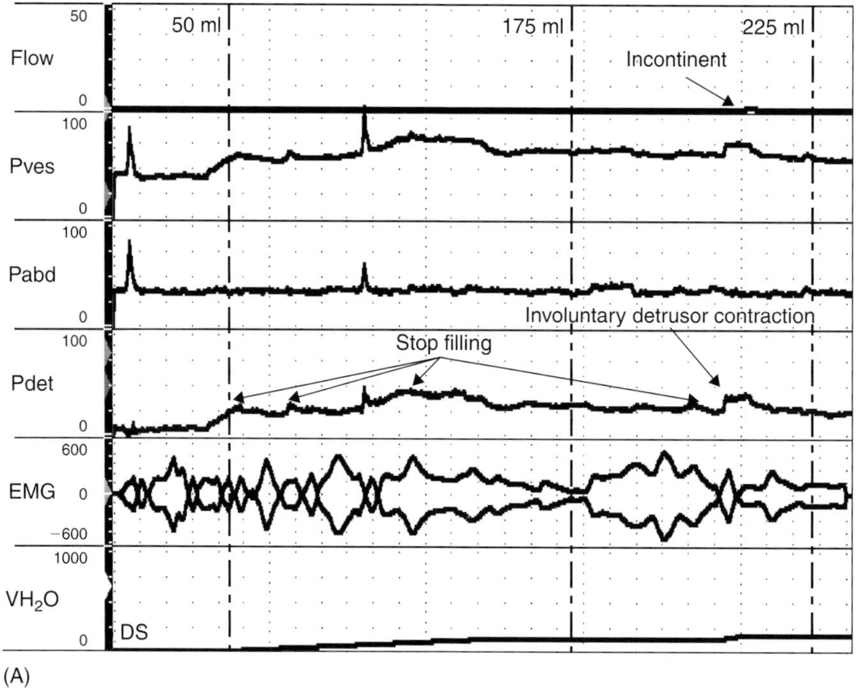

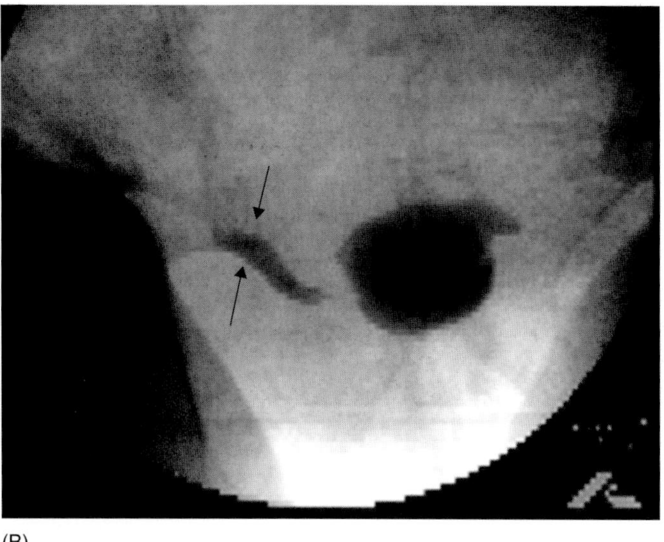

(B)

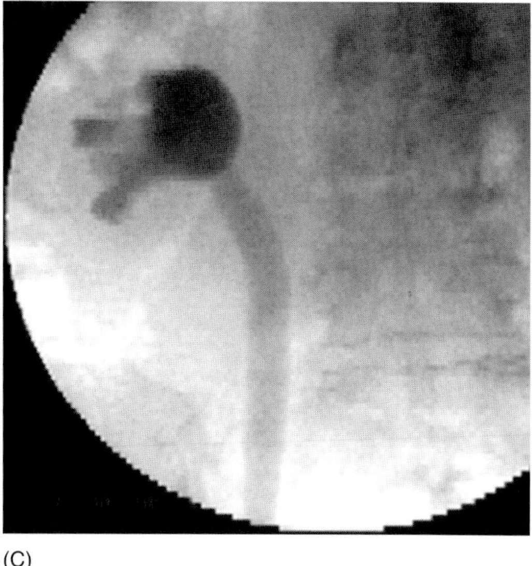

(C)

Fig. 6.4 Low bladder compliance in a 70-year-old woman who underwent multiple surgeries after she developed a colovesical and vesicovaginal fistula after synthetic pubovaginal sling. (A) Urodynamic tracing. Bladder compliance at 50, 175, and 225 ml was 50/37 = 1.35, 175/48 = 3.6, and 225/25 = 9 ml/cmH_2O, respectively (vertical dotted lines). At 225 ml, she had an involuntary detrusor contraction and was incontinent. (B) X-ray obtained at 50 ml shows right vesicoureteral reflux (arrows). (C) X-ray obtained immediately after (Fig. 4B) shows the reflux to be grade 3.

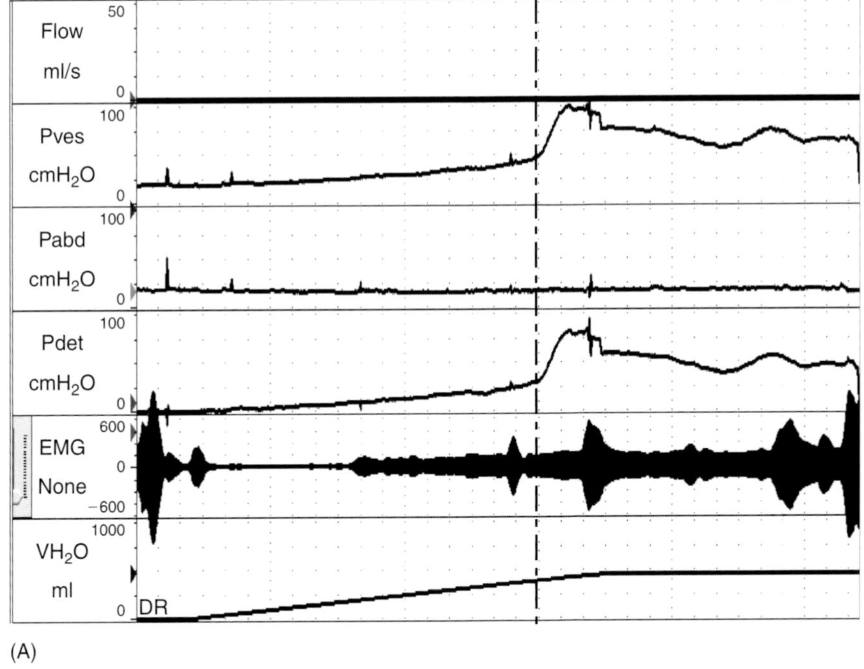

(A)

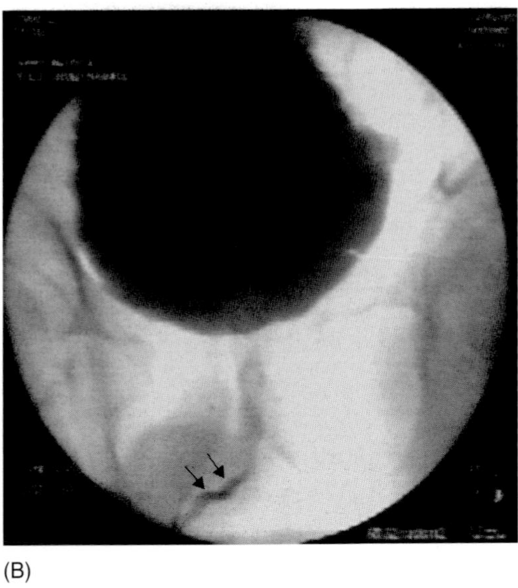

(B)

Fig. 6.5 Low bladder compliance due to longstanding Schafer grade 5 prostatic obstruction. DR is a 57-year-old man referred because of "voiding dysfunction" of at least 20 years' duration. His chief complaint is "weak stream, incomplete emptying and it's getting worse . . . and if I don't do something, it could get very serious," or so he's been told by his doctors. He ordinarily voids every 2 hours during the day and has nocturia once a night. He usually has to push and strain to void. His AUA symptom score is 22. He's been treated with a variety of alpha adrenergic antagonists without effect. Multiple bladder diaries showed an MVV = 180 ml and 24-hour volumes ranging from 1200 to 1500 ml, Q_{max} = 3 ml/s, and post-void residual (PVR) = 350 ml. (A) Urodynamic tracing. FSF = 201 ml, 1st urge = 435 ml, and severe urge occurred at 455 ml. At bladder capacity he had a voluntary detrusor contraction, but was unable to void. Bladder compliance measured just prior to the detrusor contraction (vertical dotted line) = 375/32 = 11.7 ml/cmH_2O. (B) X-ray obtained at Pdetmax shows no visualization of the prostatic urethra and a trabeculated bladder. There are shadows overlying the prostatic urethra that might be misinterpreted as contrast but are due to the compound effects of visualization of the penis and pubis. There is some dye in the bulbar and anterior urethra (arrows). The bladder has a scalloped appearance due to marked bladder trabecutations.

Videourodynamics

7

The synchronous measurement and display of urodynamic parameters with radiographic visualization of the lower urinary tract is, in our judgment, the most precise diagnostic tool for evaluating disturbances of micturition. In these studies, radiographic contrast is used as the infusant for cystometry and other urodynamic parameters including abdominal pressure, uroflow, and sphincter electromyography are recorded as well. By measuring multiple urodynamic variables, one gains a better insight into the underlying pathophysiology. Moreover, since all variables are visualized simultaneously one can better appreciate their interrelationships and identify artifacts with ease.

What are the indications for videourodynamics? The indications depend upon the threshold of the clinician for obtaining the most accurate diagnostic information. In patients who complain of urge incontinence, one hardly needs videourodynamics (or even cystometry) to diagnose detrusor overactivity, but detrusor instability may be due to urethral obstruction and only synchronous detrusor pressure/uroflow studies can diagnose obstruction with any degree of certainty. In women who complain of stress incontinence and have obvious leakage of urine during cough or valsalva, one hardly needs videourodynamics to diagnose sphincteric incontinence, but sphincteric incontinence may be accompanied by impaired detrusor contractility, detrusor overactivity, or even urethral obstruction. It may or may not be accompanied by urethral hypermobility.

All these diagnoses are most accurately made by videourodynamics and all have important implications for treatment, particularly surgical treatment. Nonetheless, videourodynamics serves no clinical purpose unless the clinician bases his therapy on the results of the study. The main purpose of urodynamic evaluation is to document the underlying cause of symptoms and to correlate them with urodynamic findings. To this end, it is essential to understand the nature of the patient's complaints and to use the urodynamic evaluation as a provocative test to mimic those symptoms. The symptoms should be clearly documented prior to beginning the urodynamic evaluation on the basis of the history, the physical examination, the voiding diary, and pad test.

The urodynamic study itself is an interactive process between an examiner and a patient. The examiner should document, at the time of the study, whether or not the patient's symptoms are reproduced and, if they are, the underlying cause should be clearly understood before completion of the study. The specific techniques for performing urodynamic studies differ according to the age and sex of the patient and the specifics of the complaints; but for all patients, before starting the urodynamic study the following information should be known:

1 What symptoms are you trying to reproduce?

2 What is the functional bladder capacity (maximum voided volume on the voiding diary)?

3 What is the post-void residual urine?

4 What is the uroflow?

5 Is there a neurologic disorder that could cause neurogenic bladder?

Urodynamic technique

A 7 F double lumen bladder and rectal catheter are passed into the bladder and rectum to measure vesical and abdominal pressure, respectively. The pressure transducers are zeroed to atmospheric pressure at the level of the symphysis pubis. Vesical pressure (Pves) and abdominal pressure (Pabd) are displayed on a computer screen and detrusor pressure (Pdet) is electronically calculated by subtracting abdominal pressure from vesical pressure and displayed on a third channel. Other channels display sphincter electromyography (EMG), infused bladder volume, voided volume, and uroflow. Fluoroscopic images are sampled periodically during filling, voiding, and provocative maneuvers such as measurement of leak point pressure (LPP). The format for display of these parameters is depicted in Figure 7.1.

For bladder filling, we use a Y connector attached to normal saline and radiopaque contrast. We adjust the amount of contrast based on the fluoroscopic appearance. We usually fill the bladder initially at a medium fill rate of 50–100 ml/min with alterations in the rate based on patient response to filling and the aforementioned goal of symptom reproduction. Normal studies in a man and woman are depicted in Figures 7.2 and 7.3.

For patients with painful bladder syndromes we fill more slowly; for those with large capacity bladders we fill rapidly. During the filling phase, the patient is instructed to neither void nor try to prevent micturition, but, rather, to report his or her sensations to the examiner. Notation is made of the first filling, first urge, and severe urge sensation volumes. The presence or absence of involuntary detrusor contractions (IDC) is noted. Patients who complain of incontinence are asked to cough, strain, or do whatever else might cause them to become incontinent. LPP is measured periodically during filling. During the cough, it is noted, either on direct visualization or by X-ray, whether or not there is any descent of the vesical neck and proximal urethra associated with urinary leakage.

For measurement of LPP, with the urethral catheter in place, we have the patient cough and strain to the point of leaking (Fig. 7.4). Straining slowly with increasing intensity allows more accurate assessment of exact LPP than does coughing, but coughing is still utilized in order to assess concomitant stress hyperreflexia. Stress hyperreflexia occurs when a cough, sneeze, or other valsalva type maneuver induces an IDC.

Clinically this is manifest either by incontinent flow, which persists long after the cough is over, or uncontrollable voiding which commences several seconds after the cough. With the urethral catheter in place, the IDC will be obviously demonstrated on the subtracted detrusor pressure channel.

If the patient complains of stress incontinence, but it is not demonstrated, we remove the urethral catheter and have the patient repeat the cough and strain maneuvers and measure the abdominal pressure at which leakage occurs.

When the patient experiences a normal urge to void, he or she is asked to do so, a voiding Pdet/Q study is done and post-void residual urine measured.

For urge and mixed incontinent patients, or during any IDC, filling, or provocative maneuvers, we assess the amplitude of the IDC; whether or not the patient is aware of the IDC; and the degree of control that the patient exhibits (see chapter 9), overactive Bladder.

In patients suspected of having a neurologic lesion, urodynamic evaluation can provide objective documentation. The presence of detrusor-external sphincter dysynergia is strong evidence in favor of a spinal cord lesion above the sacral micturition center. An acontractile bladder and an open vesical neck at rest (radiographic contrast within the urethra in the absence of a detrusor contraction) are strongly suggestive of a thoracolumbar neurologic lesion. An acontractile detrusor and absent or diminished bladder filling sensations suggest a sacral lesion.

In addition, there are certain urodynamic findings, which pose significant risk for hydronephrosis, vesicoureteral areflux, infection, and stones. These include: (1) detrusor-external sphincter dysynergia, (2) low bladder compliance, and (3) sustained high magnitude detrusor contractions.

The fluoroscopic portion of the videourodynamic evaluation allows for concomitant cystography and voiding cystourethrography at the time of cystometric and detrusor pressure/uroflow evaluation. It is utilized to evaluate overall bladder contour; degree of cystocele and urethrocele at rest and with straining; the state of the bladder neck at rest and straining (closed, beaked, or open); the presence or absence of vesicoureteral reflux, bladder, or urethral diverticula, fistula; and the site of urethral obstruction.

Suggested Reading

Blaivas JG. Pathophysiology and differential diagnosis of benign prostatic hypertrophy, *Urology* 32 (6): 5–11, 1988.

Blaivas JG. Bladder outlet obstruction in men. In Nitti VW (ed) *Practical Urodynamics*, Philadelphia: WB Saunders, 1998, pp. 156–171.

Griffiths DJ. Pressure-Flow Studies of micturition, *Urol Clin North Am*, 23 (2): 279–297, 1996.

Schafer W. Principles and clinical application of advanced urodynamic analysis of voiding function, *Urol Clin North Am*, 17: 553–566, 1990.

Schafer W, Abrams P, Liao L, Mattiasson A, Pesce F, Spangberg A, Sterling AM, Zinner NR, van Kerrebroeck P. Report on Good Urodynamic Practice, *Neurourol Urodyn* 21 (3): 261–274, 2002.

van Mastrigt R, Griffiths DJ. ICS standard for digital exchange of urodynamic study data, *Neurourol Urodyn*, 23 (3): 280–281, 2004.

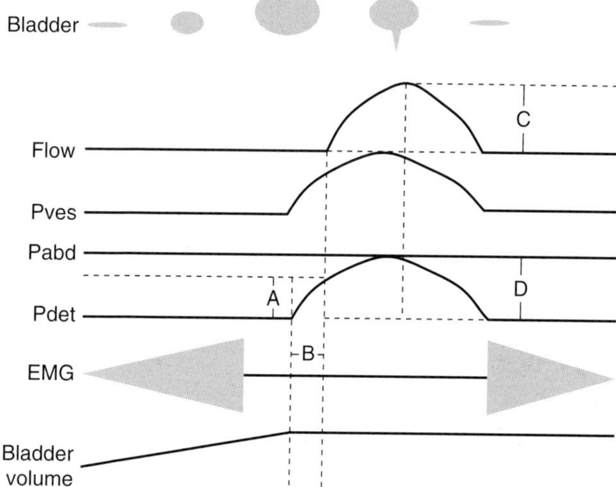

Fig. 7.1 Format for depiction of videourodynamic studies in this book. In most studies either EMG or bladder volume is displayed. A: opening detrusor pressure (the detrusor pressure at which flow begins); B: opening time; C: Q_{max}; D: Pdet@Q_{max}.

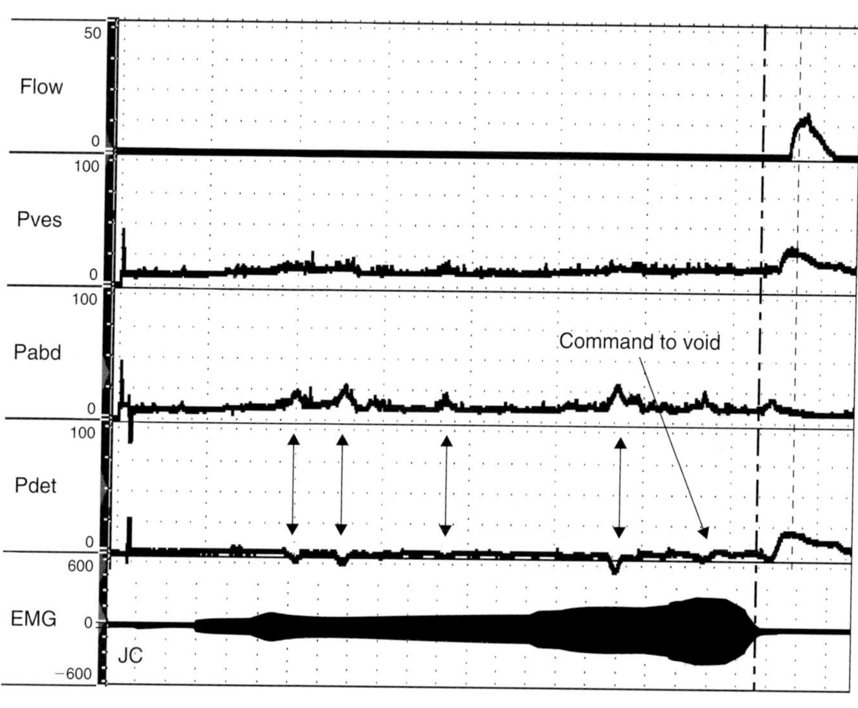

Fig. 7.2 Normal micturition in a 74-year-old man who was evaluated because of a history of urinary frequency that was determined to be caused by polyuria due to excessive fluid consumption based on his belief that "it is healthy to drink a lot of water." (A) Urodynamic tracing. First sensation of filling (FSF) = 93 ml, 1st urge = 210 ml, severe urge = 597 ml, and bladder capacity = 673 ml. Note that there are several rectal contractions (arrows) that cause an artifactual fall in Pdet. When asked to void, the EMG sphincter relaxation (vertical dotted line) occurred prior to the onset of the detrusor contraction. Q_{max} = 16 ml/s and Pdet@Q_{max} = 20 cmH_2O.

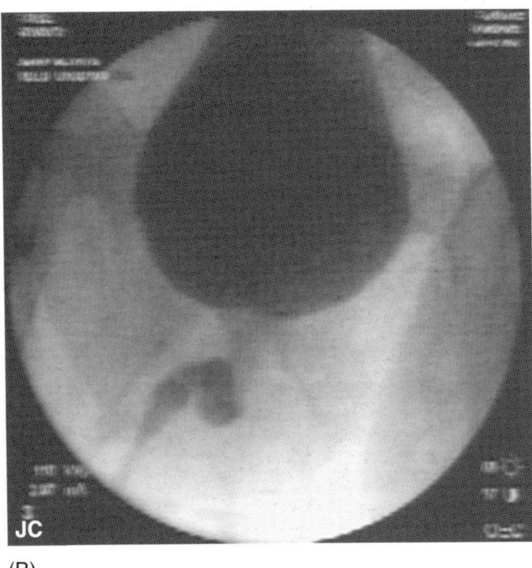

(B)

Fig. 7.2 (continued) (B) X-ray obtained during the first third of voiding shows a normally funneled bladder neck and an open urethra.

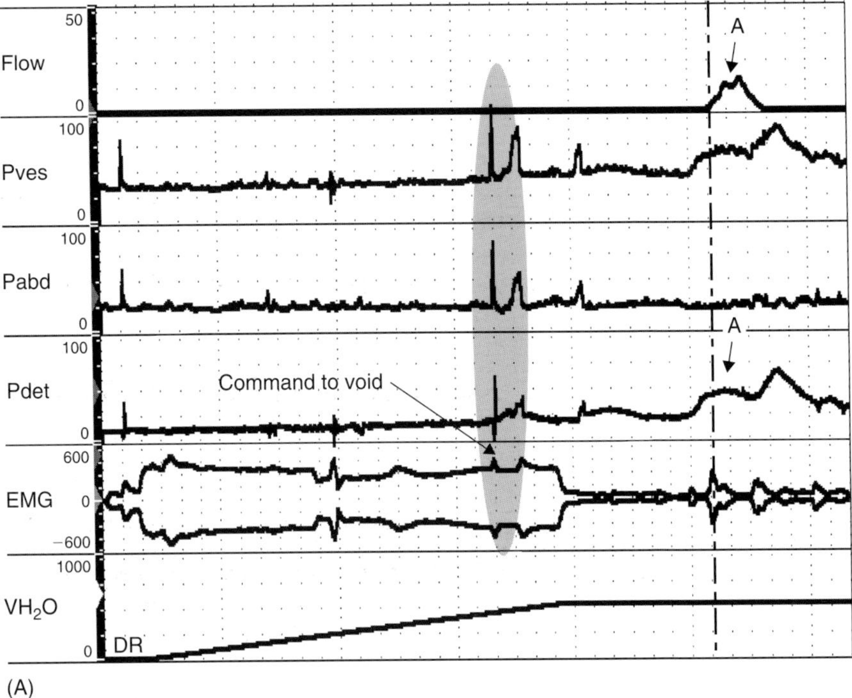

(A)

Fig. 7.3 Normal micturition in a 59-year-old woman referred for evaluation of elevated residual urine found unexpectedly during CAT scan done for abdominal pain. She denied any urologic symptoms. Uroflow was normal. (Voided volume = 230 ml, Pattern = normal, Q_{max} = 25 ml/s, and post-void residual = 0 ml.) (A) Urodynamic study. First sensation of filling (FSF) = 75 ml, 1st urge = 210 ml, severe urge = 523 ml, and bladder capacity = 533 ml. At the command to void, at first she could not relax, coughed, and then strained in an attempt to void (shaded oval). There is an artifactual rise is detrusor pressure due to unequal pressure registration in the vesical and abdominal tracings because of a calibration error seen during a cough at the far left of the tracing. Once she is able to relax, the sphincter EMG tracing becomes silent and there is a slight rise in detrusor pressure followed by a sustained detrusor contraction and near normal uroflow curve. During voiding there were several small increases in EMG activity. The first one (the vertical dotted line) momentarily prevents micturition, but as she relaxes, she voids with a normal upswing in the flow curve. The second one occurs after flow has begun to decline and appears to have no effect on flow, i.e. an artifact. On the other hand, the undulations on the flow curve near Q_{max} (arrow A) must be due to sphincter contractions that were not picked up by the EMG tracing since the Pdet tracing is smooth at this time point. Once she emptied her bladder and flow ceased, there is a further rise in detrusor pressure (an aftercontraction). After contractions are considered to be normal variants. Q_{max} = 16 ml, Pdet@ Q_{max} = 43 H_2O, Pdetmax = 50 cmH_2O, voided volume = 533 ml, and post-void residual = 0 ml.

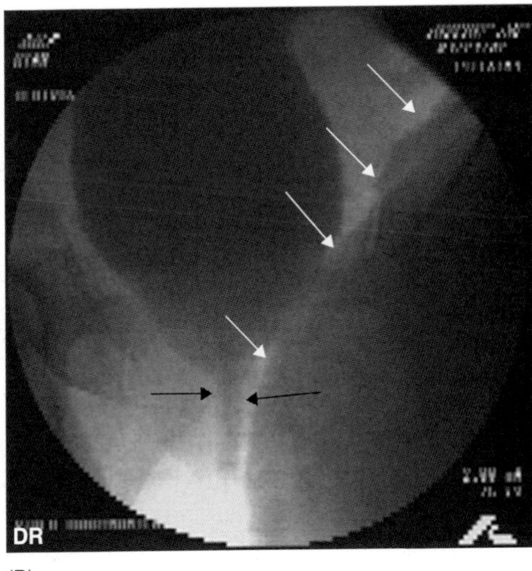

(B)

Fig. 7.3 (continued) (B) X-ray obtained during voiding shows a normal, funneled bladder neck (black arrows), and open urethra. The dark region outlined by white arrows is her thigh that is seen because of the oblique projection of the X-ray beam necessary to show the urethra in relief.

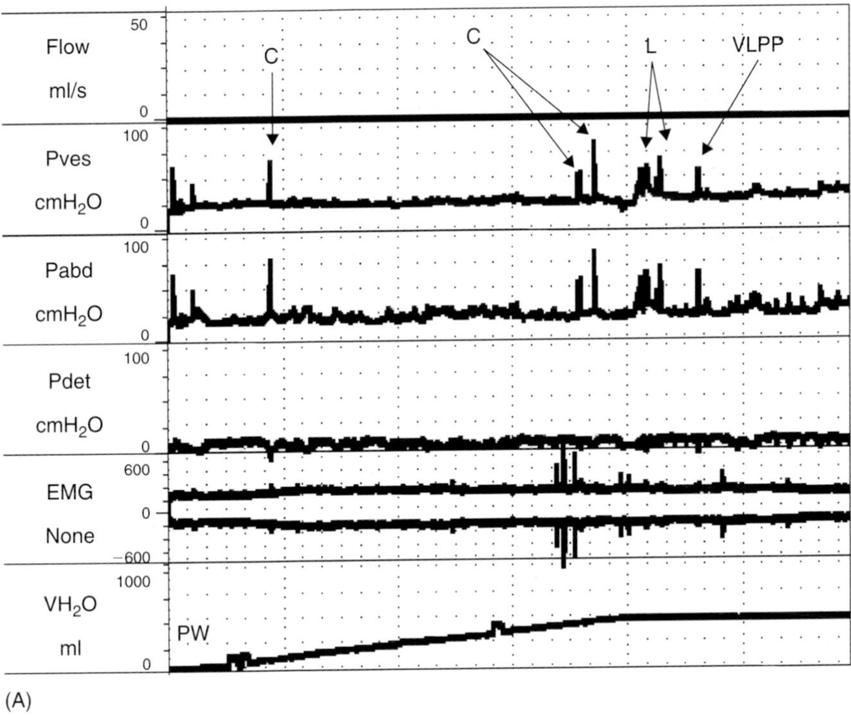

(A)

Fig. 7.4 LPP: (A) Urodynamic tracing. The bladder is filled to 150 ml with radiographic contrast and the patient is asked to cough (C), but there is no leakage. Filling is continued and there is no leakage to several more coughs (C) at a bladder volume of 240 ml. At 250 ml there is leakage visible on X-ray at Pves = 67 and 70 cmH_2O (L). The lowest pressure at which leakage occurs is 54 cmH_2O (VLPP, vesicle leak point pressure).

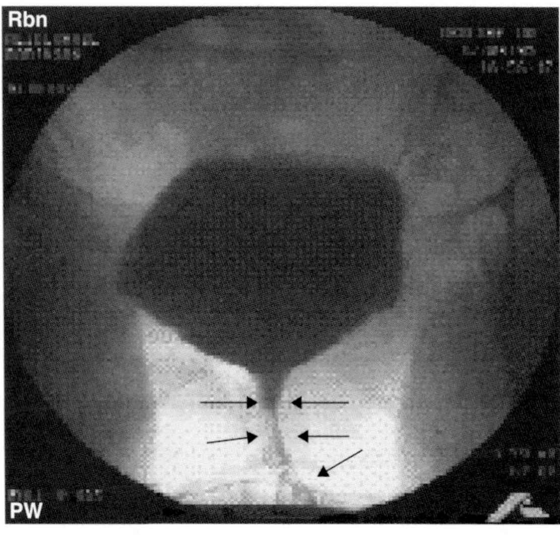

(B)

Fig. 7.4 (continued) (B) X-ray obtained at the VLPP. Note the contrast in the entire urethra and leakage into the vagina (arrows).

8 Pitfalls in Interpretation of Urodynamic Studies

Urodynamic studies are invaluable in delineating the pathophysiology of lower urinary tract symptoms, but there are many potential sources of error that may cause difficulty in interpretation of data obtained. In this chapter, general principles are set forth and illustrated with a few representative tracings. In the other chapters, whenever error is encountered, it is explained fully in the legend to the figures.

Sampling error

Sampling error is of two generic kinds. One is physiologic and the other temporal. From a physiologic standpoint, it is important to remember that urodynamic studies represent a snapshot at a single point in time, and as such, may not be representative of the patient's symptoms or pathophysiology. For example, a patient may complain of urge incontinence, which is due to detrusor overactivity, but cystometry is normal because he was able to prevent the detrusor overactivity due to his heightened awareness during the urodynamic study. Or, a patient with sphincteric incontinence may demonstrate an acontractile detrusor because she is unable to relax during the study and may show no stress incontinence because she anticipates the cough and contracts her sphincter (Fig. 8.1). In instances like these, it is important not to over- or under-interpret the studies. To this end, the patient should be asked whether or not the urodynamic study was representative of his usual symptoms and the data interpreted with this in mind.

Temporal sampling errors relate to how frequently the data points are recorded and displayed. For example, consider the tracing depicted in Figure 8.2. When the tracing is compressed so that the entire study can fit on a single page, much information is lost.

Uroflow and post-void residual urine

Uroflow and determination of post-void residual (PVR) urine are the two most commonly performed urodynamic studies and these are subject to a number of potential errors. First and foremost, it essential to determine whether or not the recorded uroflow and PVR are representative of the patient's usual voiding. How can you determine this? Ask the patient! Is this the way you usually urinate? Be specific. For example, if the flow pattern is interrupted, ask the patient if he usually stops and starts like that. If the answer is no, disregard the tracing and repeat it another time. If there is PVR urine, ask if he usually voids like that and did he feel as if he emptied his bladder. If the answer is no, disregard it.

The influence of bladder volume on uroflow is well known and while conventionally a minimum voided volume of 150ml is thought to be requisite in order to properly assess uroflow, clearly many patients' flow rates continue to increase with voided volumes above that arbitrary cut point as illustrated in Figure 4.7.

Another artifact may occur depending on the time interval over which data are sampled and displayed. To avoid reporting values of flow that are artifacts due to sudden burst of increased uroflow (usually due to jostling the flowmeter), it is recommended that only flow events lasting 2 seconds or more be reported (see Figure 4.6).

Multichannel urodynamic studies

Abdominal and vesical pressure should always go up equally during coughing and straining. If the Pves and Pabd transducers are calibrated properly and zeroed to atmosphere, when the stopcock is opened to the patient, both pressures will increase in tandem and detrusor pressure will remain unchanged. The two most common problems with unequal pressure transmission are damping (Fig. 8.3) and unequal transducer calibration (Fig. 8.4). Damping is any effect, either deliberately engendered or inherent to a system, that tends to reduce the amplitude of oscillations of an oscillatory system. In order to determine if damping is the problem, carefully examine the tracing spike during a cough. If there are more fluctuations in one of the tracings than the other, there is damping of the channel with diminished fluctuations. The two most common causes of damping are air bubbles in the line and obstruction of the catheter because it is up against the wall of the bladder or rectum. Another source of artifact occurs when, after the initial establishment of satisfactory transducer calibration, one of the catheters moves or is expelled. This is illustrated in Figures 8.4–8.5. In Figures 8.4 and 8.5, the rectal catheter moved and lost its zero. Recognition of this factor enabled the technician to reposition the rectal catheter and avoid losing valuable data during the filling and voiding phases of the study.

Yet another cause of artifact is rectal contractions. Since Pdet is electronically derived by the subtraction of Pabd from Pves, spontaneous rectal contractions cause an artifactual rise in Pdet (Fig. 8.6).

Effect of urodynamic catheter on uroflow

A catheter in the urethra may affect flow in two ways. Firstly, while the normal urethra usually allows unobstructed voiding over a 7F urodynamic catheter, this is not always the case. In some patients, the catheter itself causes obstruction. It is postulated that in such patients, urethral compliance is abnormal (low) even though the urethra is not narrow enough to cause obstruction. Secondly, the patient may not void in his or her usual fashion because of the presence of the catheter. In addition, one must always remember to take the voided volume into account when comparing the two tracings because uroflow is significantly affected by voided volume (Fig. 8.7). In Figure 8.8, the urethral catheter is clearly causing obstruction.

Bladder compliance versus involuntary detrusor contraction

In cases where there is an increase in detrusor pressure accompanying bladder filling during cystometry, distinction between low bladder compliance and involuntary contractions may be difficult. Further, both conditions may exist in the same patient. A practical method for distinguishing low bladder compliance from detrusor overactivity is to stop the water inflow in the midst of observed detrusor pressure increase. If detrusor pressure drops and then stabilizes upon suspension of water inflow, decreased bladder compliance is diagnosed (Fig. 8.9). If detrusor pressure continues to rise despite cessation of inflow, detrusor contraction is more likely.

Detrusor areflexia or absent detrusor contractions

A common cause of an erroneous diagnosis of detrusor areflexia is failure to fill the bladder to capacity. A typical example is a patient who present with urinary retention fails multiple voiding trials and is referred for evaluation. Since most filling media comes in prepackaged containers containing 600 or 1000 ml, there is a tendency amongst many clinicians to discontinue bladder filling at those volumes. In our judgment, bladder filling should continue until the patient feels a strong urge to void or an uncomfortable fullness before concluding that the bladder does not contract. Failure to do so may lead to a faulty diagnosis of detrusor areflexia (Fig. 8.10).

Electromyography artifacts

Electromyography (EMG) artifacts are so common in adults that EMG signals should be interpreted with great caution and only when there is good correlation between changes in EMG and changes in detrusor pressure and uroflow. Needle EMG is much more accurate and sensitive than patch electrodes, but they are rarely used because of patient discomfort.

Patch electrodes should be applied to a clean, dry skin surface in the perineum and it should be assured that proper grounding has been established. Since there are no absolute units of measurement that are important, the gain should be adjusted so that the EMG tracing can be visualized properly. A weak EMG signal may result from electrodes being placed too far from the sphincter or if the gain is too low. Loss of EMG signal occurs when electrodes become wet. EMG signals will go off scale when one or more electrodes falls off the patient. In order to rule out a major malfunction of the EMG unit, a simulation test is performed using a patch placed upon the forearm of the patient or technician. Using a scale of about (±) 400, deflection of half-scale should be obtainable by slight movement of the forearm. Common EMG artifacts are depicted in Figures 8.11 and 8.12.

Pitfalls in radiographic interpretation

The video component of video-urodynamic studies adds anatomic perspective, but is subject to many pitfalls. First and foremost, it is essential that the radiographic picture is correlated exactly with the urodynamic tracing, and the urodynamic tracing be annotated to describe what the patient was trying to do. For example, the three images depicted in Figure 8.13 all look like detrusor-external sphincter dyssynergia (DESD), but in fact one has an acquired voiding dysfunction, one has impaired detrusor contractility and one, is, in fact DESD.

Another pitfall relates to obtaining the proper view of the urethra. When the urethra is viewed in the anterior–posterior (AP) position, its anatomy is obscured, but when obliqued sufficiently, the shape of the urethra becomes obvious (Figs. 8.14 and 8.15). If the X-rays are obtained in the sitting position, it is often not possible to oblique the patient sufficiently because the excursion of the C-arm is limited by the patient's knees. Further, it is possible (and usual) that the X-ray beam is not perpendicular to the long axis of the patient. This results in the bladder appearing much lower than it really is (Fig. 8.15). The reason for this is, that it is often difficult to visualize the urethra unless the beam is tilted upward.

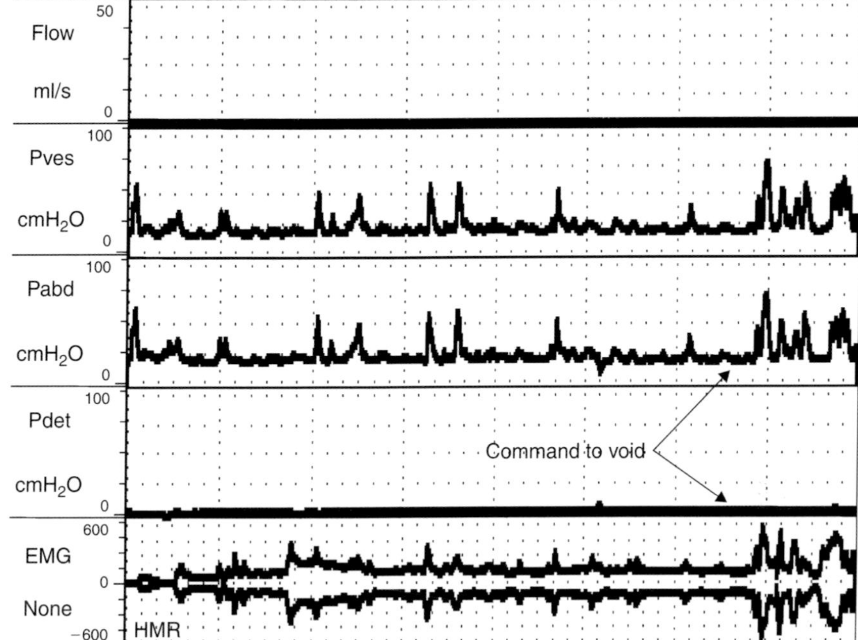

Fig. 8.1 Physiologic sampling error. Type 1 overactive bladder (OAB). This 38-year-old woman complains of urinary frequency, urgency, and mixed stress and urge incontinence, documented by bladder diary and pad test. The urodynamic tracing, however, not only fails to confirm detrusor overactivity, but she does not even generate a voluntary detrusor contraction when asked to try to void. During multiple coughs and straining, there is no stress incontinence either.

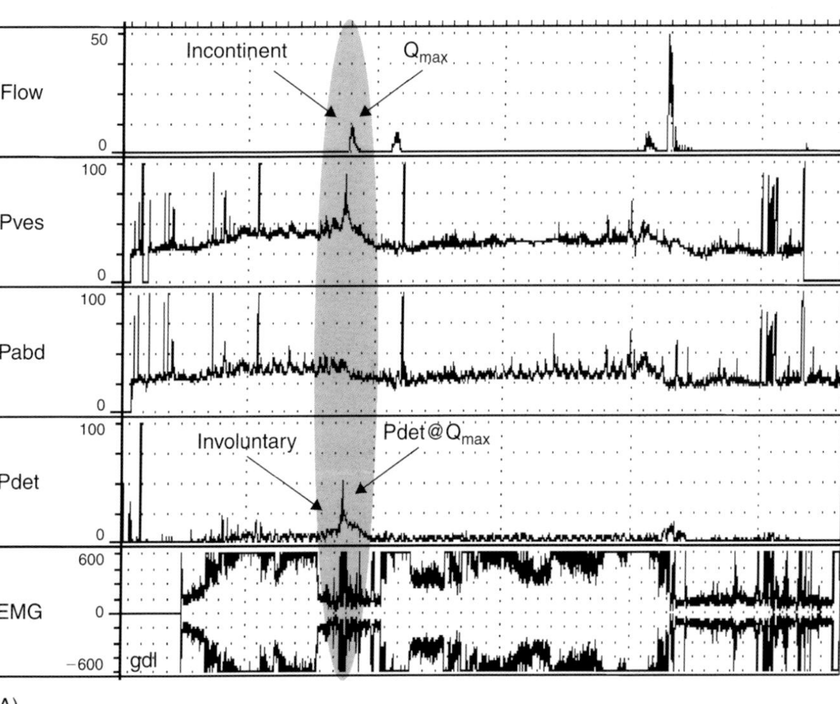

Fig. 8.2 Temporal sampling error. (A) This tracing displays an entire urodynamic study in one screen and, thus compresses the data, making it difficult to properly interpret. There is an involuntary detrusor contraction and an incontinent episode depicted in the shaded oval. At first glance, it appears that $Pdet@Q_{max} = 50\,cmH_2O$ and $Q_{max} = 11\,ml/s$. This is consistent with uretrial obstruction.

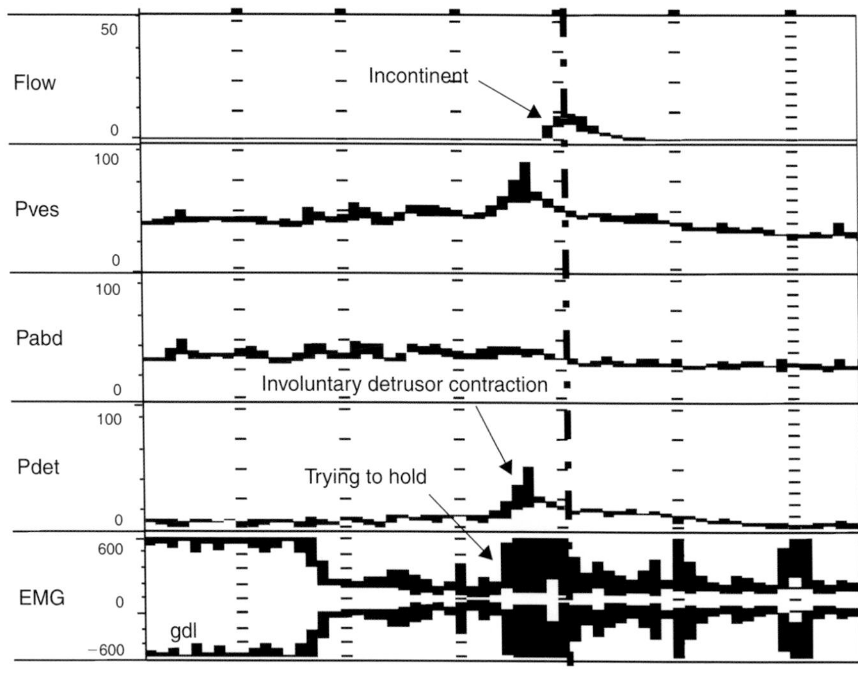

Fig. 8.2 (continued) (B) Expanded view of the involuntary detrusor contraction marked by the shaded oval. She perceived the contraction as an urge to void and temporarily prevented incontinence by contracting the sphincter, but once she fatigued, she was incontinent. On this expanded view, it becomes apparent that the high detrusor pressure (50 cmH_2O) occurred prior to flow, while she was voluntarily trying to hold. Pdet@Q_{max} and Q_{max} are marked by the vertical black line: Pdet@Q_{max} = 15 cmH_2O, Q_{max} = 10 cmH_2O, and PVR = 0. Thus, the apparent obstruction is an artifact due to data compression.

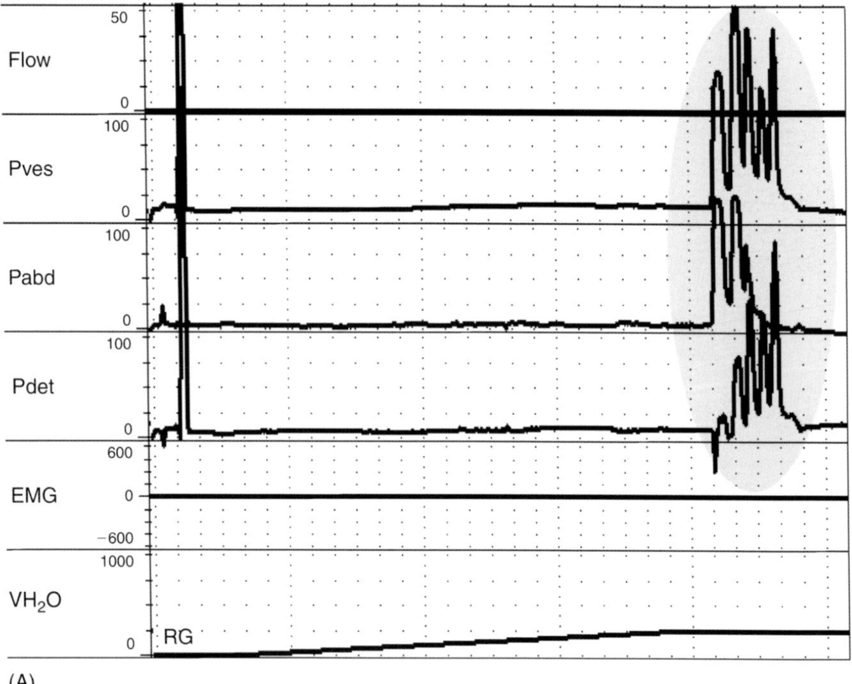

Fig. 8.3 Damping. (A) This patient has an acontractile bladder and when asked to void, she strains. There is an artifactual rise in Pdet, explained in Figure 8.3B.

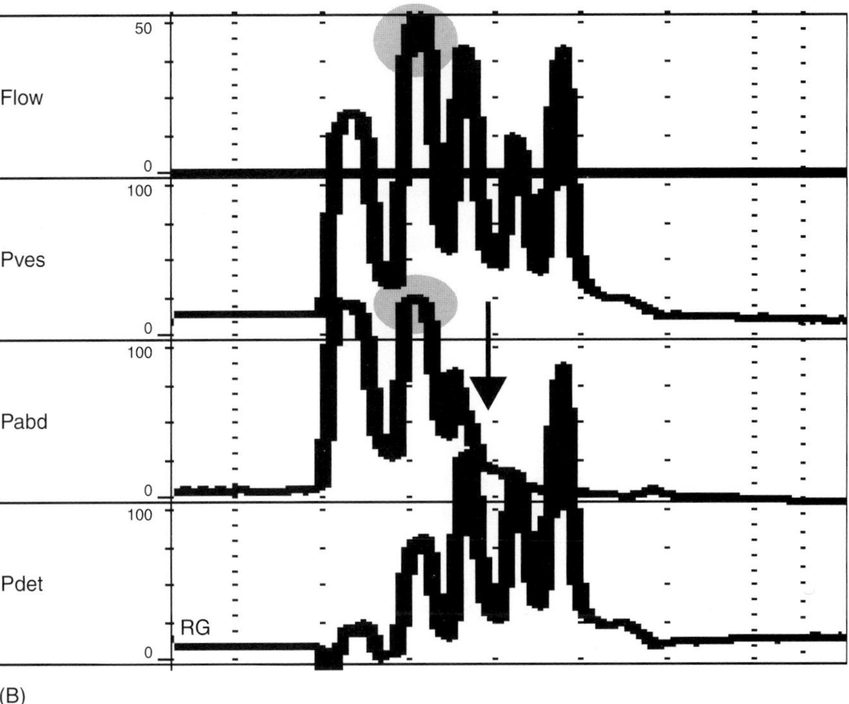

Fig. 8.3 (continued) (B) Expanded view of the area included in the shaded oval in Figure 8.2A. The artifactual rise if detrusor pressure is due to damping, presumably due to tiny air bubbles in the Pabd tubing or transducer. The net effect is that the spikes of pressure are not fully recorded. This is evident in the shaded ovals that show a flattened appearance in the Pabd tracing compared to the spikes in the Pves tracing. This causes Pabd to be artifactually lower than Pves resulting in an artifactual increase in Pdet. At the arrow, the Pabd catheter fails to register the pressure at all. This could be caused by air buffer in the system or catheter lodged against the rectal wall.

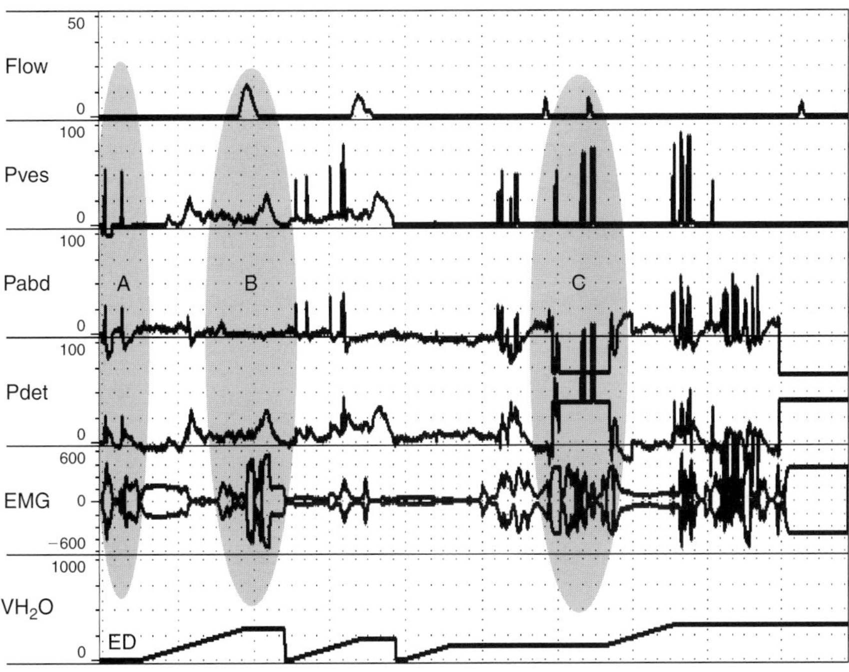

Fig. 8.4 Unequal pressure transmission (and a potpourri of other artifacts). Before bladder filling is begun, when the patient coughs, vesical pressure rises much higher than abdominal pressure and detrusor pressure is artifactually elevated (shaded oval A). Thereafter, whenever there is a rise in Pves > Pabd, Pdet artifactually rises. In the area marked by the shaded oval B, she is incontinent during an involuntary detrusor contraction that is barely measurable. In the midst of the contraction, she was asked to stop. She contracts her sphincter (increased EMG activity), interrupts the stream (Q falls to 0), and Pdet rises as the bladder is contracting against the closed sphincter. The bladder is refilled and she is asked to repeatedly cough. Each time, Pves > Pabd and Pdet is artifactually increased. During one of the coughs, the Pabd catheter is expelled and Pabd falls well below 0, artifactually raising Pdet (shaded oval C).

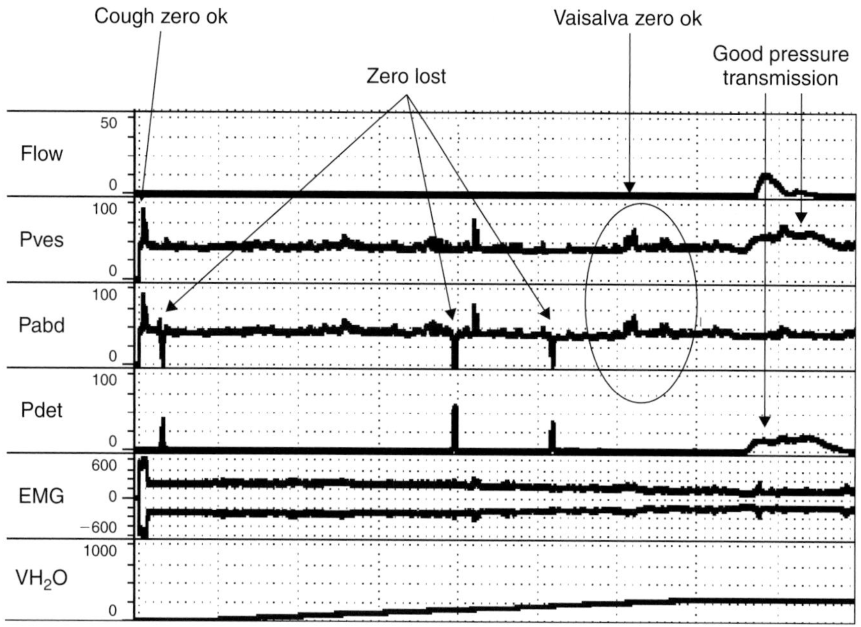

Fig. 8.5 Artefacts due to catheter movement. In this woman, each time she coughed, the rectal catheter was expelled and rectal pressure fell to zero and detrusor pressure was artifactually increased. This was immediately recognized and the catheter re-inserted.

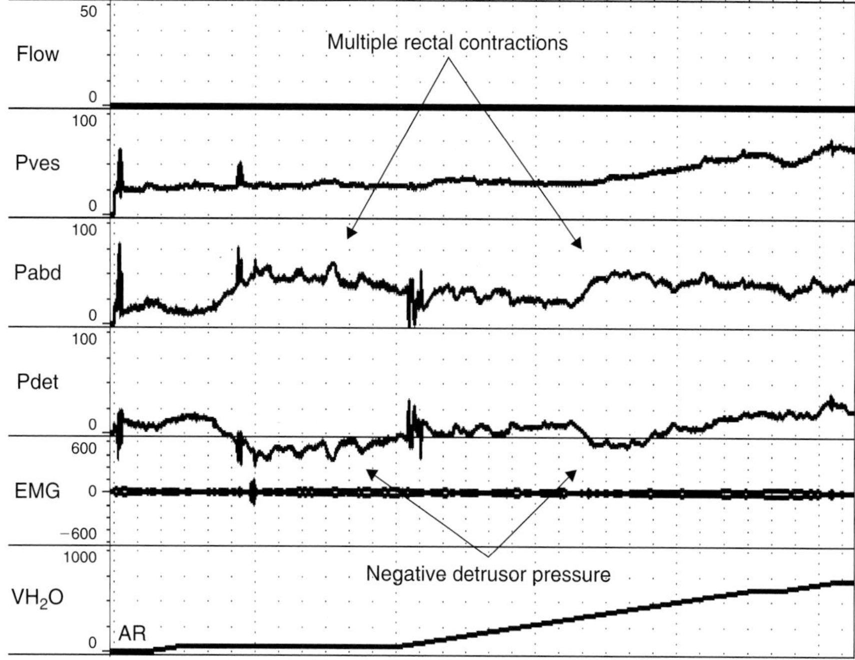

Fig. 8.6 Artifact due to rectal contractions that cause a negative deflection in detrusor pressure. Pves tracing shows a gradual rise in pressure characteristic of low bladder compliance.

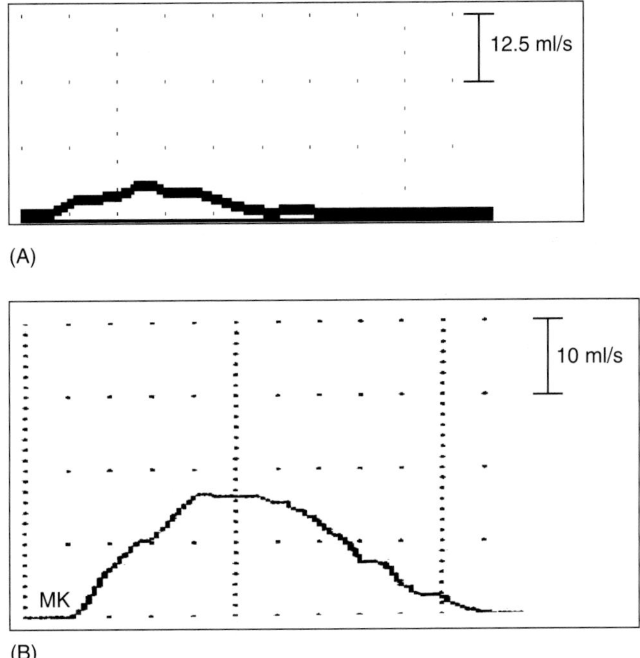

Fig. 8.7 Effect on uroflow of 7F urodynamic catheter (see Fig. 10.7). There are three potential sources of error in the uroflow obtained with the 7F urodynamic catheter in place. Firstly, the patient had a strong urge to void and voided with only 104 ml in his bladder, too low a volume for accurate assessment. Secondly, the catheter itself may cause obstruction and, finally, the patient may not sufficiently relax in the setting of the urodynamic examination. (A) Uroflow obtained with 7F urodynamic catheter in place. VOID = 6/78/26. (B) Uroflow obtained prior to urodynamic study without a urethral catheter in place. VOID = 16/190/5.

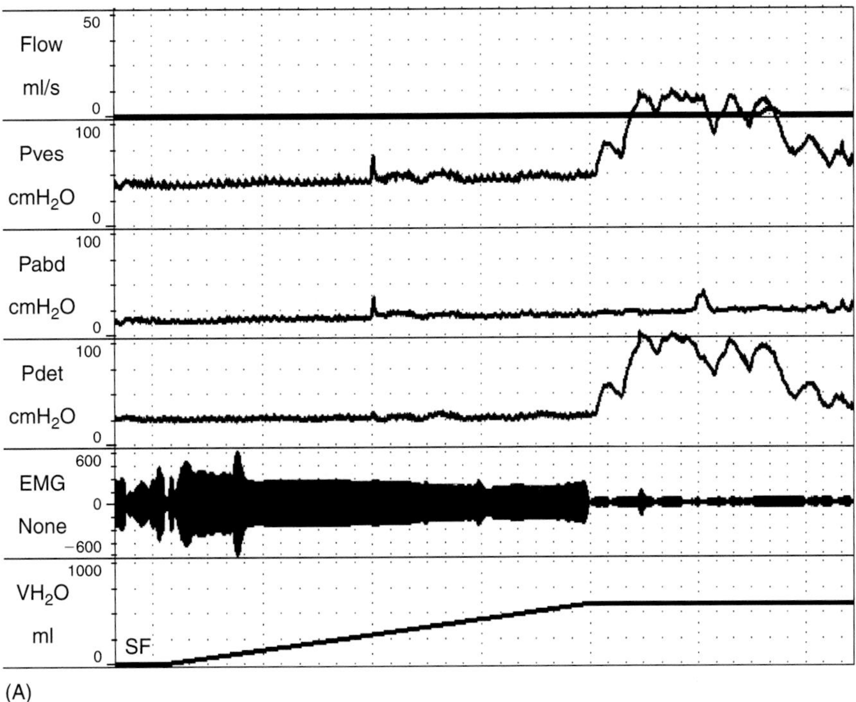

Fig. 8.8 Urodynamic catheter causing urethral obstruction. (A) Urodynamic tracing shows Schafer grade 5 urethral obstruction. Pdet/Q study: pressure flow study Pdet = 106cmH_2O, and Q_{max} = 3ml/s. Note that there is a sustained detrusor contraction and relaxation of the external urethral sphincter during the contraction.

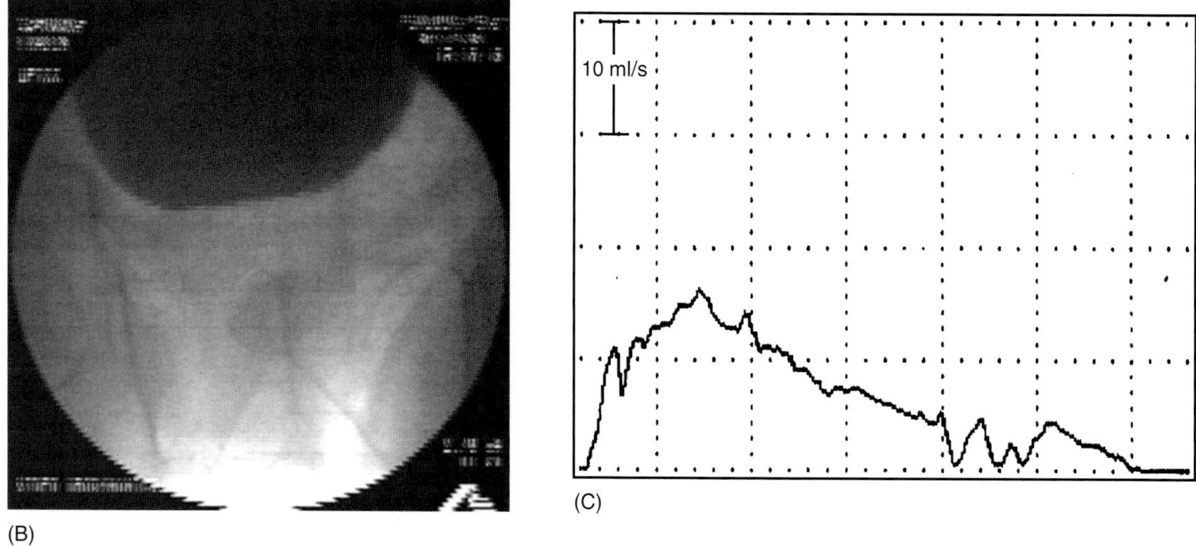

Fig. 8.8 (continued) (B) X-ray obtained at Q_{max} shows what appears to be a bladder neck obstruction because no contrast is seen past the bladder neck. (C) Unintubated uroflow. VOID: 15/440/44.
Comment: During the videourodynamic study, the patient relaxed his sphinter and had a strong, sustained detrusor contraction, yet Q_{max} was only 3 ml/s. Immediately after the study he voided normally. The only explanation for this is obstruction from the catheter.

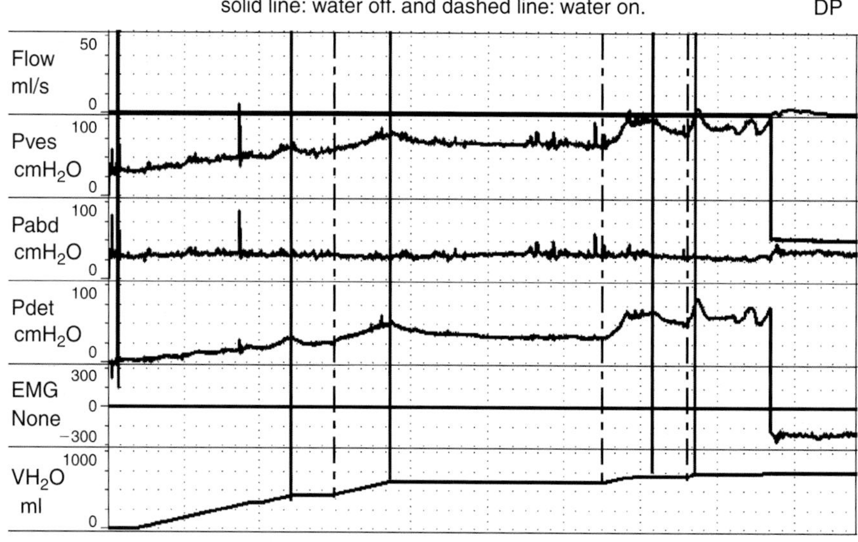

Fig. 8.9 Distinguishing low bladder compliance from detrusor contraction. Each of the rises in Pdet looks like a detrusor contraction, but when bladder filling is stopped, Pdet falls proving that the pressure rises are due to low bladder compliance.

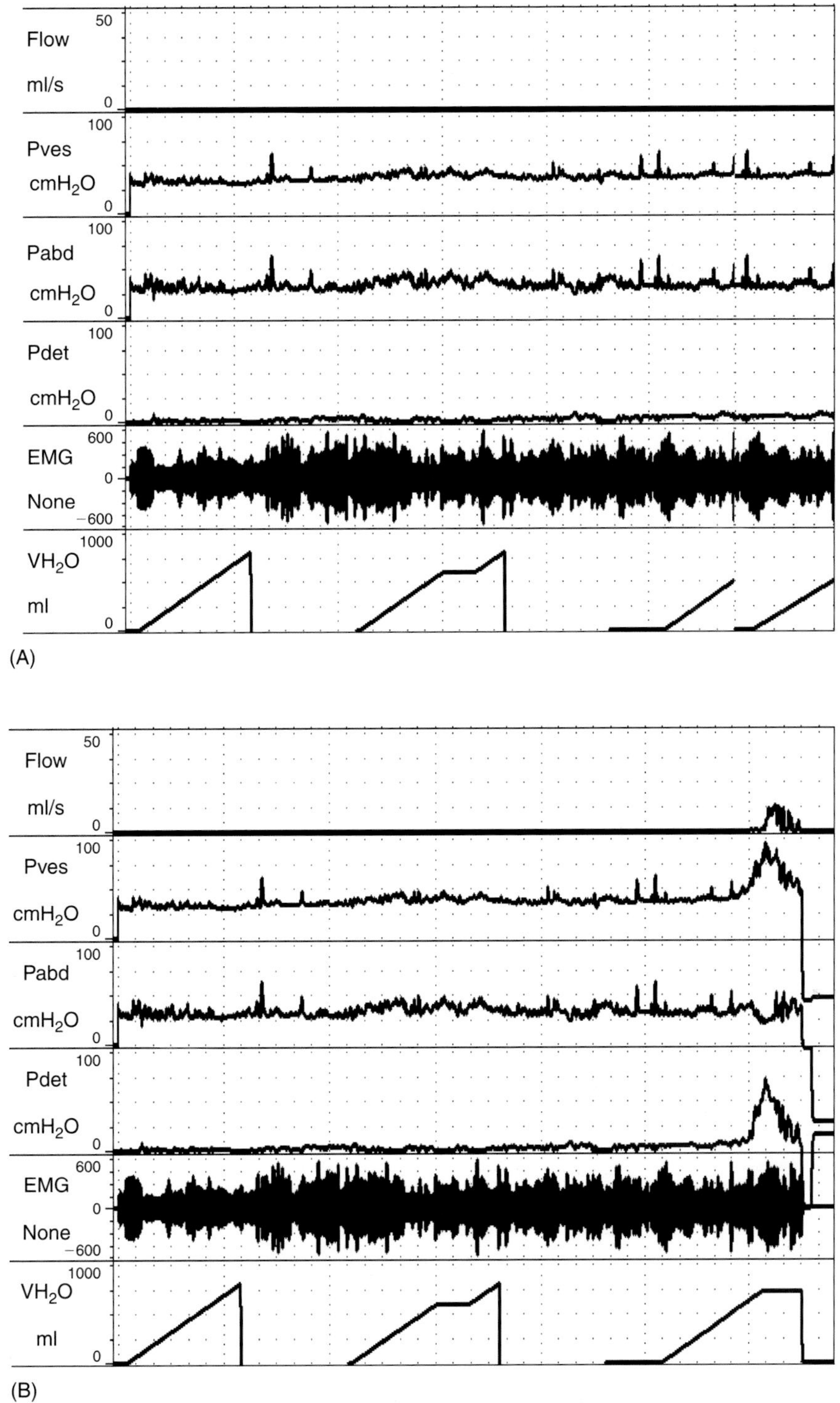

Fig. 8.10 This asymptomatic man was found to have a large PVR (>3,000 ml) during a pre-employment examination. He underwent several urodynamic studies that reported an areflexic detrusor and the patient was placed on self-catheterization. (A) Urodynamic study done several months later appears to show an acontractile detrusor with a bladder capacity in excess of 3 l. (B) Bladder filling was continued until he had a strong urge to void and he had a voluntary detrusor contraction. The Pdet/Q study documented Schafer grade 3 obstruction.

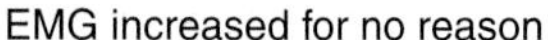

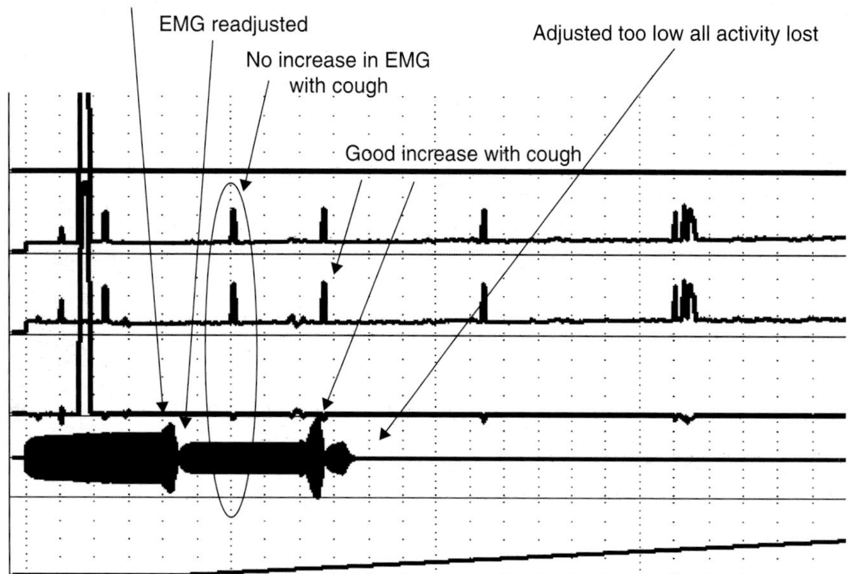

Fig. 8.11 Common EMG artifacts.

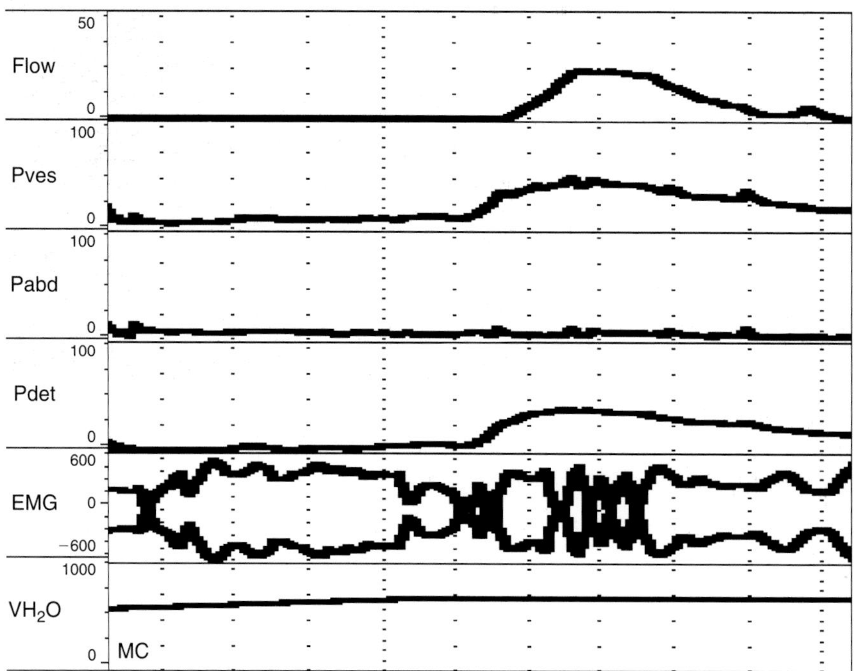

Fig. 8.12 EMG artifact (expanded view of the Fig. 10.12C). Note that this patient has a sustained detrusor contraction and normal uroflow. Both the detrusor contraction and uroflow have smooth curves, yet there are multiple increases in EMG activity that suggest contractions of the striated urethral sphincter. If these were sphincter contractions, there should be synchronous changes in detrusor pressure and uroflow.

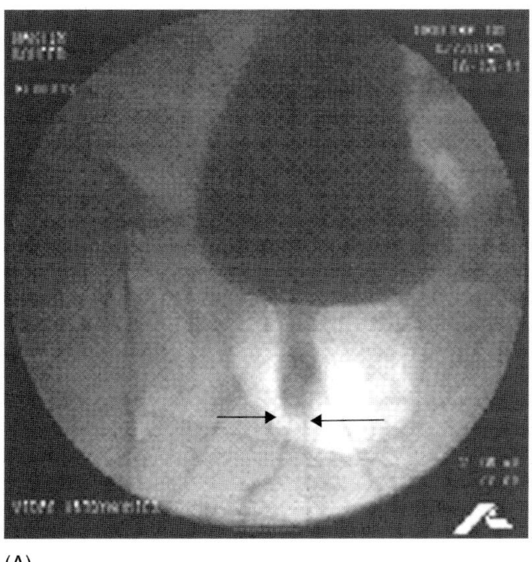
(A)

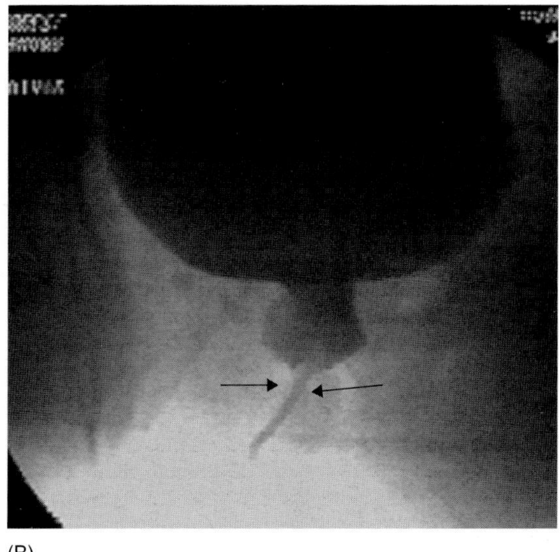
(B)

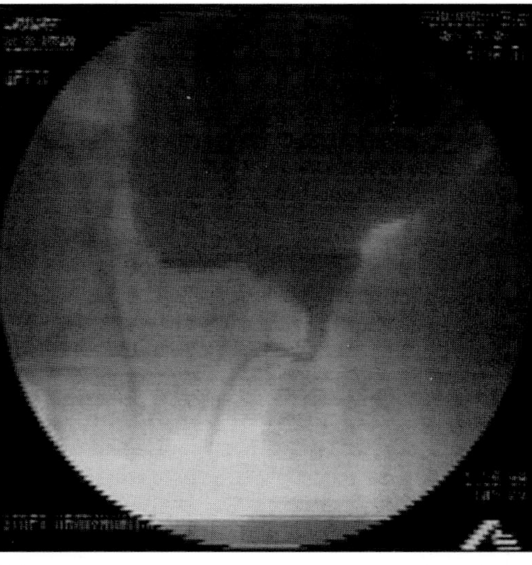
(C)

Fig. 8.13 DESD (Fig. 14.1B). (A) X-ray obtained at Pdetmax shows the classic picture of DESD – complete obstruction at the membranous urethra (arrows) and a "Christmas tree" shaped bladder. (B) Surgical defect after transurethral resection of the prostate ("TURP defect") simulating DESD. The X-ray was exposed at Q_{max} and shows a dilated prostatic urethra and a narrowed membranous and bulbar urethra, but urodynamic tracing showed impaired detrusor contractility. (C) Acquired voiding dysfunction simulating DESD (see Fig. 13.7D). X-ray obtained during voiding shows a dilated prostatic urethra and narrowed membranous urethra (arrows) due to subconscious contraction of the external sphincter (Fig. 10.14B).

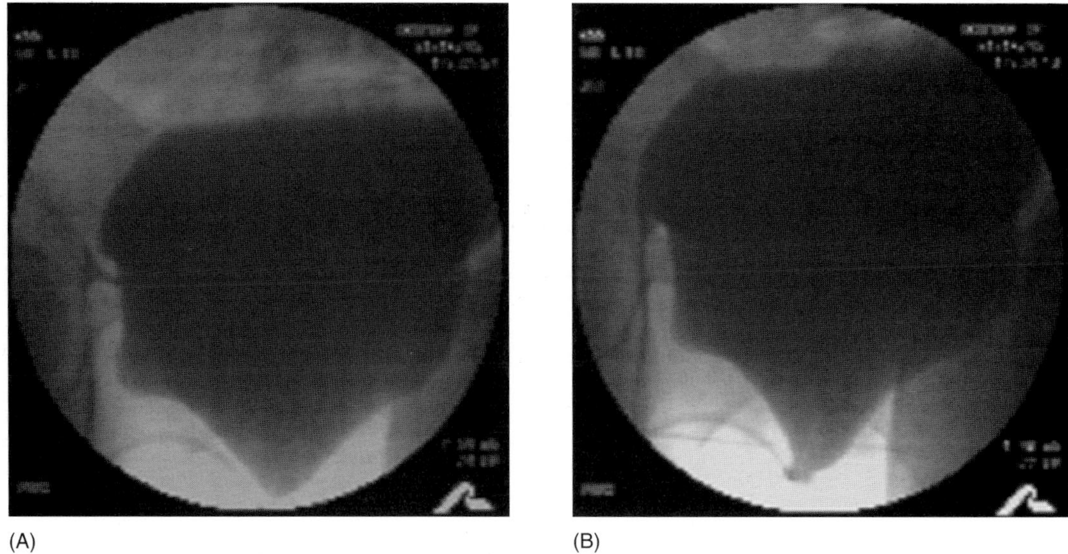

(A) (B)

Fig. 8.14 Effect of radiographic view on visibility of the urethra. In a woman with sphincteric incontinence. (A) In the AP projection, the urethra is obscured by a small cystocele. (B) When the X-ray projection is obliqued, rotational descent of the urethra and sphincteric incontinence is apparent.

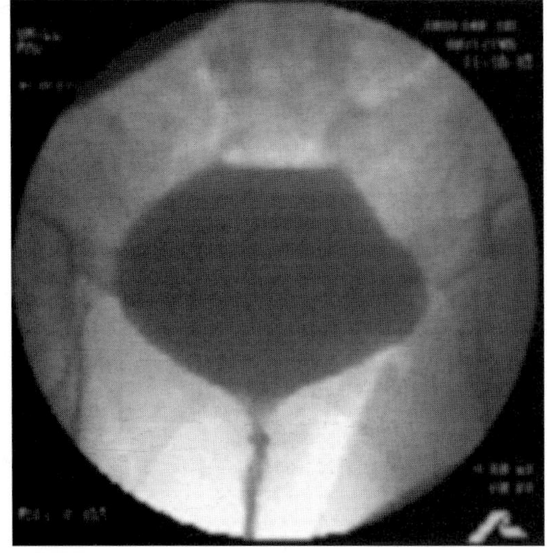

Fig. 8.15 X-ray exposed during voiding in the AP position shows a focal dilation due to the distal urethra seen on end. Note that about half of the bladder appears to be below the pubis. This is an artifact due to the fact that the X-ray beam was tilted upward in order to try to get a better view of the urethra.

9 Overactive Bladder

Overactive bladder (OAB) is defined by the International Continence Society (ICS) as "urgency, with or without urge incontinence, usually with frequency and nocturia . . . if there is no proven infection or other etiology." [1] From a practical standpoint, though, we believe this definition to be much too restrictive and, in contradistinction to the ICS definition, we consider OAB to be a symptom complex caused by one or more of the following conditions: detrusor overactivity, sensory urgency, and low bladder compliance. Sensory urgency is a term, abandoned by the ICS, which refers to an uncomfortable need to void that is unassociated with detrusor overactivity. Conditions causing and/or associated with OAB are diverse and include urinary tract infection, urethral obstruction, pelvic organ prolapse, neurogenic bladder, sphincteric incontinence, urethral diverticulum, bladder stones/foreign body, and bladder cancer [2–13]. In patients with OAB, diagnostic evaluation should be directed at early detection of these conditions because in many instances the symptoms are reversible if the underlying etiology is successfully treated.

Detrusor overactivity. Detrusor overactivity is a generic term that refers to the presence of involuntary detrusor contractions during cystometry, which may be spontaneous or provoked. The ICS further describes two patterns of detrusor overactivity: terminal and phasic. **Terminal detrusor overactivity** is defined as a single involuntary detrusor contraction occurring at cystometric capacity, which cannot be suppressed, and results in incontinence usually resulting in bladder emptying (Fig. 9.1). **Phasic detrusor overactivity** is defined by a characteristic waveform, and may or may not lead to urinary incontinence (Fig. 9.2). Involuntary detrusor contractions are not always accompanied by sensation. Some patients have no symptoms at all. Others void uncontrollably without any awareness. Still others may detect them as a first sensation of bladder filling or a normal desire to void. The ICS classifies detrusor overactivity as either idiopathic or neurogenic. By definition, neurogenic activity and idiopathic detrusor overactivity are distinguished not by specific symptoms or urodynamic characteristics, but rather by the presence or absence of a neurologic lesion or disorder. For example, a spinal cord injury patient with involuntary bladder contractions is said to have detrusor hyperreflexia (neurogenic detrusor), whereas an elderly male with such a finding secondary to prostatic obstruction is said to have detrusor instability. We believe, though, that the term idiopathic detrusor overactivity is somewhat of a misnomer. While in some cases the origin of the involuntary detrusor contractions is unknown, in other cases they are caused by, or at least are associated with, a variety of non-neurogenic clinical conditions, the same as listed

Table 9.1 Causes of detrusor overactivity.

Idiopathic detrusor overactivity
Neurogenic detrusor overactivity
Supraspinal neurologic lesions
Stroke
Parkinson's disease
Hydrocephalus
Brain tumor
Traumatic brain injury
Multiple sclerosis
Suprasacral spinal lesions
Spinal cord injury
Spinal cord tumor
Multiple sclerosis
Myleodysplasia
Transverse myelitis
Diabetes mellitus
Non-neurogenic detrusor overactivity
Bladder infection
Bladder outlet obstruction
Men: prostatic and bladder neck, strictures
Women: pelvic organ prolapse, post surgical, urethral, diverticulum, primary bladder neck, stricture
Bladder tumor
Bladder stones
Foreign body
Aging

above for OAB. For that reason, we prefer to classify detrusor overactivity three ways – idiopathic, neurogenic, and non-neurogenic. A list of specific causes of detrusor overactivity can be found in Table 9.1.

There is no lower limit for the amplitude of an involuntary detrusor contraction but confident interpretation of low pressure waves depends on high quality urodynamic technique and is enhanced by corroborating factors such as a concomitant urge to void, sudden relaxation of the sphincter electromyography (EMG), opening of the bladder neck, and incontinence (Fig. 9.3).

Data regarding the prevalence and urodynamic characteristics of involuntary detrusor contractions in various clinical settings, as well as in neurologically intact versus neurologically impaired patients, are scarce. In 1985, Coolsaet proposed a standardized method of evaluating detrusor overactivity in which detrusor pressure during involuntary detrusor contraction, bladder volume at which the contraction occurs, awareness of and ability to abort the contraction, presence or absence of urinary incontinence during the contraction, and ability to abort contraction-related incontinent flow are assessed [2]. These parameters have been used to compare urodynamic characteristics of involuntary detrusor contractions amongst a variety of etiologies [3]. The ability to abort the contractions was significantly higher among continent patients with frequency/urgency (77%) compared with patients who experienced urge incontinent (46%) and neurologically impaired patients (38%). The utility of urodynamic evaluation may therefore lie in the assessment of these parameters, rather than in the mere documentation of the presence or absence of detrusor overactivity. A urodynamic classification of patients with OAB based on the presence of detrusor overactivity, patient awareness, and ability to abort the involuntary contraction was recently proposed [4]. They defined four types of OAB. In type 1, the patient complains of OAB symptoms, but no involuntary detrusor contractions are demonstrated (Fig. 9.4). In type 2, there are involuntary detrusor contractions, but the patient is aware of them and can voluntarily contract his or her sphincter, prevent incontinence, and abort the detrusor contraction (Fig. 9.5). In type 3, there are involuntary detrusor contractions, the patient is aware of them and can voluntarily contract his or her sphincter and momentarily prevent incontinence, but is unable to abort the detrusor contraction and once the sphincter fatigues, incontinence ensues (Fig. 9.6). In type 4, there are involuntary detrusor contractions, but the patient is neither able to voluntarily contract the sphincter nor abort the detrusor contraction and simply voids involuntarily (Fig. 9.7). This classification system serves two purposes. Firstly, it is a shorthand method of describing the urodynamic characteristics of the OAB patient. Secondly, it provides a substrate for therapeutic decision making. For example, a patient with type 1 and 2 OAB exhibits normal neural control mechanisms and, at least theoretically, is an excellent candidate for behavioral therapy. It is likely that over time (with or without treatment), an individual patient can change from one type to another. Further, this classification only relates to the storage stage and can co-exist with normal voiding, bladder outlet obstruction, and/or impaired detrusor contractility.

Suggested Reading

1 Abrams P, Cardozo L, Fall M, Griffiths D, Rosier P, Ulmsten U, van Kerrebroeck P, Victor A, Wein A. The standardisation of terminology of lower urinary tract function: report from the standardisation subcommittee of the International Continence Society. *Neurourol Urodyn*, 21: 167–178, 2002.

2 COOLSAET, BrLA. Bladder compliance and detrusor activity during the collection phase. Neuroural and Urodynamic, 4: 263–273, 1985.

3 Romanzi LJ, Groutz A, Heritz DM, Blaivas JG. Involuntary detrusor contractions: correlation of urodynamic data to clinical categories. *Neurourol Urodyn*, 20: 249–257, 2001.

4 Flisser AJ, Wamsley K, Blaivas JG. Urodynamic classification of patients with symptoms of overactive bladder. *J Urol*, 169: 529–533, 2003.

5 Hebjorn S, Andersen JT, Walter S, Dam AM. Detrusor hyperreflexia: a survey on its etiology and treatment. *Scand J Urol Nephrol*, 10: 103–109, 1976.

6 Awad SA, McGinnis RH. Factors that influence the incidence of detrusor instability in women. *J Urol*, 130: 114–115, 1983.

7 Webster GD, Sihelnik SA, Stone AR. Female urinary incontinence: the incidence, identification and characteristics of detrusor instability. *Neurourol Urodynam*, 3: 325, 1984.

8 Resnick NM, Yalla SV, Laurino E. The pathophysiology of urinary incontinence among institutionalized elderly persons. *New Engl J Med*, 320: 1–7, 1989.

9 Fantl JA, Wyman JF, McClish DK, Bump RC. Urinary incontinence in community dwelling women: clinical, urodynamic, and severity characteristics. *Am J Obstet Gynecol*, 162(4): 946–951, 1990.

10 Groutz A, Blaivas JG, Romanzi LJ. Urethral diverticulum in women: diverse presentations resulting in diagnostic delay and mismanagement. *J Urol*, 164: 428–433, 2000.

11 Fusco F, Groutz A, Blaivas JG, Chaikin DC, Weiss JP. Videourodynamic studies in men with lower urinary tract symptoms: a comparison of community based versus referral urological practices. *J Urol*, 166: 910–913, 2001.

12 Chou ECL, Flisser AJ, Panagopoulos G, Blaivas JG. Effective treatment for mixed incontinence with a pubovaginal sling. *J Urol*, 170: 494–497, 2003.

13 Segal JL, Vassallo B, Kleeman S, et al. Prevalence of persistent and de novo overactive bladder symptoms after the tension-free vaginal tape. *Obstet Gynecol*, 104(6): 1263–1269, 2004.

14 Artibani W. Diagnosis and significance of idiopathic overactive bladder. *Urology*,50(Suppl): 25–32, 1997.

15 Blaivas JG. The neurophysiology of micturition: a clinical study of 550 patients. *J Urol*, 127: 958–963, 1982.

16 Coolsaet BRLA, Blok C. Detrusor properties related to prostatism. *Neurourol Urodynam*, 5: 435, 1986.

17 Gormley EA, Griffiths DJ, McCracken PN, et al. Effect of transurethral resection of the prostate on detrusor instability and urge incontinence in elderly males. *Neurourol Urodyn*, 12: 445–453, 1993.

18 Hyman MJ, Groutz A, Blaivas JG. Detrusor instability in men: correlation of lower urinary tract symptoms with urodynamic findings. *J Urol*, 166: 550–553, 2001.

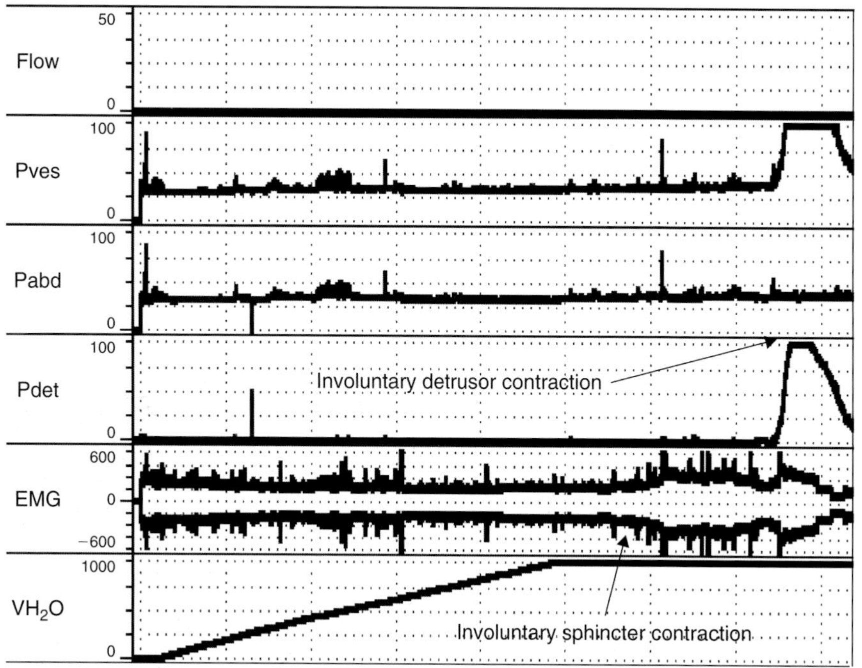

Fig. 9.1 Terminal detrusor overactivity in a man with type 1 detrusor-external sphincter dyssynergia (EMG relaxes after onset of detrusor contraction). During this examination he was incontinent and voided to completion, but the examination was performed in the supine position, so uroflow was not measured.

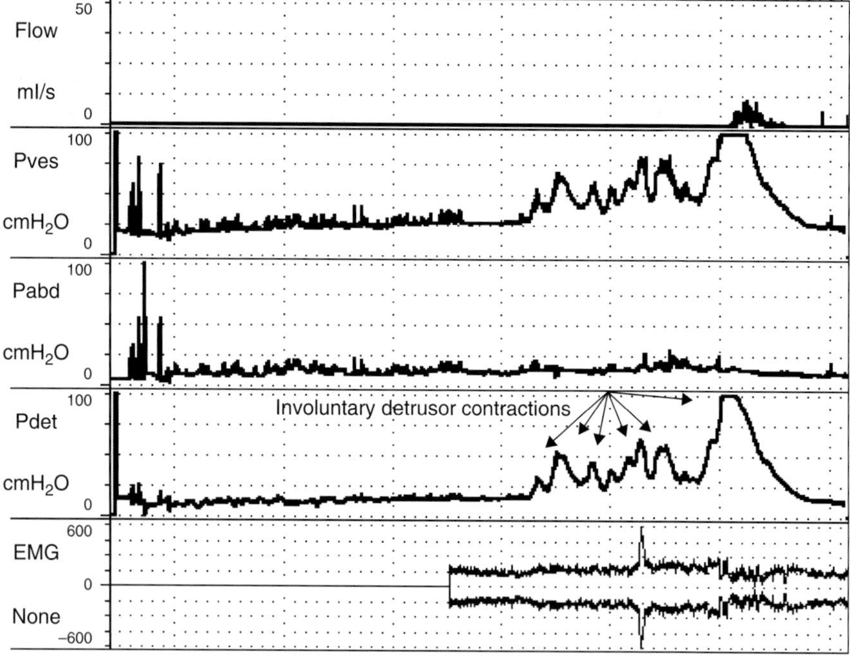

Fig. 9.2 Phasic detrusor overactivity in a 53-year-old man with prostatic obstruction.

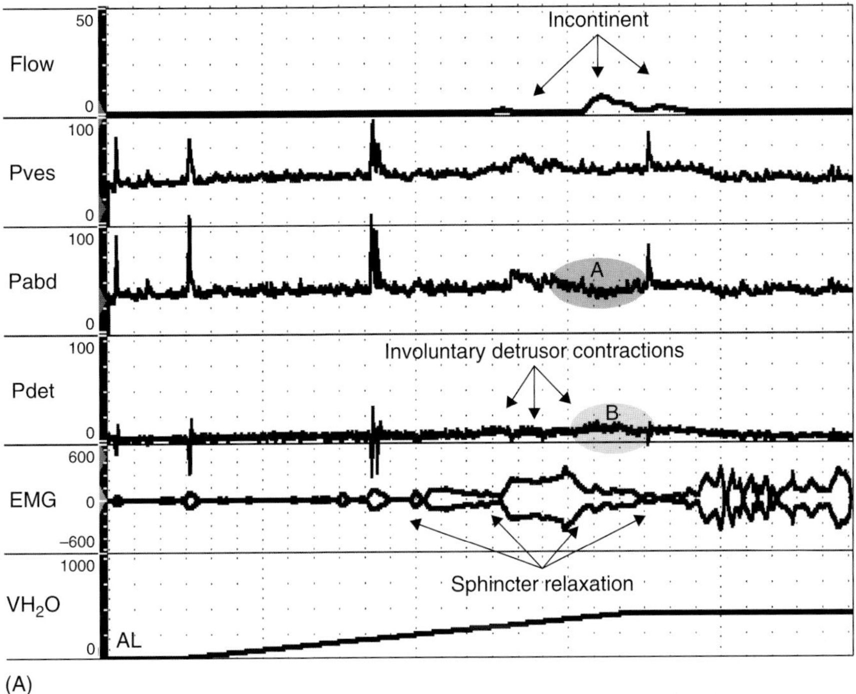

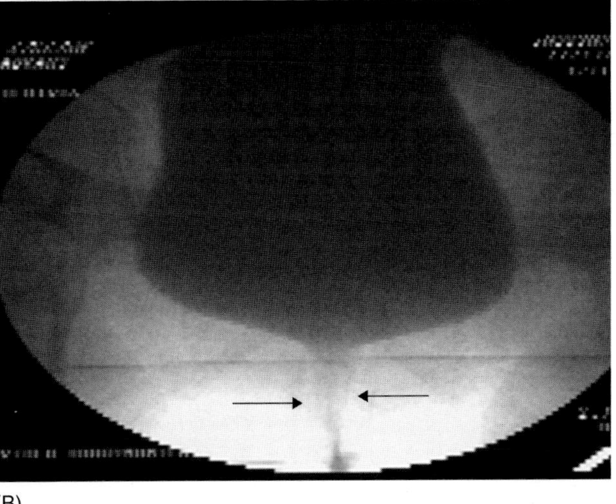

Fig. 9.3 Low magnitude detrusor overactivity. (A) Urodynamic tracing. Just looking at the urodynamic tracing, one would be hard pressed to diagnose detrusor overactivity. However, each rise in Pdet was preceded by an urge to void, relaxation of the striated sphincter, opening of the vesical neck, and incontinence. At the shaded oval A there is an inexplicable fall in Pabd. This causes an artifactual increase in detrusor pressure (shaded oval B). The observation of incontinence concurrent with this artifactual rise in Pdet indicates that a low amplitude contraction was disguised within the detrusor tracing and made to seem of higher amplitude owing to the fall in Pabd. The generally low flow in this study is due to impaired detrusor contractility. (B) X-ray obtained during voiding shows normal urethral configuration, but the urethra is not well visualized because of the low flow.

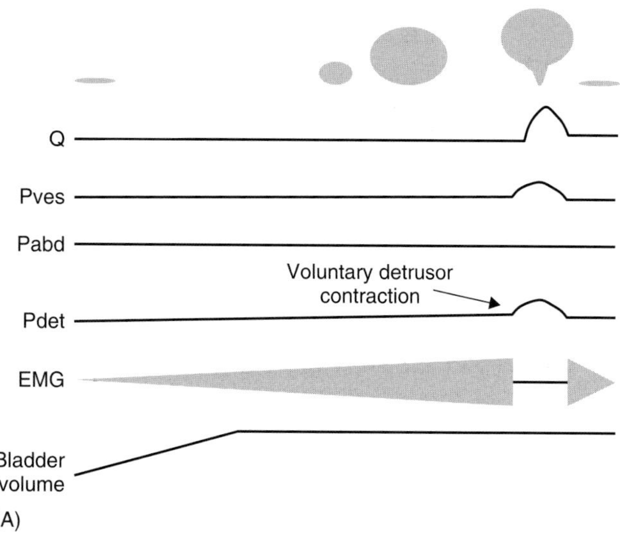

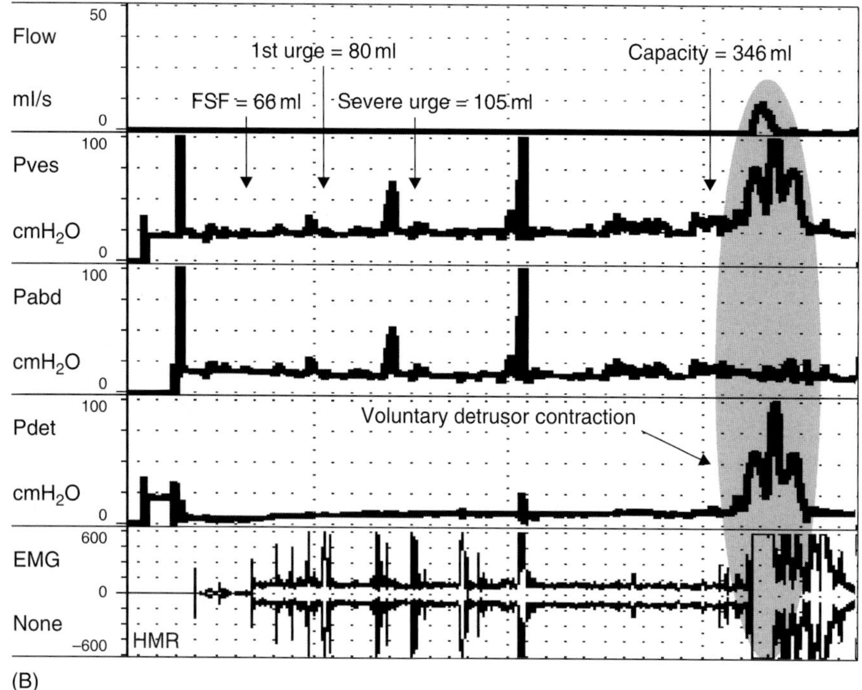

Fig. 9.4 (A) A schematic depiction of type 1 OAB. The patient complains of OAB symptoms, but there are no involuntary detrusor contractions. (B) Type 1 OAB: This is a 54-year-old woman with mild exacerbating-remitting multiple sclerosis who complains of urinary frequency, urgency, and urge incontinence. Urodynamic tracing. FSF = 66 ml, 1st urge = 80 ml, severe urge = 105 ml, and bladder capacity = 346 ml. There were no involuntary detrusor contractions. She had a voluntary detrusor contraction at 346 ml. The apparent increase in EMG activity during the detrusor contraction is artifact. VOID: 20/346/0, pressure flow: Pdet@ Q_{max} = 25 cmH_2O, Q_{max} = 14 ml/s, and Pdetmax = 60 cmH_2O.

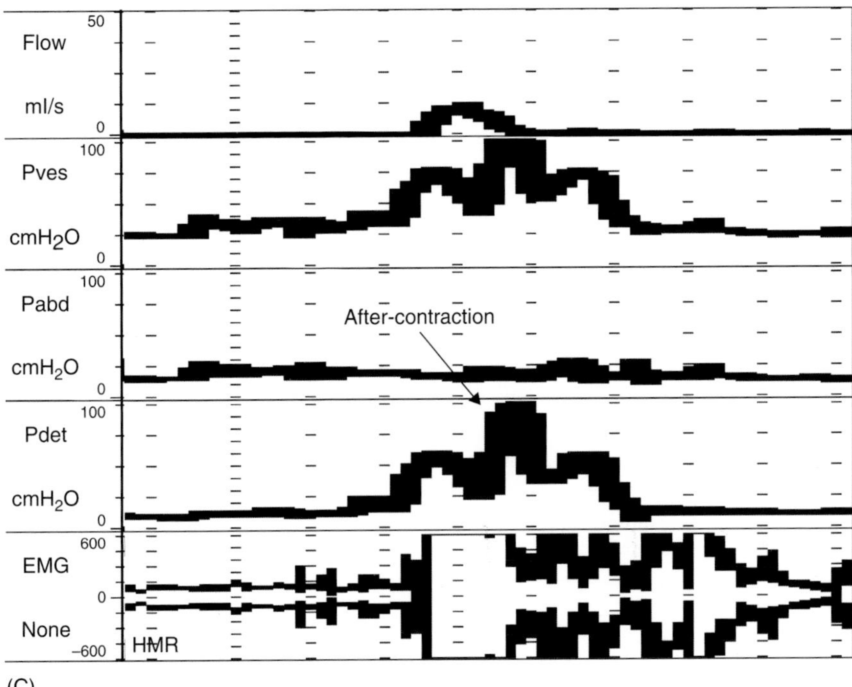

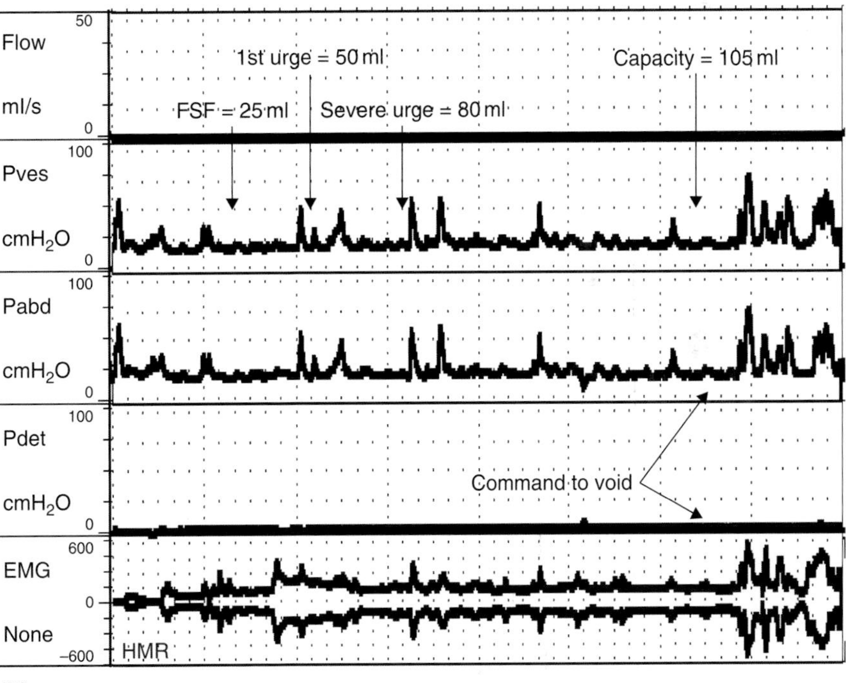

Fig. 9.4 (continued) (C) This is a magnified view of the tracing obtained during voluntary micturition (shaded oval in figure B). The apparent increase in EMG activity is an artifact. Two observations confirm this. Firstly, despite the increase in EMG activity, the flow curve has a smooth bell shaped curve. Secondly, she completely empties her bladder. The rise in detrusor pressure immediately after voiding is an after-contraction that has no pathologic significance. (D) Type 1 OAB: This 38-year-old woman complains of urinary frequency and urgency, but the urodynamic tracing fails to confirm detrusor overactivity. When asked to void, she strains, but does not generate a detrusor contraction.

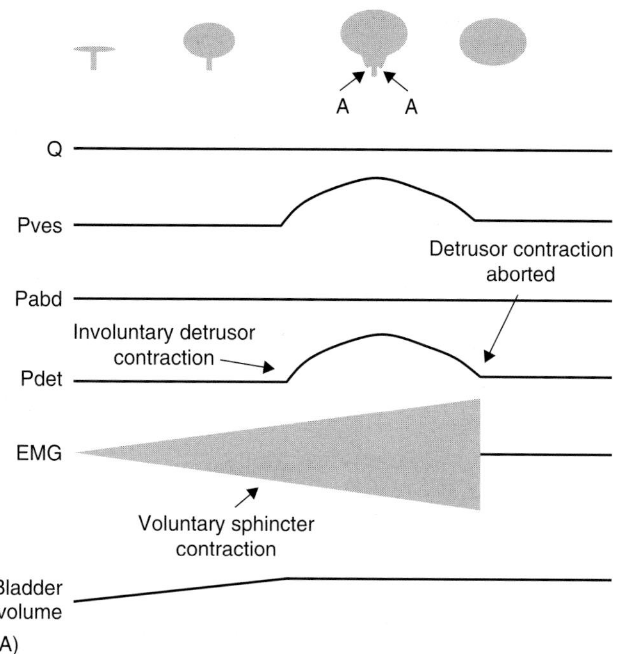

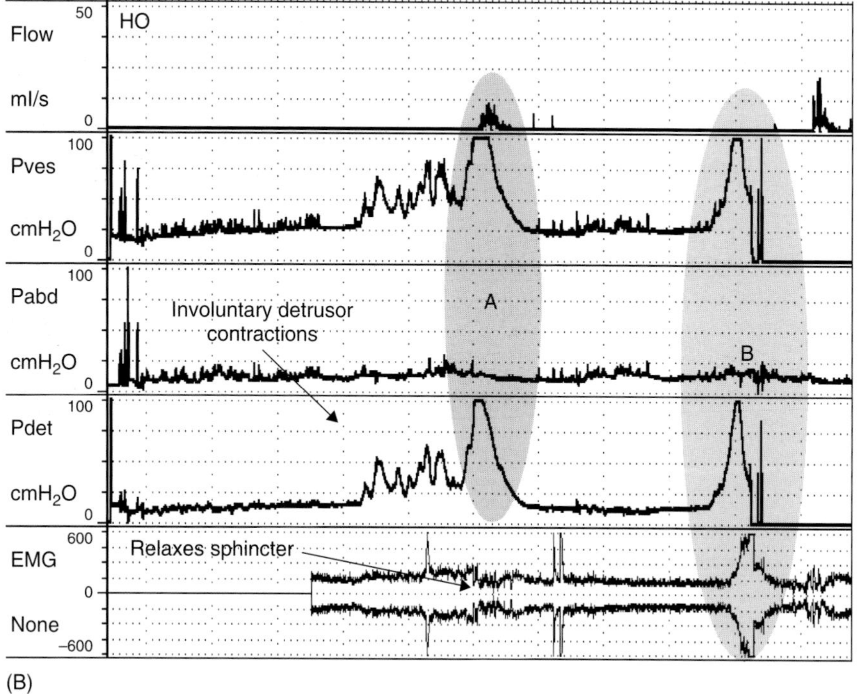

Fig. 9.5 Type 2 OAB. (A) Schematic depiction of type 2 OAB. The impending onset of an involuntary detrusor contraction is sensed by the patient who immediately contracts the striated sphincter. This is manifest as increased EMG activity. At this point, the urethra is dilated in its proximal urethra with obstruction in the distal third by the sphincter contraction (arrows A). Through a reflex mechanism, the detrusor contraction is aborted and continence maintained. (B) Type 2 OAB and prostatic obstruction in a 53-year-old man with a 20-year history of refractory urgency, urge incontinence, and enuresis. He had previously been treated with alpha-adrenergic antagonists, anticholinergics, and transrectal thermotherapy. VOID: 16/251/50.

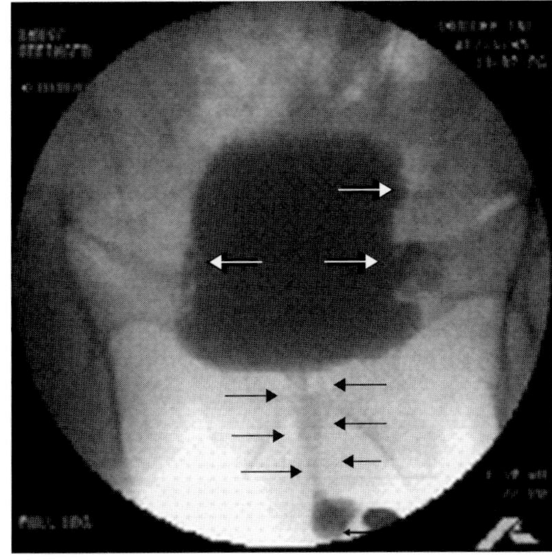

(C)

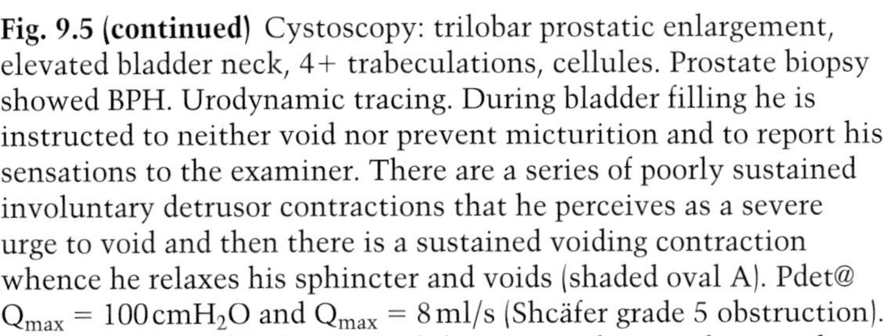

Fig. 9.5 (continued) Cystoscopy: trilobar prostatic enlargement, elevated bladder neck, 4+ trabeculations, cellules. Prostate biopsy showed BPH. Urodynamic tracing. During bladder filling he is instructed to neither void nor prevent micturition and to report his sensations to the examiner. There are a series of poorly sustained involuntary detrusor contractions that he perceives as a severe urge to void and then there is a sustained voiding contraction whence he relaxes his sphincter and voids (shaded oval A). Pdet@ $Q_{max} = 100\,cmH_2O$ and $Q_{max} = 8\,ml/s$ (Shcäfer grade 5 obstruction).

The bladder is filled again and there is another involuntary detrusor contraction. This time he is instructed to try to hold. He contracts his sphincter, obstructing the urethra, the detrusor contraction subsides, and he is not incontinent (shaded oval B). (C) X-ray obtained at Q_{max} shows a narrowed and faintly visualized prostatic urethra (black arrows) characteristic of prostatic obstruction. The bladder is trabeculated and there are several small and medium sized diverticula (white arrows). (D) X-ray obtained as he contracts his sphincter to prevent incontinence (shaded oval B in figure B). One would expect the contrast to stop at the distal prostatic urethra, but since he has prostatic obstruction that narrows the proximal urethra, no contrast is seen in the urethra at all.

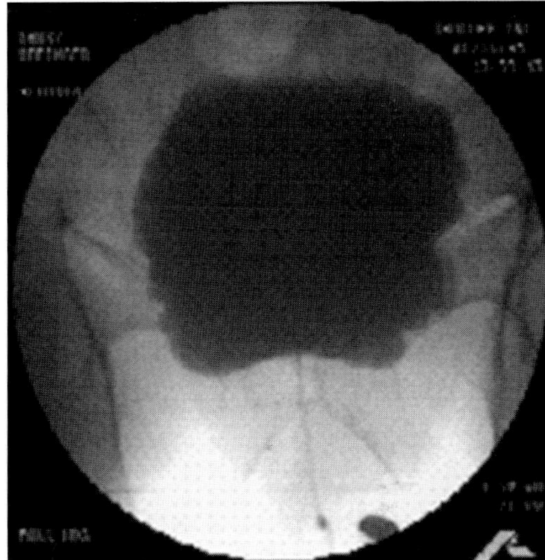

(D)

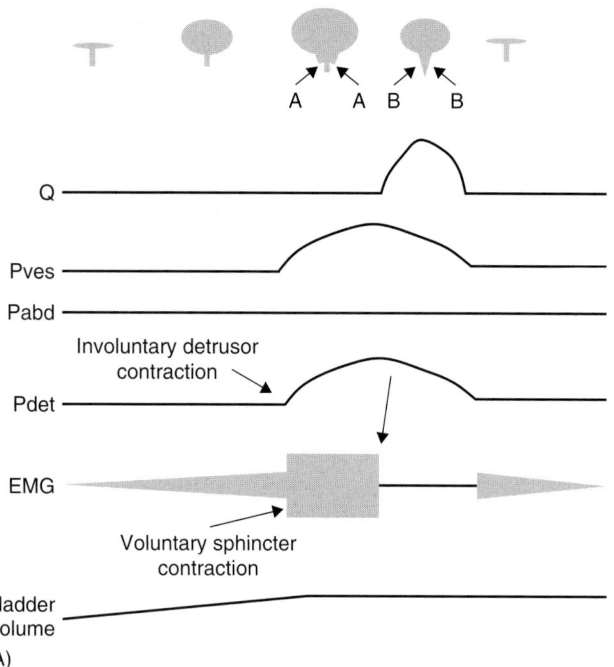

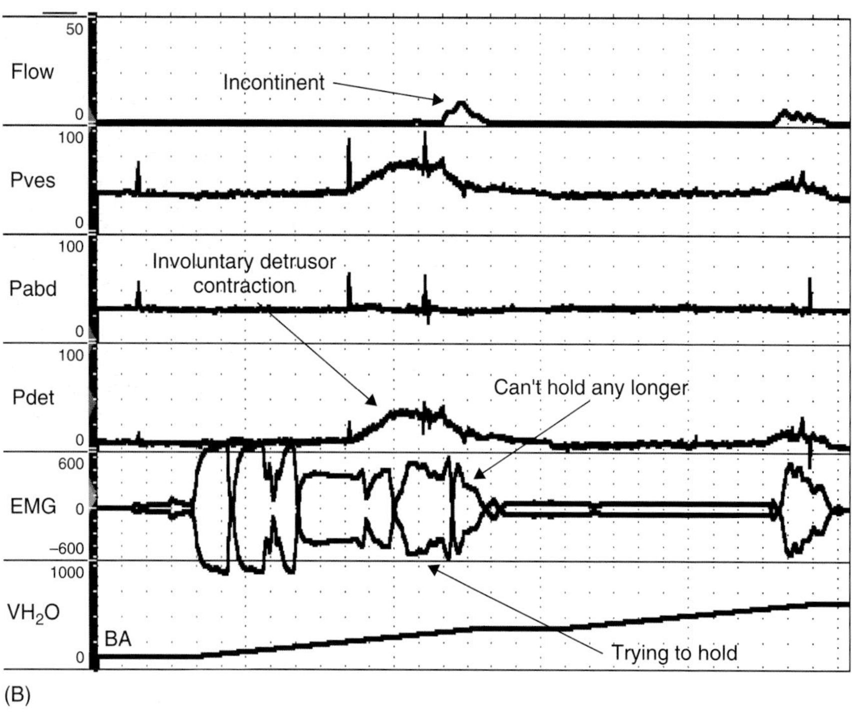

Fig. 9.6 Type 3 OAB. (A) Schematic depiction of type 3 OAB. The patient experiences an involuntary detrusor contraction. As soon as he senses the detrusor contraction, he voluntarily contracts his sphincter (increased EMG activity) in an attempt to prevent incontinence. At this point, the urethra is dilated in its proximal urethra with obstruction in the distal third by the sphincter contraction (arrows A), momentarily maintaining continence. Once the sphincter fatigues, the urethra opens and incontinence ensues (arrows B). (B) Type 3 OAB in a 42-year-old woman with refractory urge incontinence. Her symptoms began 18 months previously, coincident with the onset of an *E. coli* cystitis and have progressively worsened ever since. Neurologic evaluation was normal. She had failed all available anticholinergics and neuromodulation. Botox was not yet available. She subsequently underwent augmentation enterocystoplasty using detubularized ileum and remained continent without urgency and voiding without the need for intermittent catheterization.

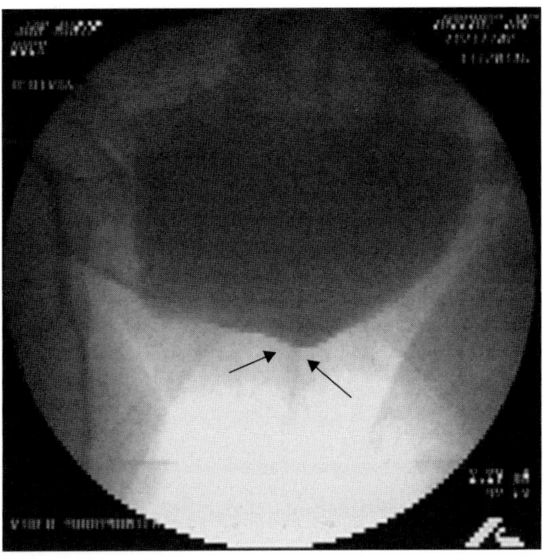

(C)

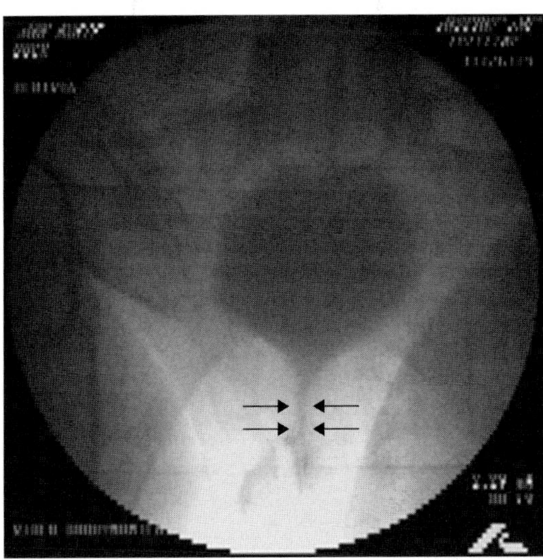

(D)

Fig. 9.6 (continued) Urodynamic tracing. A strong urge is felt at a bladder volume of 50 ml and she contracts her sphincter to prevent incontinence. At a volume of 275 ml, she develops an involuntary detrusor contraction and is able to continue contracting her sphincter, preventing incontinence. At 350 ml, she can no longer hold and she voids involuntarily. (C) X-ray obtained while she is contracting her sphincter during the involuntary detrusor contraction, preventing incontinence. Note that the bladder neck is closed (arrows). (D) X-ray exposed (once the sphincter relaxes and she is incontinent) shows a normally funneled urethra (arrows).

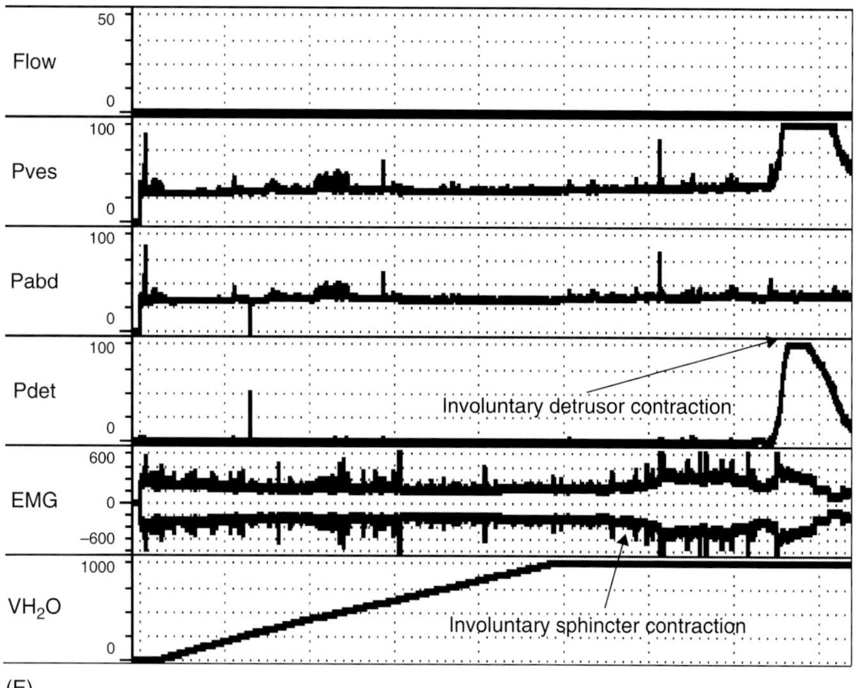

(E)

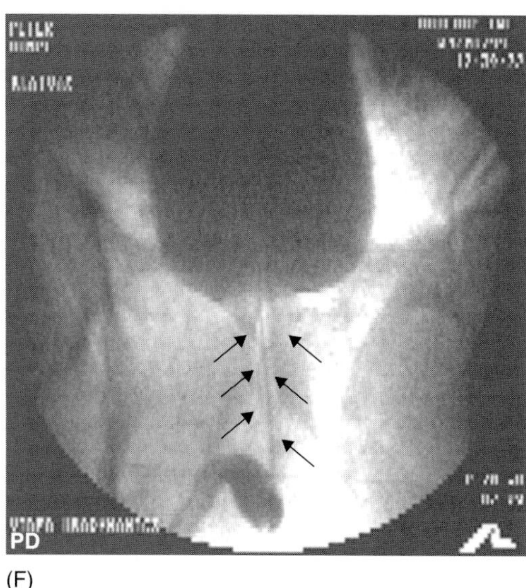

(F)

Fig. 9.6 (continued) (E) Type 3 OAB in a 56-year-old man with LUTS, OAB, and urge incontinence. Urodynamic tracing. At a bladder volume of 160ml there was an involuntary detrusor contraction. He momentarily contracted his sphincter, but could not abort the detrusor contraction and was incontinent. Pdet@Q_{max} = 135 and Q_{max} = 4ml/s (Schäfer grade 6 urethral obstruction). He subsequently underwent suprapubic prostatectomy and was asymptomatic at his latest follow-up 4 years postoperatively. (F) X-ray obtained at Q_{max} shows a narrowed prostatic urethra (arrows).

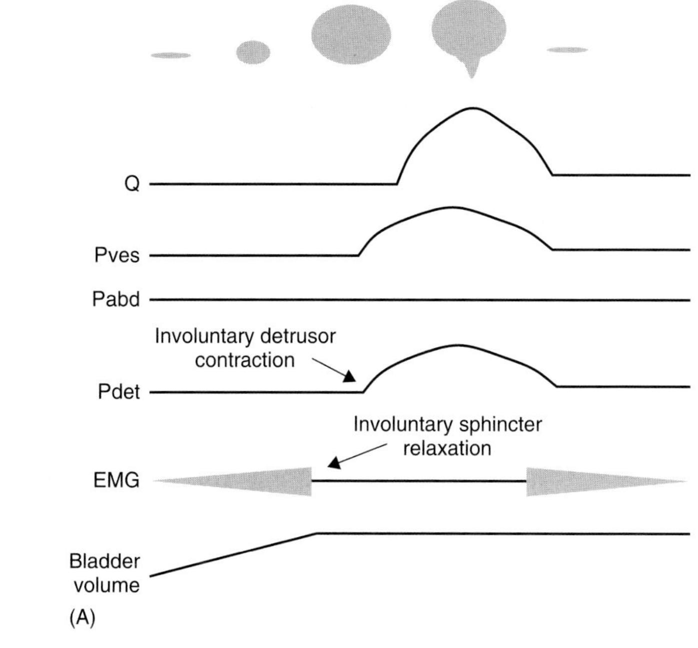

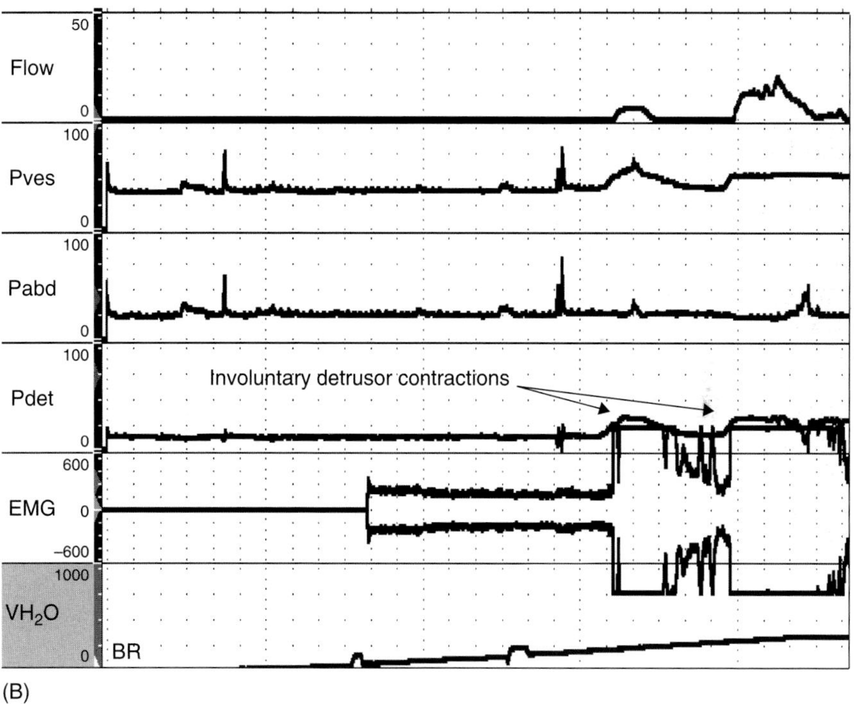

Fig. 9.7 Type 4 OAB. (A) Schematic depiction of type 4 OAB. There is an involuntary detrusor contraction, but the patient has no awareness and can neither contract the sphincter nor abort the stream. The urodynamic tracing is identical to a normal micturition reflex. (B) Type 4 OAB in an otherwise normal woman with refractory urge incontinence. Urodynamic tracing. There are two involuntary detrusor contractions; each time she voids involuntarily without control. The apparent increase in EMG activity is artifact, likely due to poor contact of the EMG, electrodes, possibly due to urine leakage.

Benign Prostatic Hyperplasia, Bladder Neck Obstruction, and Prostatitis

10

Introduction

In the vernacular of urology, the terms benign prostatic hyperplasia (BPH) and prostatic obstruction have been used interchangeably since their inception. In fact, they are not synonymous and a new lexicon has emerged [1]. Enlargement of the prostate gland by BPH or inflammation is termed benign prostatic enlargement (BPE), but, of course, it may be enlarged by prostatic cancer as well. Urinary tract symptoms are termed lower urinary tract symptoms (LUTS), an ingenious use of language. From a physiologic viewpoint, the cause of LUTS is multifactorial, comprising at least five conditions: (1) urethral obstruction, (2) impaired detrusor contractility, (3) detrusor overactivity, (4) sensory urgency, and (5) nocturnal polyuria and polyuria [2]. The latter, of course, are not due to lower urinary tract abnormalties and will not be discussed further.

LUTS may be sub-divided into voiding or storage symptoms as first described by Wein [3]. Storage symptoms include urinary frequency, urgency, urge incontinence, nocturia, and some kinds of pain. Voiding symptoms include hesitancy, straining, decreased stream, dysuria, and post-void dribbling. Conventional wisdom asserts that voiding symptoms are caused by prostatic obstruction and storage symptoms are caused by lower urinary tract inflammation or detrusor overactivity. Despite the logic implied herein, most clinical studies find no such correlation [4–9]. It is not even known, for example, whether urethral obstruction is the primary mechanism by which BPH causes symptoms. Likewise, there appears to be little relationship between symptoms, symptoms scores and commonly used indices of obstruction, and impaired detrusor contractility such as uroflow, post-void residual (PVR) urine, nomograms, and mathematical formulas.

The relationship between benign prostatic hyperplasia (BPH), benign prostatic enlargement (BPE) and benign prostatic obstruction (BPO) has never, to our satisfaction, been adequately defined. Suffice it to say, there are many men with BPE who do not have BPO and many men with small prostates who do have BPO. Further, most men with LUTS have a multifactorial pathophysiology accounting for their symptoms [2]. Only about two-thirds of men with LUTS have diagnosable BPO and about 50% have detrusor overactivity. A detailed compilation of urodynamic abnormalities in men with LUTS is depicted in Table 10.1 and Figure 10.1 [2].

Table 10.1 Urodynamic abnormalities in men with LUTS [2].

Storage abnormalities	Men (%)	Voiding abnormalities	Men (%)
Detrusor overactivity	47	Prostatic obstruction	69
Large capacity	10	Impaired detrusor contractility	20
Low bladder compliance	10	Acontractile detrusor	8
Low bladder capacity	2	Normal	3

Even in patients with documented prostatic obstruction, it is evident that factors other than the mechanical effects of prostatic bulk play an important role. These include detrusor muscle strength and tone, bladder wall compliance, smooth muscle function of the bladder neck and prostatic urethra, striated muscle function of the prostate-membranous urethra, and interstitial factors such as elastin and collagen type. The physiologic dysfunction associated with LUTS is a composite of the effects of all these factors, not simply the effects of mechanical obstruction caused by the mass of glandular tissue.

Mechanical (static) obstruction

Enlargement of the glands which surround the prostatic urethra results in urethral compression, causing mechanical obstruction. Pathologically, BPH develops, as nodules comprising both epithelial and stromal elements of the glands lining the proximal prostatic urethra. These nodules enlarge and coalesce within the anterior, posterior, and lateral walls of the prostate, forming lobular masses of various shapes and sizes. The anterior lobe is usually only minimally involved, thus BPH is often designated as bilobar (lateral lobe enlargement only) or trilobar (both lateral and posterior lobe enlargement). Some patients will have only posterior, median lobe hyperplasia which may be obstructive. In these cases of BPH, the lateral lobes may be only minimally enlarged while the median lobe grows infravesically to obstruct the bladder neck. This explains why there is a variable correlation between prostatic size and the degree of obstruction.

Smooth muscle (dynamic) obstruction

The human prostate contains an abundance of alpha-1 adrenergic receptors, which modulate the contractility of prostatic smooth muscle. Stimulation of these receptors by norepinephrine and other alpha-adrenergic agonists results in contraction of the smooth muscle and compression of the prostatic urethra, increasing the resistance to urinary flow. Thus, the dynamic component of BPH may be viewed as a result of the increased smooth muscle tone of the bladder neck, prostatic adenoma, and prostatic capsule.

Differential diagnosis

All men have prostates, of course, but only about two-thirds of men with LUTS have prostatic obstruction and many have other comorbid conditions including bacterial cystitis, non-specific cystitis (e.g. radiation or interstitial cystitis), papillary transitional cell carcinoma, transitional cell carcinoma in situ, and prostate cancer. In addition, bladder or ureteral calculi may induce storage symptoms. Emptying and storage symptoms may also occur with detrusor–external sphincter dyssynergia (DESD), primary bladder neck obstruction, and urethral stricture.

Urodynamic evaluation

The only definitive method of distinguishing the possible causes of LUTS in men is cystometry and voiding detrusor pressure/uroflow studies. Neither simple uroflow nor simple cystometry can make the necessary distinctions between urethral obstruction, impaired detrusor contractility, detrusor overactivity, and sensory urgency [10]. Concomitant fluoroscopic imaging (videourodynamics) pinpoints the site of obstruction.

Bladder outlet obstruction and impaired detrusor contractility are defined by the relationship between detrusor pressure and uroflow – a high pressure and low flow indicate obstruction (Fig. 10.2) and a low pressure (or poorly sustained detrusor contraction) and low flow indicates impaired detrusor contractility (Fig. 10.3). Multiple nomograms have been described to interpret pressure flow studies (PFS) [11–14]. The nomograms plot detrusor pressure at maximum flow (Pdet@Q_{max}) versus synchronous maximum flow rate (Q_{max}). We prefer the Schafer nomogram to the others because it provides a simple 6 point obstruction scale and a 5 point detrusor contractility scale (Fig. 10.4). Figures 10.5–10.11 depict Schafer grades 0–6 prostatic urethral obstruction.

Primary bladder neck obstruction

Primary bladder neck obstruction is an uncommon but not rare condition seen mostly in young and middle-aged men [15]. The etiology is unknown but it is most likely the result of neuromuscular overactivity and failure of the bladder neck to open wide during detrusor contraction. The usual presenting symptoms are urinary frequency and urgency. Obstructive symptoms are usually not as prominent. The diagnosis can only be established by videourodynamics and cystoscopy. The videourodynamic criteria include high Pdet@Q_{max}, low Q_{max}, narrowing of the bladder neck on fluoroscopic imaging, and relaxation of external sphincter electromyography (EMG) during micturition (Fig. 10.13). The urodynamic appearance of bladder neck contracture (due to prior prostatic surgery) is identical to primary bladder neck obstruction. Only cystoscopy can distinguish the two entities. In the great majority of cases, bladder neck incision or resection is curative (Fig. 10.12), but occasionally there may be persistent obstruction (Fig. 10.13).

Acquired voiding dysfunction

In acquired voiding dysfunction (AVD), there are involuntary (and often subconscious) contractions of the external urethral sphincter during voiding that are nearly identical to DESD (see Chapter 12, Figs. 7–9). The distinction between AVD and DESD is based on both clinical and urodynamic findings. Firstly, DESD is always due to a neurologic lesion that interrupts the pathways between the brain stem and sacral micturition center. In the absence of such a lesion (spinal cord injury, transverse myelitis, multiple sclerosis, etc.), the diagnosis should not be made. Secondly, in DESD, the contraction of the external sphincter (and increase in EMG) activity always occurs prior to the onset of the detrusor contraction, whereas, in AVD, the detrusor contraction occurs first and is preceded by sphincter relaxation (and EMG silence). Once the detrusor contraction starts, the patient subconsciously contracts the sphincter (Fig. 10.14).

Bladder diverticula

Bladder diverticula are another cause of LUTS in men. In most cases, bladder diverticula are associated with prostatic obstruction (Figs. 10.11 and 10.15). In such cases, treatment of the obstruction usually suffices. Sometimes, though, there is no diagnosable obstruction and surgical excision of the bladder diverticulum is necessary (Fig. 10.16).

The neurogenic bladder and BPH

Neurogenic bladder dysfunction often generates symptoms that are attributed to prostatic obstruction particularly in men after stroke, Parkinson's disease, and multiple sclerosis. The distinction between prostatic obstruction and neurogenic bladder can only be made with videourodynamics (Fig. 10.6, PD/CVA (Parkinson's disease/cerebrovascular accident) chapter; Fig. 10.17), but sometimes even the most sophisticated studies cannot make these distinctions with certainty (Fig. 10.18). In our judgment, empiric treatment of men with BPH and any of these neurologic conditions is unwise and often results in poor results. Empiric prostatectomy is particularly hazardous and often results in unsatisfactory outcomes.

Chronic pelvic pain syndrome/prostatitis

Chronic pelvic pain syndrome (CPPS)/prostatitis is an enigmatic condition frustrating to both patients and doctors alike. In our judgment videourodynamics plays a vital role in the diagnosis and treatment of such patients for several reasons. Firstly, many of the symptoms of CPPS can be due to primary bladder neck obstruction and/or detrusor overactivity. Secondly, the filling phase of the cystometrogram is an excellent method for assessing the relationship between bladder filling and the patient's pain. Finally, the patient may have an AVD that is either the cause of, or the result of, his symptoms (Fig. 10.14).

Suggested Reading

1 Abrams P. New words for old: lower urinary tract symptoms for prostatism, *Br Med J*, 308: 929–930, 1994.

2 Fusco F, Groutz A, Blaivas JG, Chaikin DC, Weiss JP. Videourodynamic studies in men with lower urinary tract symptoms: a comparison of community based versus referral urological practices, *J Urol*, 166: 910–913, 2001.

3 Wein AJ. Classification of neurogenic voiding dysfunction, *J Urol*, 125: 605, 1981.

4 Ezz el Din K, De Wildt MJAM, Rosier PFWM, Wijkstra H, Debruyne FMJ, De LA Rosette JJMCH. The correlation between urodynamic and cystoscopic findings in elderly men with voiding complaints, *J Urol*, 155: 1018–1022, 1996.

5 Javle P, Jenkins SA, West C, Parsons KF. Quantification of voiding dysfunction in patients awaiting transureteral prostatectomy, *J Urol*, 156: 1014–1019, 1996.

6 Schacterie RS, Sullivan MP, Yalla SV. Combinations of maximum urinary flow rate and American Urological Association symptom index that are more specific for identifying obstructive and non-obstructive prostatism, *Neurourol Urodynam*, 15: 459–472, 1996.

7 Sirls LT, Kirkemo AK, Jay J. Lack of correlation of the American urological association symptom 7 index with urodynamic bladder outlet obstruction. *Neurourol Urodynam*, 15: 447–457, 1996.

8 Van Ventrooij GEPM, Boon TA. The value of symptom score, quality of life score, maximal urinary flow rate, residual volume and prostate size for the diagnosis of obstructive benign prostatic hyperplasia: a urodynamic analysis, *J Urol*, 155: 2014–2018, 1996.

9 Witjes WPJ, De Wildt MJAM, Rosier PFWM, Caris CTM, Debruyne FMJ, De La Rosette JMCH. Variability of clinical and pressure-flow study variables after 6 months of watchful waiting in patients with lower urinary tract symptoms and benign prostatic enlargement, *J Urol*, 156: 1026–1034, 1996.

10 Chancellor MB, Blaivas JB, Kaplan SA, Axelrod S. Bladder outlet obstruction versus impaired detrusor contractility: role of uroflow, *J Urol*, 145: 810–812, 1991.

11 Abrams PH, Griffiths DH. The assessment of prostatic obstruction from urodynamic measurements and from residual urine, *Br J Urol*, 51(2): 129–134, 1979.

12 Rollema HJ, Van Mastrigt R. Improved indication and followup in transurethral resection of the prostate using the computer program CLIM: a prospective study, *J Urol*, 148(1): 111–115; discussion 115–116, 1992.

13 Schafer W. Basic principles and clinical application of advanced analysis of bladder voiding function, *Urol Clin N Am*, 17: 553–566, 1990.

14 Schafer W. In Vahlensiek and Rutishauser (eds) *Benign Prostate Diseases*, New York: Georg Thieme Verlag Stuttgart, 1992 ISBN 0-86577-468-4 (TMP, New York).

15 Norlen LJ, Blaivas JG. Unsuspected proximal urethral obstruction in young and middle-aged men, *J Urol*, 135: 972–976, 1986.

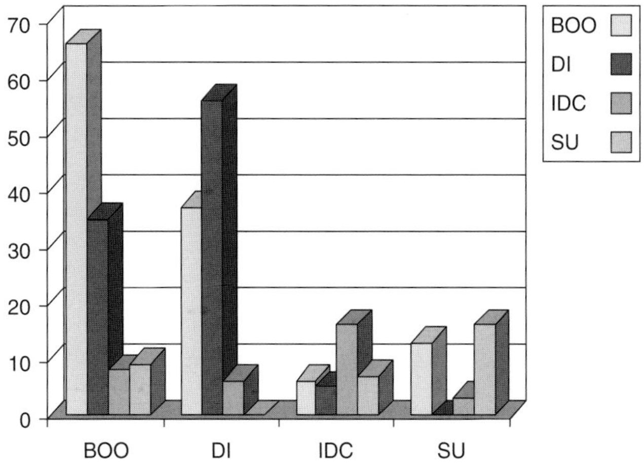

Fig. 10.1 Urodynamic abnormalities in men with LUTS. BOO = bladder outlet obstruction, DI = detrusor overactivity, IDC = impaired detrusor contractility, and SU = sensory urgency.

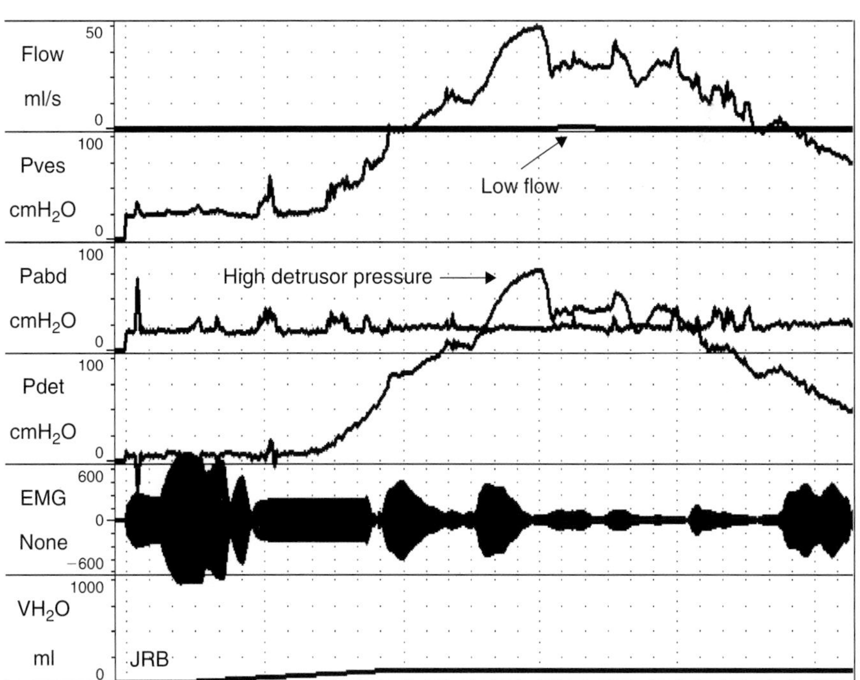

Fig. 10.2 Urethral obstruction. Prostatic obstruction in a 73-year-old man with Parkinson's disease. Urodynamic study. Q_{max} = 1 ml/s, Pdet@Q_{max} = 150 cmH_2O, Pdetmax = 187 cmH_2O, voided volume = 33 ml, and PVR = 88 ml.

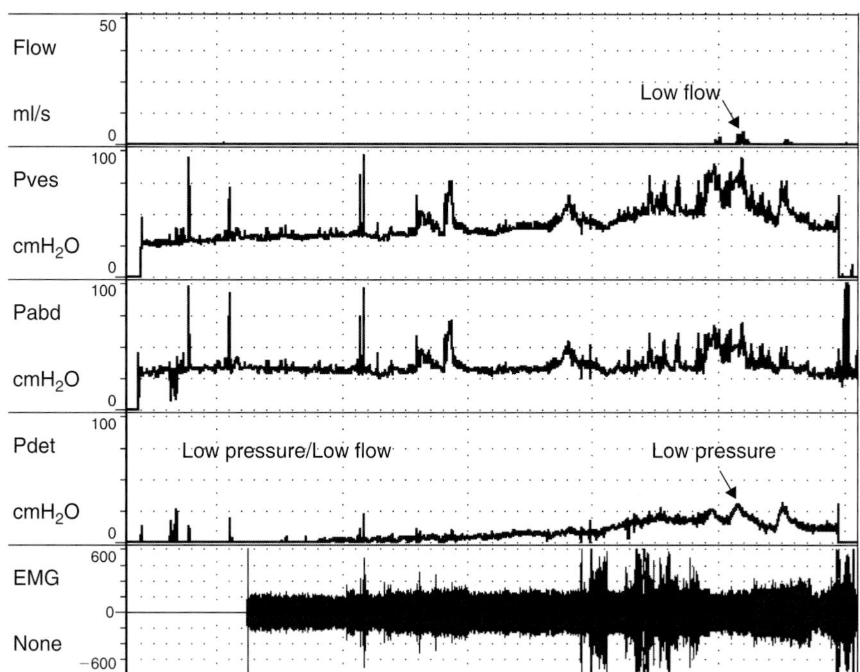

Fig. 10.3 Impaired detrusor contractility (low pressure, low flow). Pdet@ Q_{max} = 28 cmH_2O, Q_{max} = 2 ml/s, and Pdet@P_{max} = 28 cmH_2O.

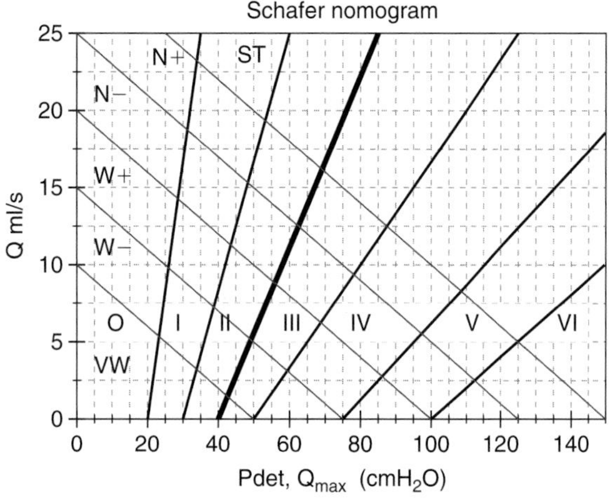

Fig. 10.4 Schafer nomogram showing 6 point obstruction scale and 5 point detrusor contractility. O–VI refers to increasing grades of obstructions. VW to ST refer to increasing detrusor strength. VW = very weak; W− + W+ = weak; N− and N + normal; ST very strong.

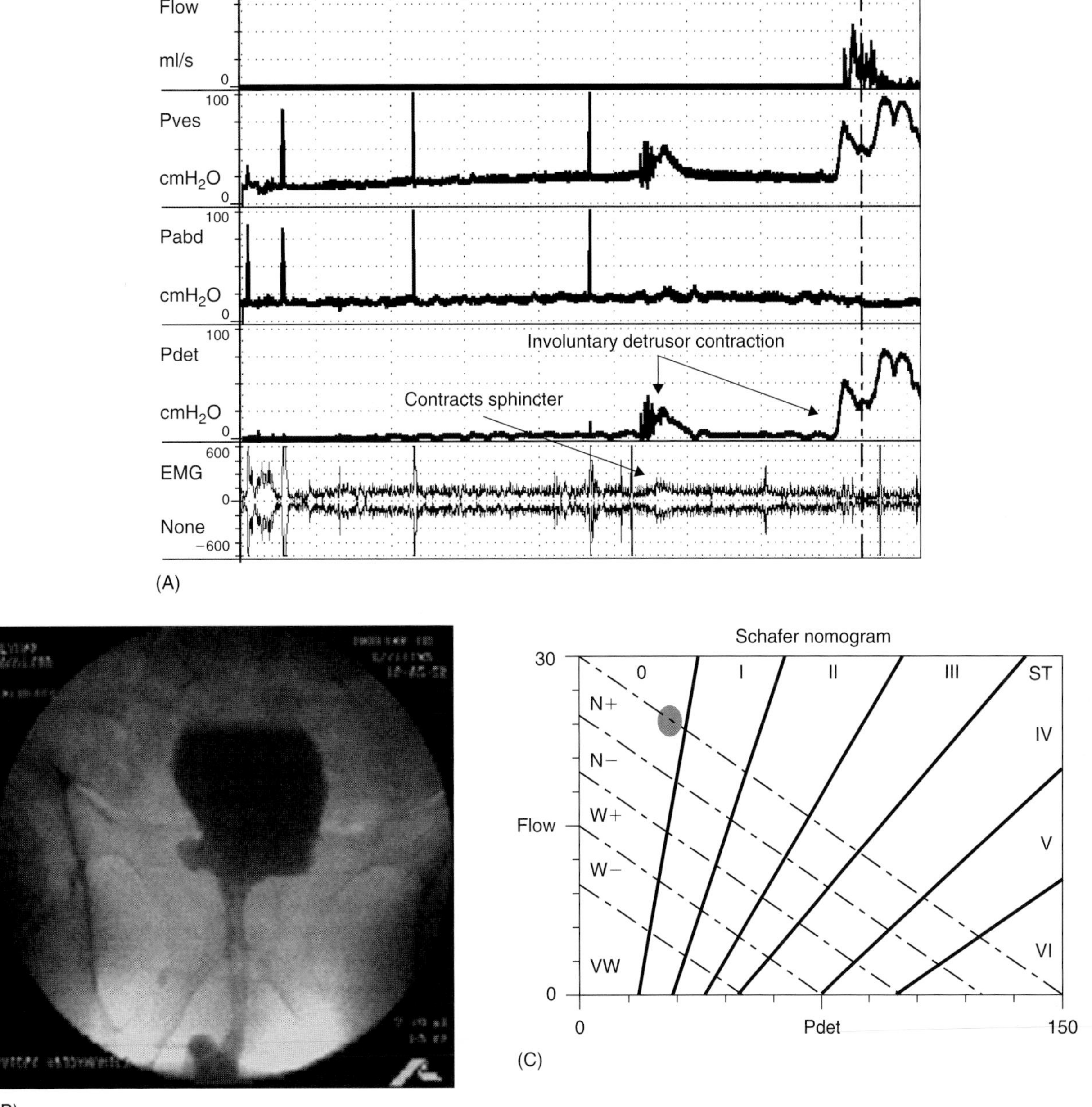

Fig. 10.5 (A) Schafer grade 0 (no obstruction) Pdet@Q_{max} = 27 cmH_2O; Q_{max} = 26 ml/s (vertical dotted line). (B) Voiding cystourethrogram (VCUG) showing wide open urethra during maximum flow. (C) Schafer nomogram plotting Q_{max} versus Pdet@Q_{max} yielding grade 0 voiding with excellent (N+) detrusor contractility.

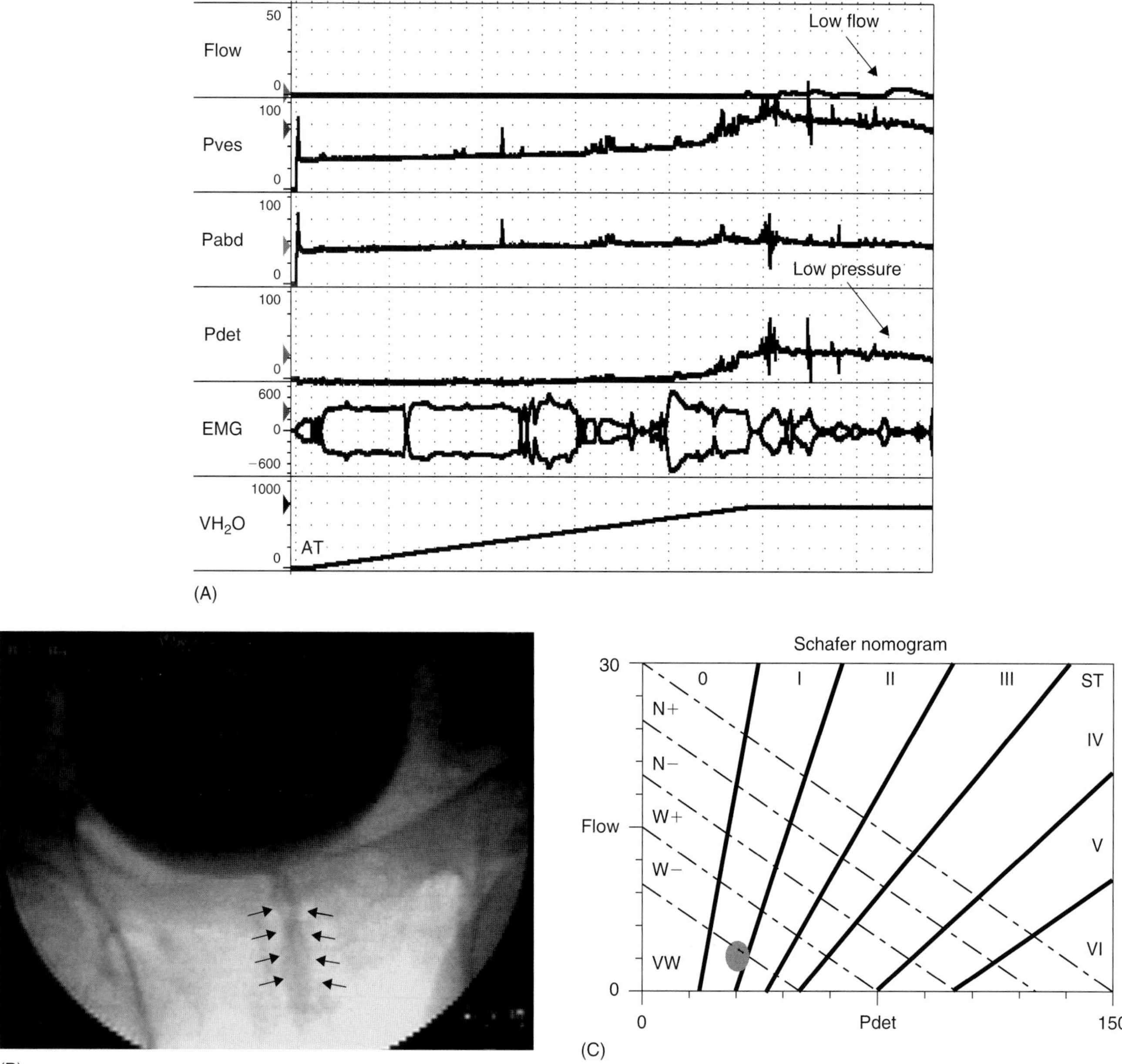

Fig. 10.6 Schafer grade 1 and impaired detrusor contractility (VW) in a 58-year-old man complaining of urinary frequency, urgency, occasional urge incontinence, hesitancy, and weak stream. (A) Urodynamic study. FSF (first sensation of filling) = 272 ml, 1st urge = 491 ml, severe urge = 620 ml, bladder capacity = 710 ml, Q_{max} = 6 ml/s, Pdet@ Q_{max} = 28 cmH_2O, and Pdetmax = 41 cmH_2O. (B) X-ray obtained at Q_{max} shows a narrowed prostatic urethra (arrows). (C) Nomogram reveals unobstructed voiding (grade 1) with very weak detrusor contractility.

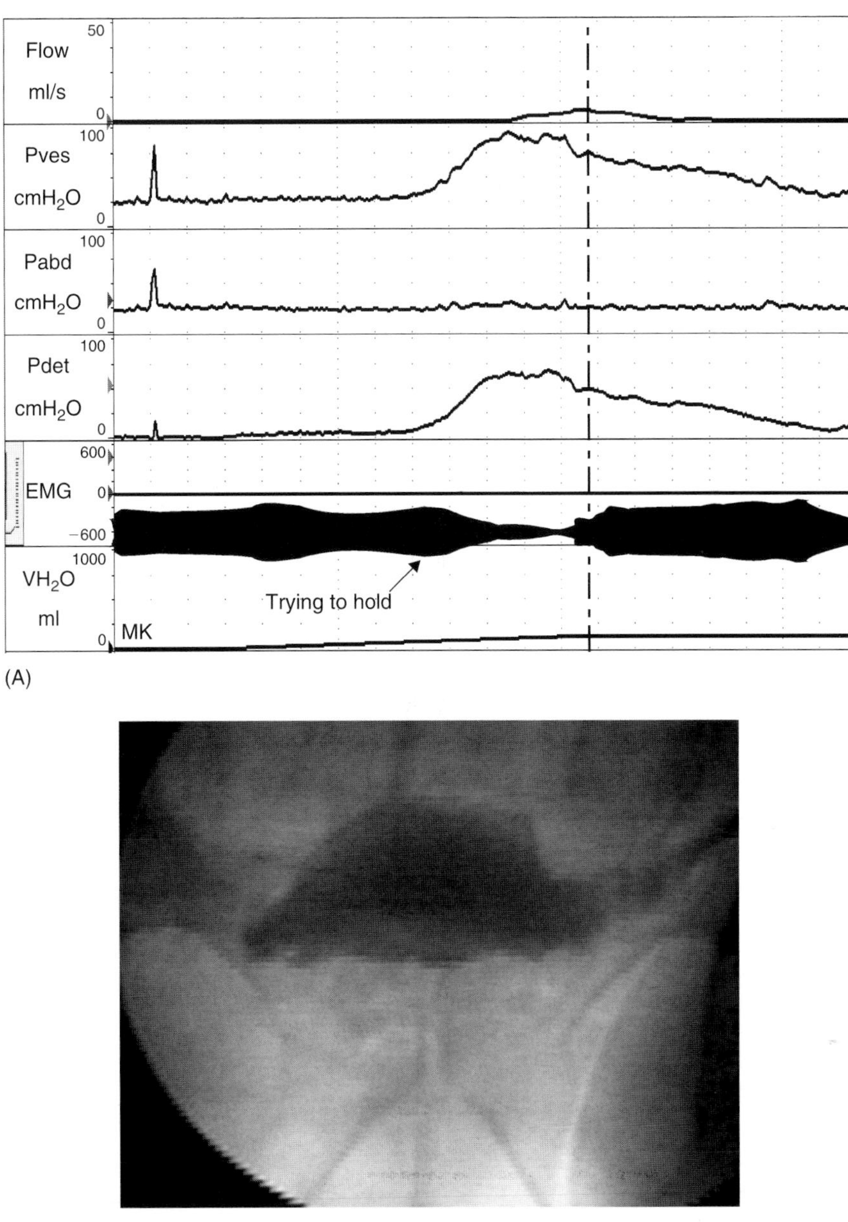

Fig. 10.7 Grade 2 obstruction and type 3 detrusor overactivity. MK is a 70-year-old man with a 10-year history of gradually worsening day and nighttime urge incontinence . He ordinarily voids every 4 hours during the day. He is awakened from sleep about every 1–2 hours. Ten years ago he was started on tamsulosin and 3 years ago underwent empiric thermotherapy, both without benefit. On examination, the prostate was 1+ in size. A 24-hour pad test showed 93 ml of urine loss. Cystoscopy showed bilobar prostatic occlusion, a 4+ trabeculated bladder, and a single large mouthed diverticulum. The urodynamic study (see below) showed borderline urethral obstruction, but the unintubated flow was perfectly normal. After this urodynamic study, he was treated with all of the commercially available overactive bladder (OAB) medications, with and without all of the available alpha adrenergic antagonists, all without effect. He subsequently underwent TURP also without benefit. He declined further treatments, but is still being followed. (A) Urodynamic tracing. At a bladder volume of 100 ml, he had a severe urge to void and tried to hold back by contracting his sphincter (Arrow A), but had an involuntary detrusor contraction that he could not abort and voided to completion. Q_{max} = 6 ml/s, Pdet@Q_{max} = 48 cmH_2O (vertical dotted line), Pdetmax = 66 cmH_2O, voided volume = 78 ml, and PVR = 26 ml. (B) X-ray obtained while he was contracting his sphincter in an attempt to prevent incontinence shows a trabeculated bladder and no contrast in the urethra.

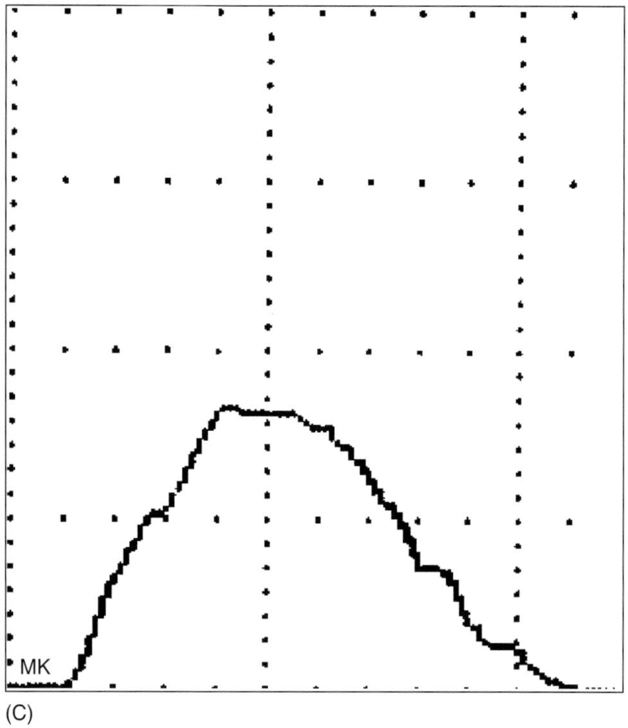

Fig. 10.7 (continued) (C) Uroflow obtained just prior to the urodynamic study. VOID: 16/190/5.

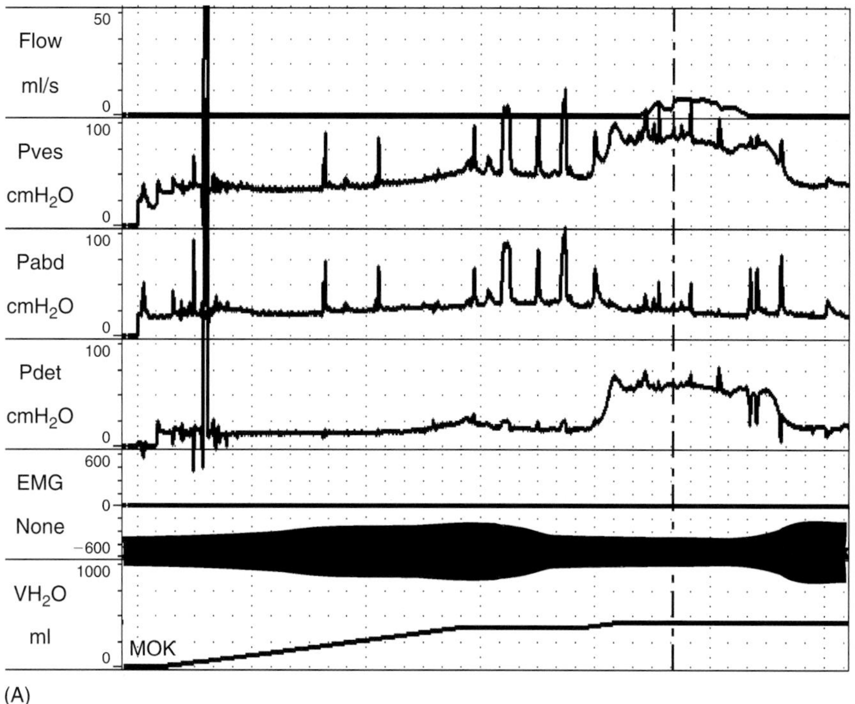

Fig. 10.8 Grade 3 prostatic obstruction. MOK is an 80-year-old man who developed urinary retention after undergoing TUR of multiple large, superficial bladder tumors. This urodynamic study showed Schafer grade 3 prostatic obstruction. He was then treated with tamsulosin and voided satisfactorily thereafter. (A) Urodynamic tracing. Q_{max} = 8 ml (vertical dotted line), Pdet@Q_{max} = 59 cmH_2O, Pdetmax = 59 cmH_2O, voided volume = 325 ml, and PVR = 98 ml. This corresponds to grade 3 obstruction on the Schafer nomogram (Fig. 10.8(C)).

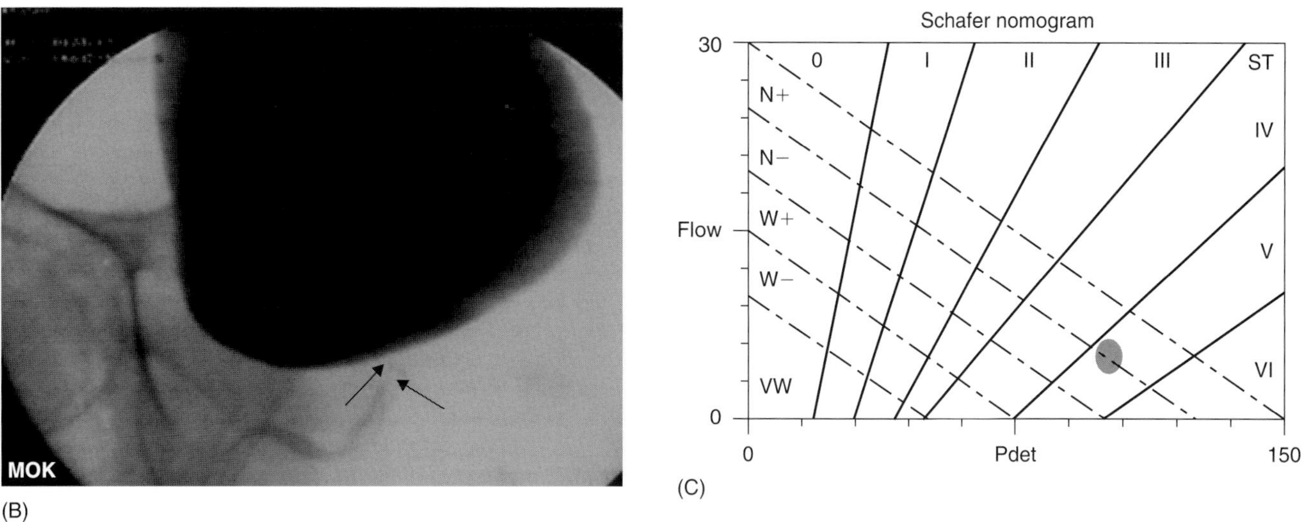

Fig. 10.8 (continued) (B) X-ray obtained at Q_{max} shows obstruction at the bladder neck and proximal prostatic urethra (arrows). (C) Schafer grade 3 obstruction.

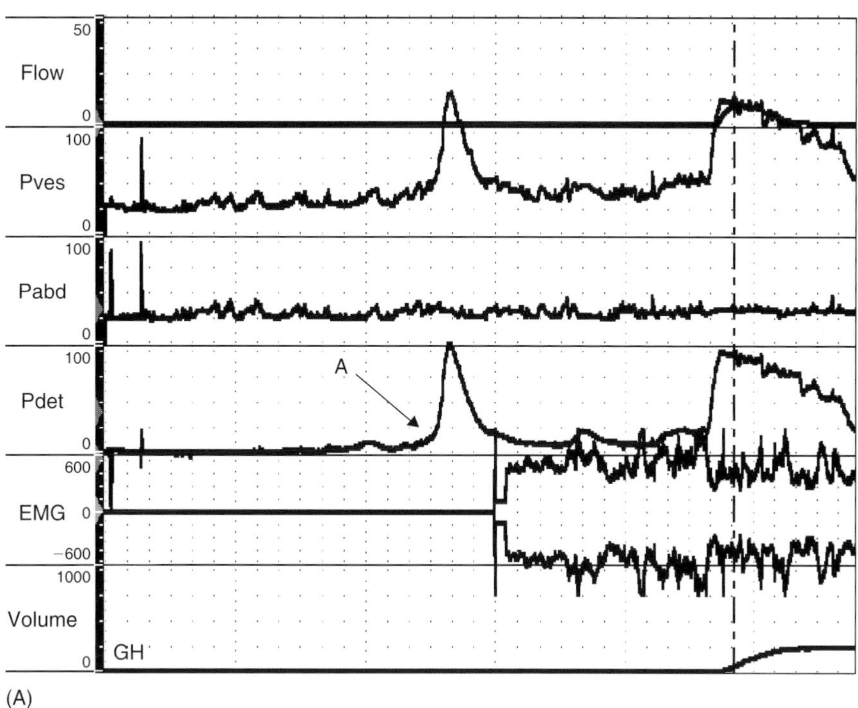

Fig. 10.9 Grade 4 prostatic urethral obstruction and type 2 detrusor overactivity in a diabetic man. GH is a 68-year-old man with juvenile onset, type 1 insulin dependent diabetes who complains of urinary frequency, decreased stream, urgency, and urge incontinence. After TURP his obstruction was relieved, but his OAB symptoms persisted for about 2 months and then subsided. (A) Urodynamic tracing. At a bladder volume of about 150 ml, he had an involuntary detrusor contraction (arrow A) that he was aware of and able to completely abort preventing incontinence. The EMG tracing was not on at that time. The bladder was then filled until he sensed the need to void and he had a voluntary detrusor contraction, voiding 244 ml. Pdet@Q_{max} = 99 cmH_2O (vertical dotted line), Q_{max} = 10 ml/s, and PVR = 6 ml. This corresponds to Schafer grade 4 obstruction.

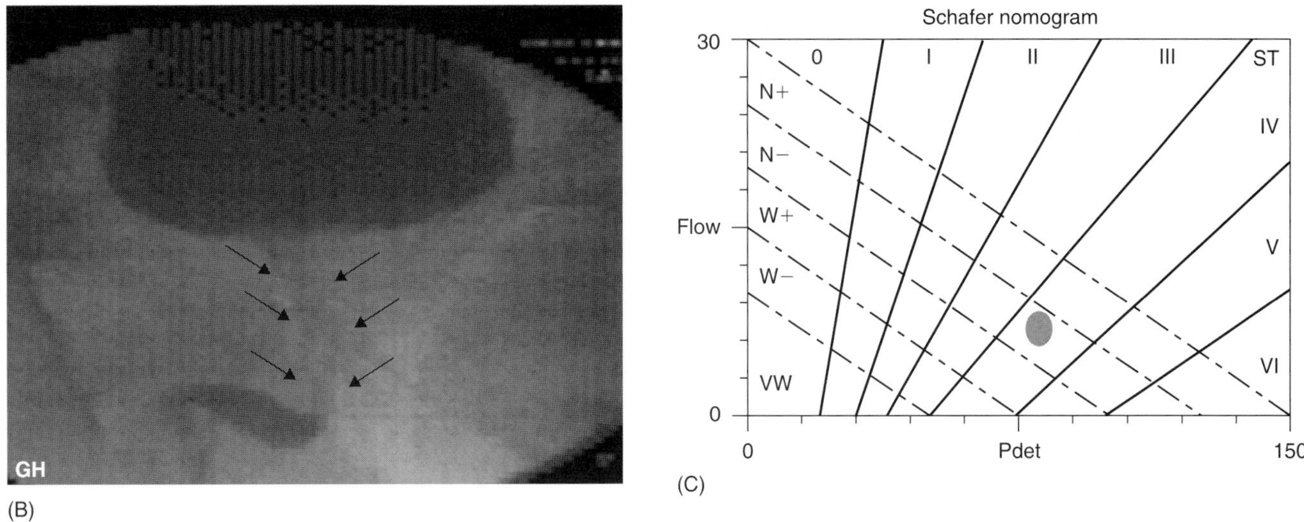

Fig. 10.9 (continued) (B) X-ray obtained at Q_{max} demonstrated diffuse narrowing of the prostatic urethra (arrows). (C) Schafer nomogram (grade 4 obstruction).

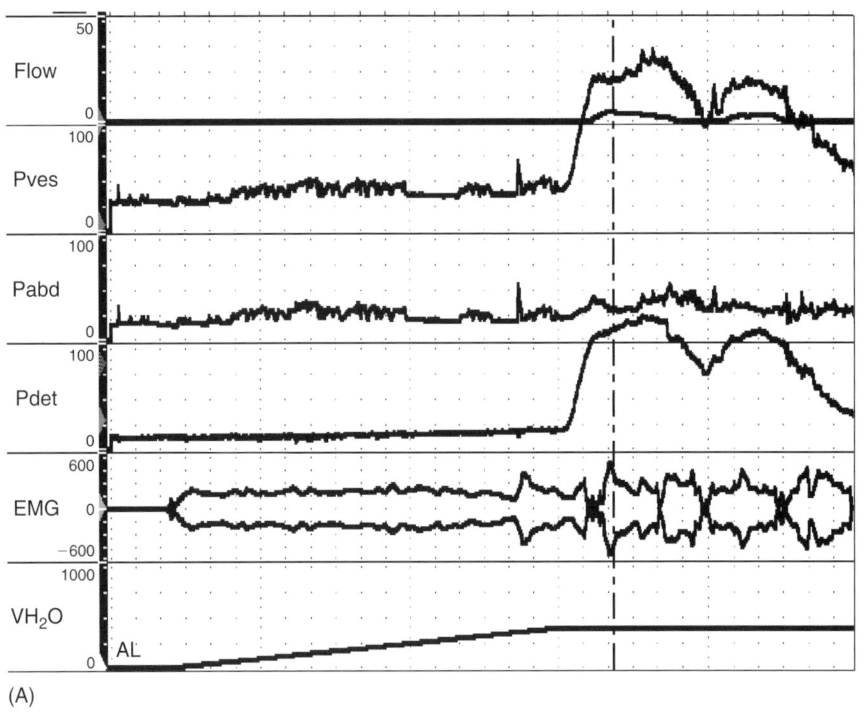

Fig. 10.10 Grade 5 prostatic obstruction. AL is a 63-year-old widowed accountant who developed urinary retention and was treated with an indwelling catheter and tamsulosin for 5 days, following at which time this urodynamic study was done. (A) Urodynamic tracing. At a bladder volume of approximately 400 ml, he had a voluntary detrusor contraction. Q_{max} = 5 ml/s (vertical dotted line), Pdet@Q_{max} = 117 cmH_2O, Pdetmax = 123 cmH_2O, voided volume = 215 ml, and PVR = 174 ml. This corresponds to a grade 5 obstruction on the Schafer nomogram.

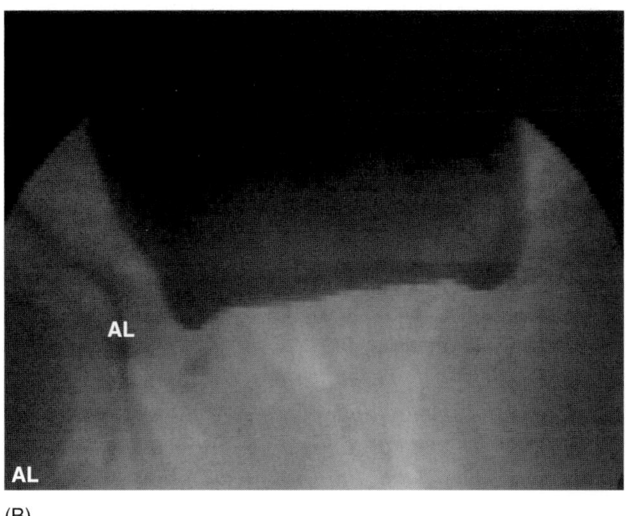

(B)

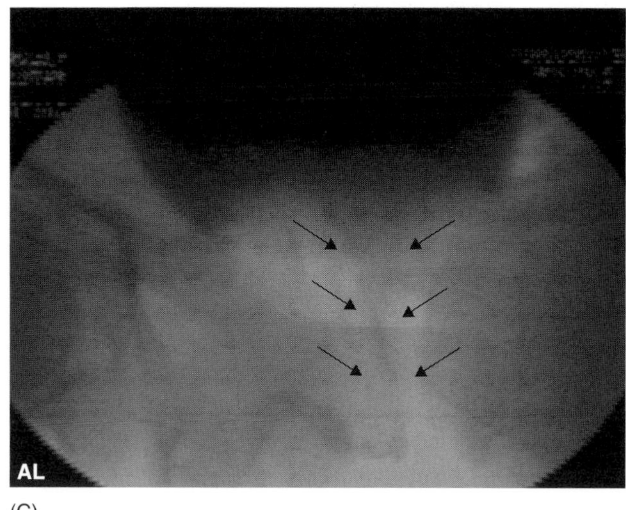

(C)

(D)

Fig. 10.10 (continued) (B) X-ray obtained just prior to voiding shows a flattened bladder base characteristic of BPO. (C) X-ray obtained at Q_{max} (Fig. 10.10(A)) reveals the prostatic urethra to be elongated and barely visible (arrows). (D) Schafer nomogram (grade 5 obstruction).

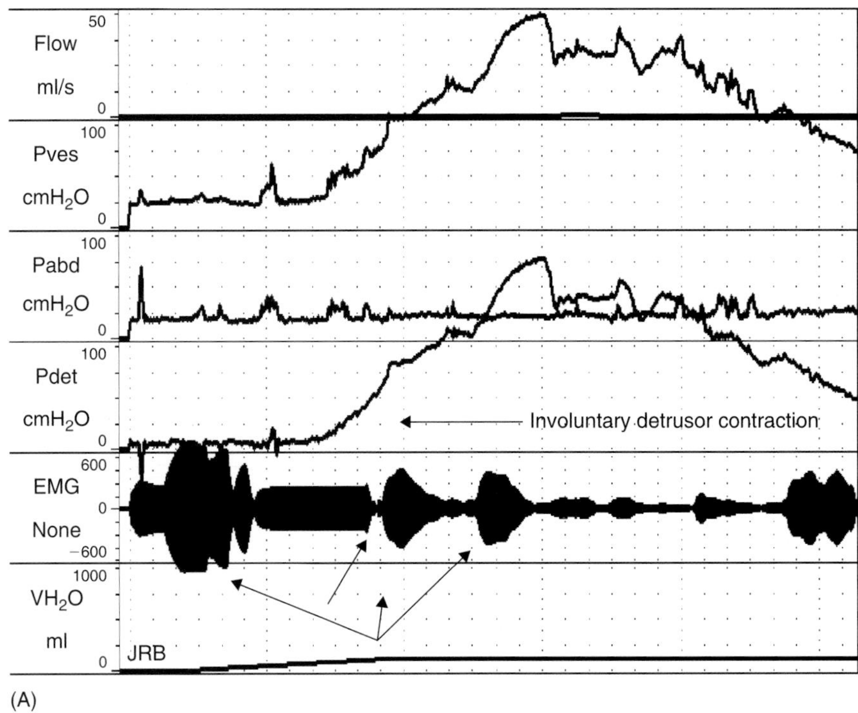

(A)

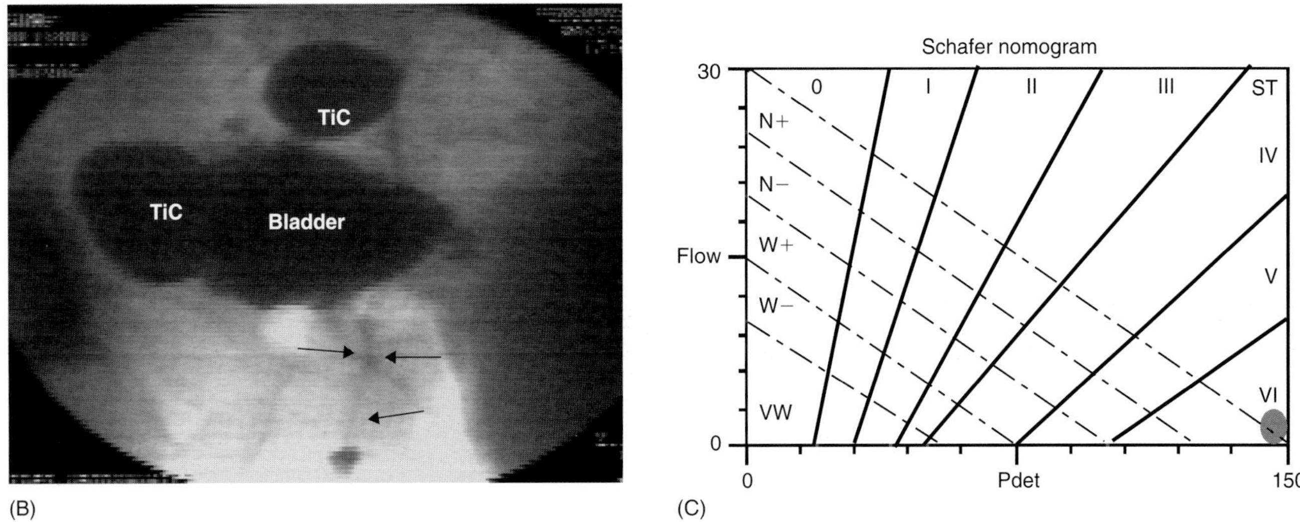

(B) (C)

Fig. 10.11 Delayed relaxation of the sphincter, detrusor hyperreflexia (type 3 OAB), prostatic obstruction (Schafer grade 6), and multiple bladder diverticula in a 73-year-old man with Parkinson's disease. His chief complaint is urinary frequency, urgency, and urge incontinence on a daily basis. PVR (post-void residual) was 0 and he was empirically treated with tolterodine, subsequently developing urinary retention. (A) Urodynamic tracing. 1st urge at 50 ml, severe urge at 121 ml synchronous with an involuntary detrusor contraction. Note the sporadic bursts of EMG activity as he was trying to prevent incontinence and he contracted his striated sphincter (arrows). At first he was able to prevent incontinence, but once the sphincter fatigued he voided involuntarily with a low flow. Q_{max} = 1 ml/s, Pdet@Q_{max} = 150 cmH_2O, $Pdet_{max}$ = 187 cmH_2O, voided volume = 33 ml, and PVR = 88 ml. (B) X-ray obtained at Q_{max} shows scant visualization of the prostatic and bulbar urethra (arrows), indicative of prostatic urethral obstruction, and two bladder diverticula (Tic). (C) Schafer 6 obstruction. Detrusor pressure and maximum uroflow plotted on the Schafer nomogram.

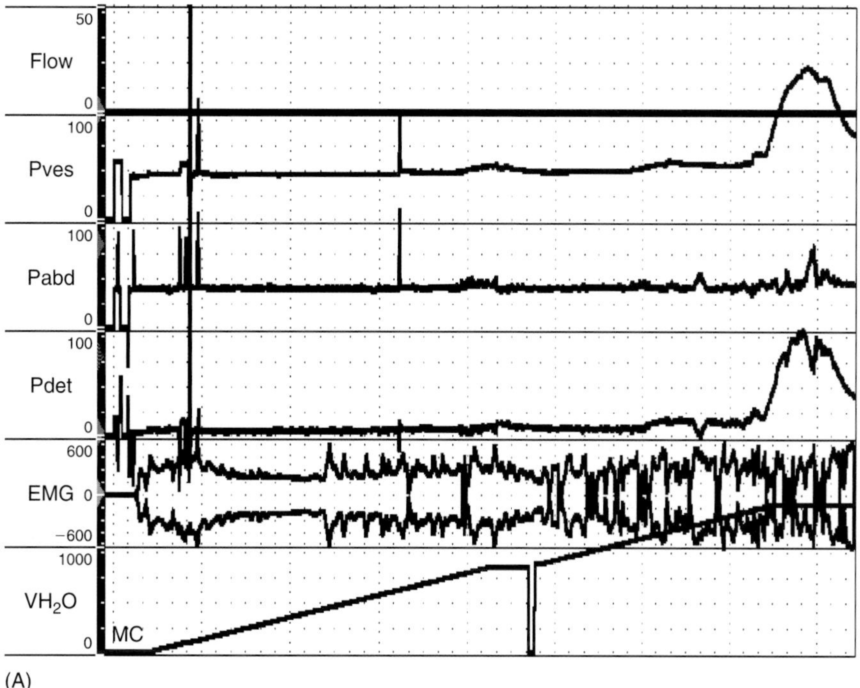

(A)

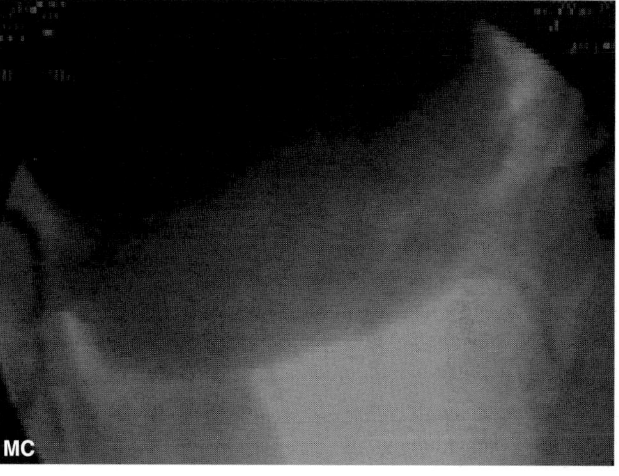

(B)

Fig. 10.12 Primary bladder neck obstruction. MC is a 31-year-old man who has been on intermittent catheterization BID for about 2 years after he was found to have renal failure (creatinine = 7 mg/dl) during an evaluation of the sudden onset of pedal edema. At first he was treated with an indwelling catheter, then intermittent catheterization 4–5 times daily. He had been found to have residual urines as high as several liters. He underwent serial urodynamics and cystoscopy and was told that "there is no blockage." (A) Urodynamic tracing. During bladder filling he was repeatedly asked to try to void once the infused volume reached about 750 ml (he had no urge to void). Finally, at a bladder volume of about 1400 ml, he had a voluntary detrusor contraction. Pdet = 100 cmH_2O, Q_{max} was too low to be detected by flowmeter. This corresponds to Schafer grade 6 obstruction. (B) X-ray obtained during voiding. Flow was too low to allow visualization of the urethra.

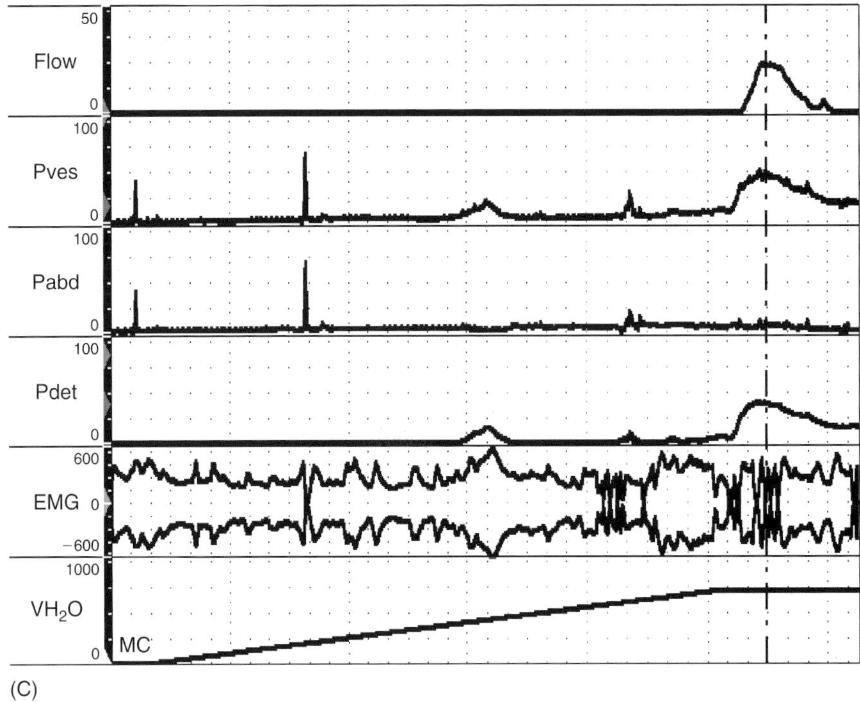

(C)

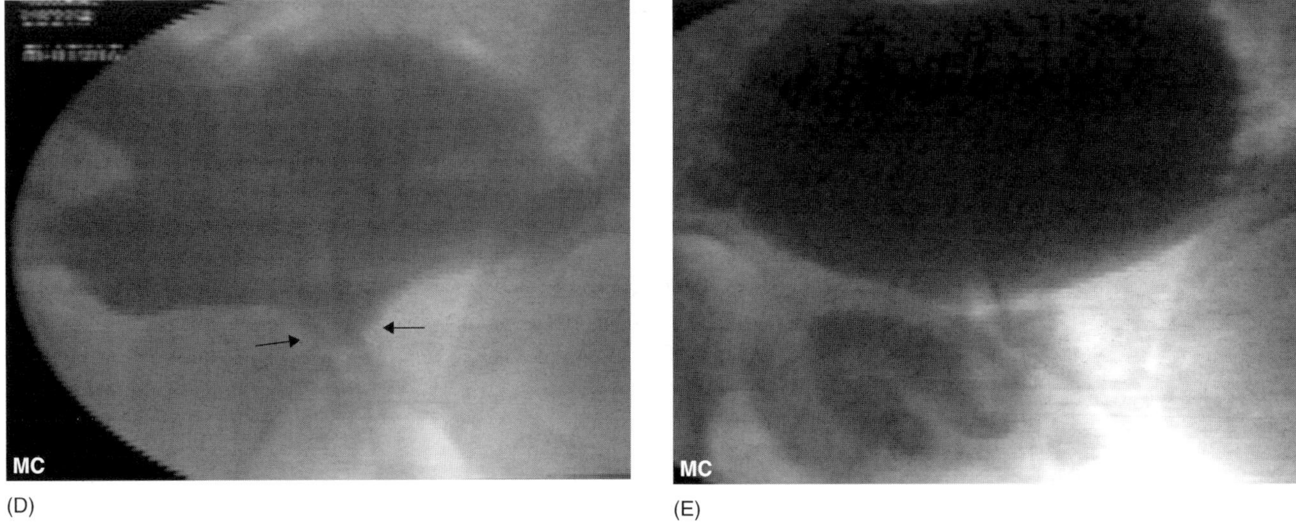

(D) (E)

Fig. 10.12 (continued) (C) Urodynamic tracing done 5 months after TURP. His creatinine had only come down to 2.0 mg/dl associated with continued bilateral hydronephrosis. Q_{max} = 24 ml/s, Pdet@Q_{max} = 39 cmH_2O, Pdetmax = 41 cmH_2O, voided volume = 566 ml, and PVR = 147 ml. (D) X-ray obtained during bladder filling shows a "TURP defect"(arrows) and an irregular bladder. (E) X-ray obtained during voiding visualizes the entire anterior urethra, but the prostatic urethra is not seen well despite the excellent uroflow.

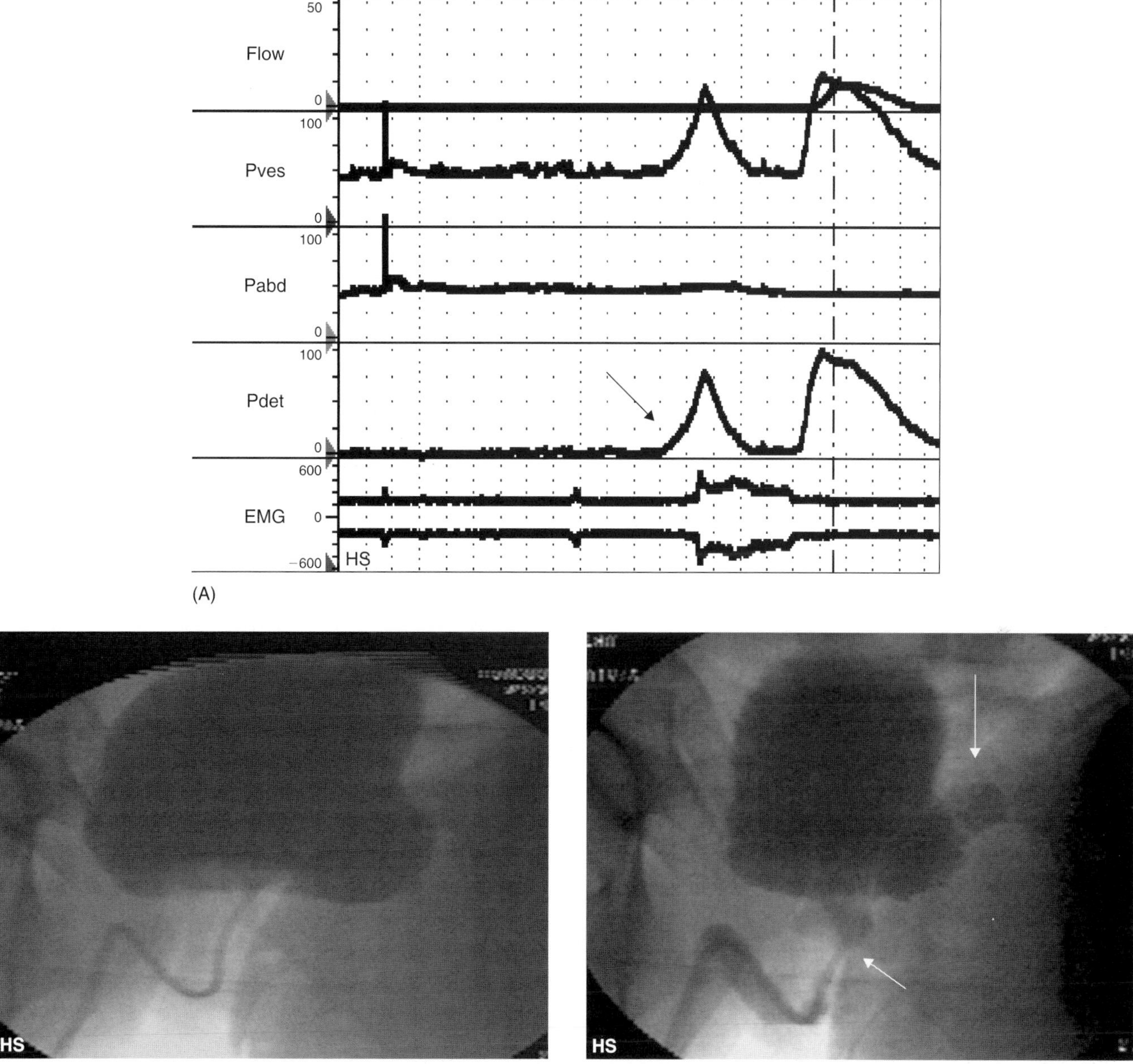

Fig. 10.13 Grade 4 distal prostatic urethral obstruction, type 2 OAB, small bladder diverticulum. HS is a 51-year-old man with a chief complaint of persistent urinary urgency and urge incontinence 4 years after bladder neck resection for primary bladder neck obstruction. (A) Urodynamic tracing. During bladder filling, there is an involuntary detrusor contraction that is perceived as an urge to void (arrow). He contracts his sphincter, prevents incontinence, and aborts the detrusor contraction (type 2 OAB). He then has a voluntary detrusor contraction, relaxes his sphincter, and voids voluntarily (vertical dotted line). Pedt@Q_{max} = 91 cmH_2O and Q_{max} = 11 ml/s. This corresponds to grade 4 obstruction on the Schafer nomogram. (B) X-ray obtained at bladder capacity discloses that, despite the history of prior bladder neck resection, there is no TURP defect. (C) X-ray obtained at Q_{max} (vertical line on the urodynamic tracing) demonstrates a narrowing at the distal prostatomembranous urethra (small arrow) as well as a small bladder diverticulum (large arrow).

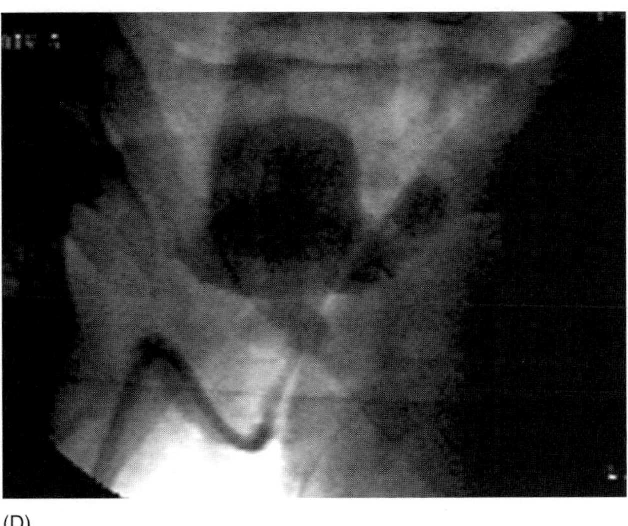

(D)

Fig. 10.13 (continued) (D) X-ray obtained just prior to the termination of voiding confirms good emptying despite the high grade obstruction.

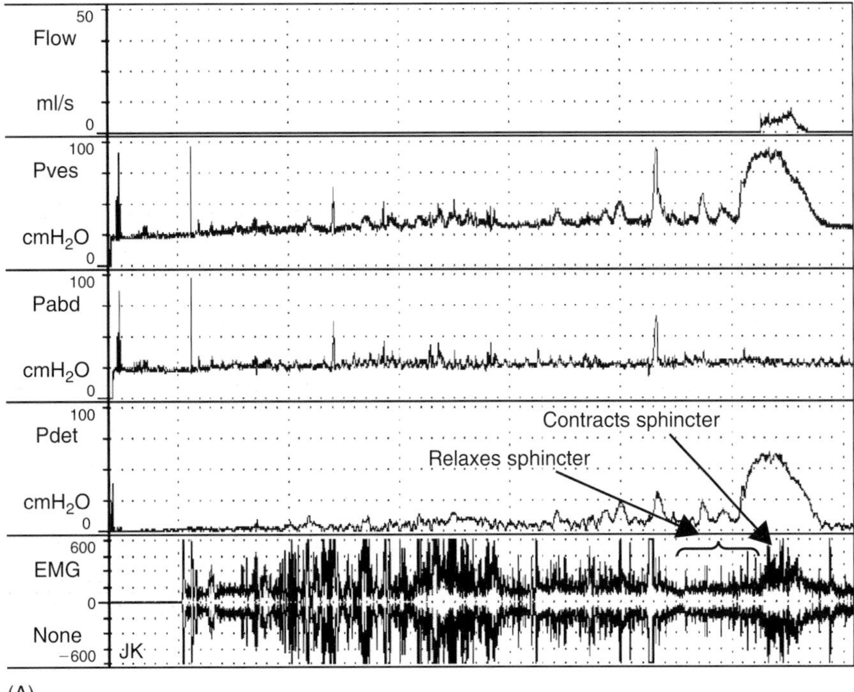

(A)

Fig. 10.14 AVD. The patient is a 31-year-old medical equipment salesman with a decade long history of "prostatitis" treated empirically by a number of urologists. His symptoms included urinary frequency, Q 1/2–1 hour urgency, nocturia 5 times, a slightly decreased stream, and chronic pelvic pain. American Urological Association (AUA) Sx score = 33. On examination, the prostate was small, smooth, non-tender, and had benign feeling. (A) Urodynamic tracing. Throughout filling he attempts to void and has multiple low magnitude detrusor contractions. However, during each such contraction, he contracts his external sphincter, preventing micturition. Finally, at the arrow, with his sphincter relaxed, he has a voluntary detrusor contraction but almost immediately contracts his sphincter and voids with an obstructed detrusor pressure/uroflow curve. Pdet@Q_{max} = 46 cmH_2O and Q_{max} = 6 ml/s (Schafer grade 3 obstruction).

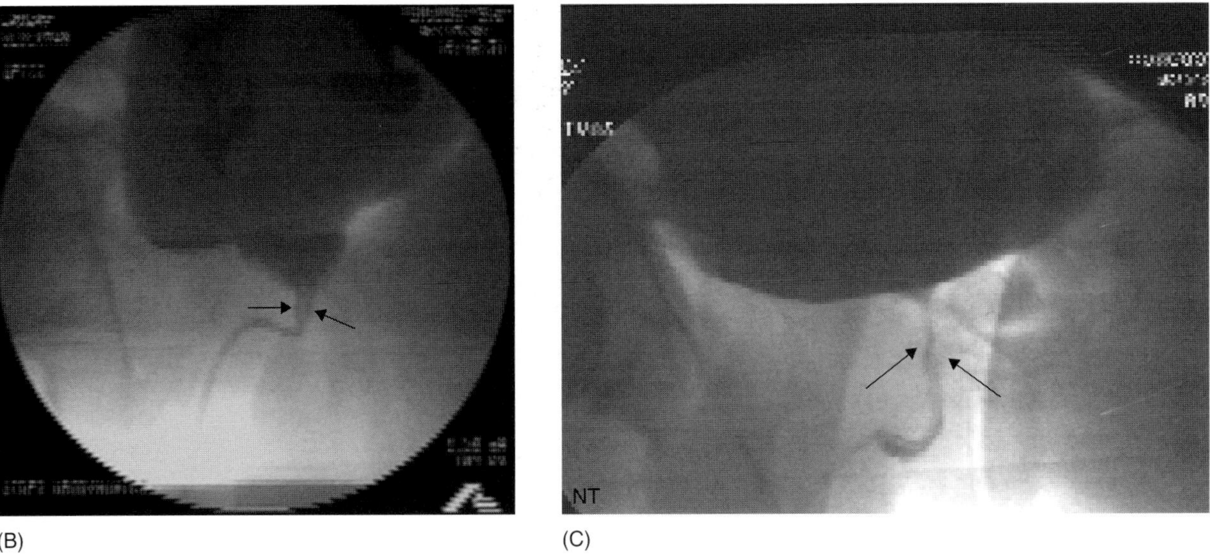

Fig. 10.14 (continued) (B) X-ray obtained during voiding shows a dilated prostatic urethra and narrowed membranous urethra arrows due to subconscious contraction of the external sphincter. (C) X-ray obtained during the first part of micturition shows a mid-prostatic urethral narrowing (arrows).

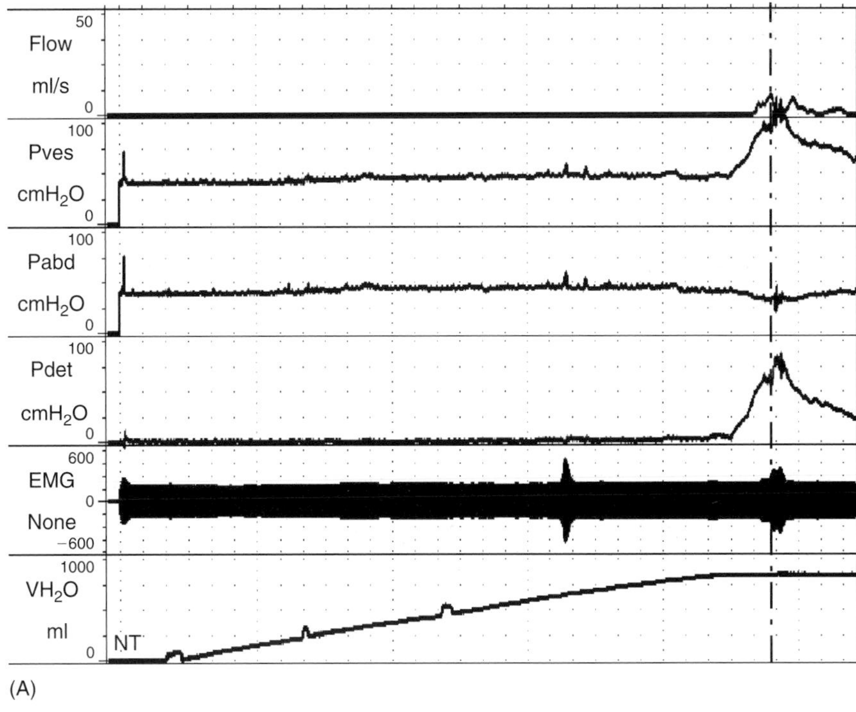

Fig. 10.15 NT is a 34-year-old man with recurrent urinary tract infections for the past year characterized by dysuria, difficulty in voiding, perineal discomfort, and strong urinary odor but without fever or chills. Bladder sonography revealed a large PVR (post-void residual). Cystoscopy demonstrated an elevated vertical neck, small bladder diverticulum at the dome, no trabeculations. He was treated with three types of alpha adrenergic antagonists without effect (except for retrograde ejaculation) and then treated with intermittent self-catheterization. (A) Urodynamic tracing. He did not feel an urge to void until a bladder volume of about 800 ml and then had a sustained voluntary detrusor contraction. Q_{max} = 10 ml/s and Pdet@Q_{max} = 59 cmH_2O (vertical dotted line). This corresponds to Schafer grade 3 obstruction. Pdetmax = 87 cmH_2O and voided volume = 152 ml. In the midst of voiding, he (involuntarily) contracts his sphincter (increased EMG activity, vertical dotted line). Detrusor pressure rises to 87 cmH_2O and uroflow falls to nearly 0. This demonstrates nicely the inverse relationship between detrusor pressure and uroflow and is an example of an AVD superimposed upon underlying prostatic obstruction. PVR = 691 ml.

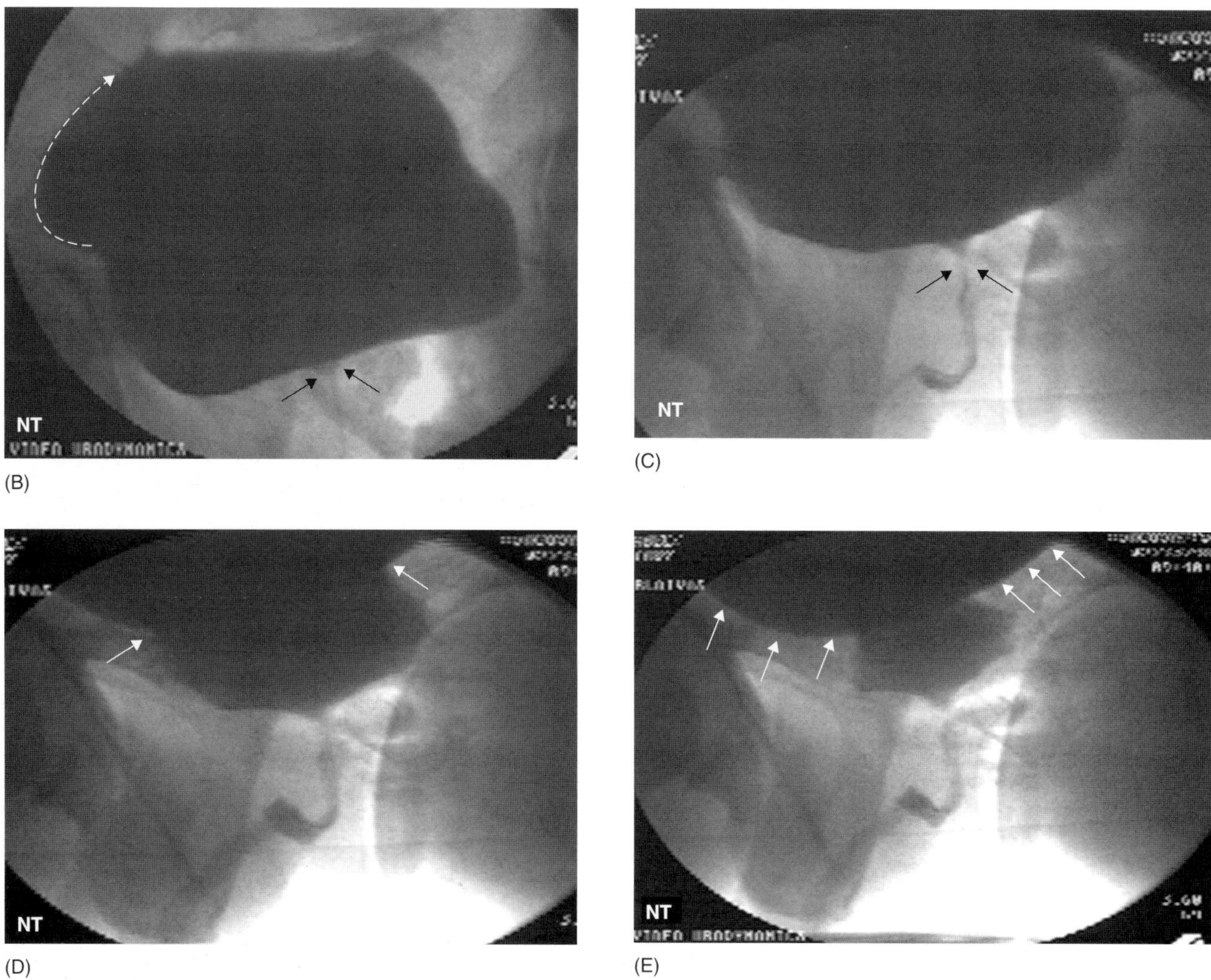

Fig. 10.15 (continued) (B) X-ray obtained during bladder filling shows an open vesical neck at rest (arrows) and a bulge at the upper right side of the bladder (dotted line) that, on later films, proved to be a large bladder diverticulum. (C) X-ray obtained during the first part of micturition shows a mid-prostatic urethral narrowing (arrows). (D) X-ray obtained at Q_{max} shows that the mid-prostatic urethra is still the narrowest part of the urethra and as he voids, the bladder diverticulum becomes larger (arrows). (E) And larger!

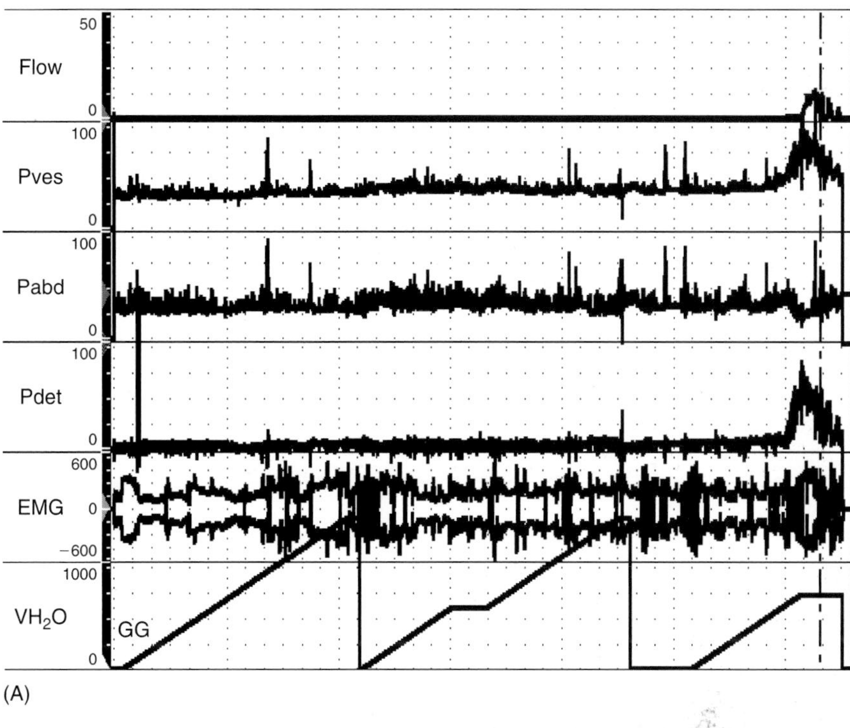

(A)

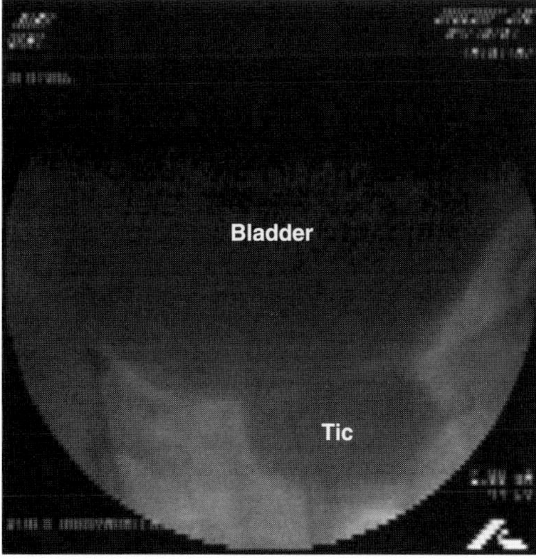

(B)

Fig. 10.16 (A) Multiple large bladder diverticula and Schafer grade 2 voiding (mild obstruction). Pdet@Q_{max} = 50 cmH_2O and Q_{max} = 12 ml/s. (B) This X-ray, obtained during voiding, at first glance appears to show a dilated prostatic urethra. In fact, the urethra is obscured by a large bladder diverticulum (discovered at surgery) that extended behind and below the prostate.

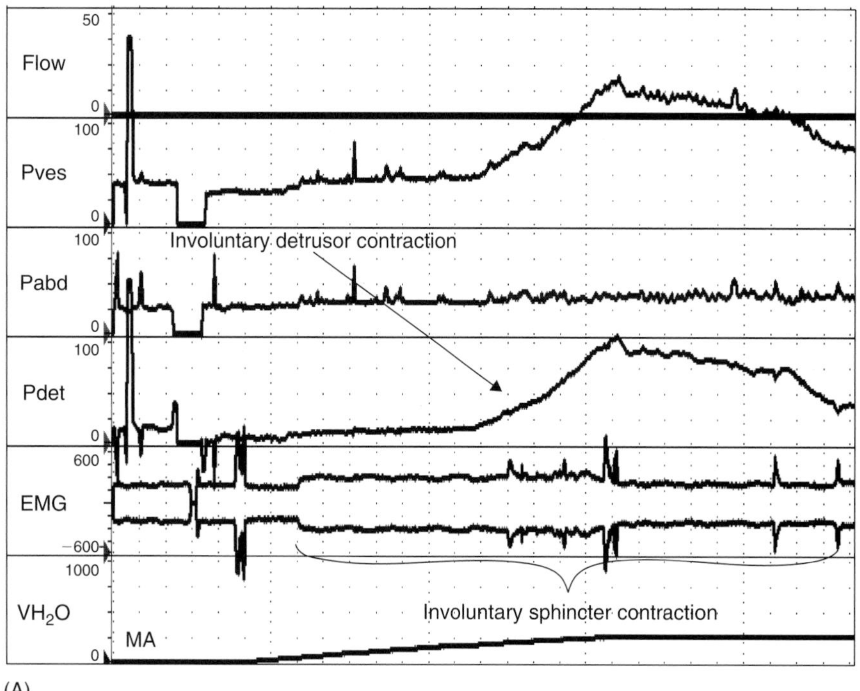

(A)

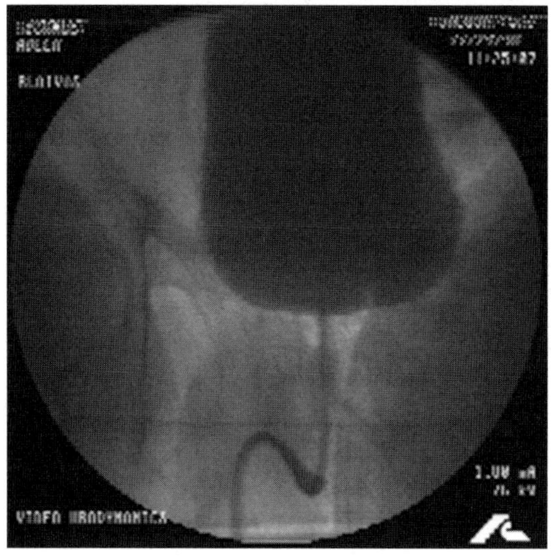

(B)

Fig. 10.17 DESD and prostatic urethral obstruction in a 52-year-old man with spastic paraparesis owing to radiation myelitis (lymphoma). (A) Urodynamic study. FSF (first sensation of filling) = 200 ml, 1st urge = 205 ml, severe urge = 217 ml, an involuntary detrusor contraction occurred at a bladder volume of 264 ml. Q_{max} = 0.7 ml/s, Pdet@Q_{max} = 92 cmH_2O, Pdetmax = 108 cmH_2O, voided volume = 16 ml, and PVR = 224 ml. (B) X-ray obtained at Pdetmax demonstrates some contrast in the bulbar urethra, but none at all in the prostatomembranous urethra. It is impossible from this study to determine to what degree the patient's symptoms are due to prostatic obstruction versus DESD.

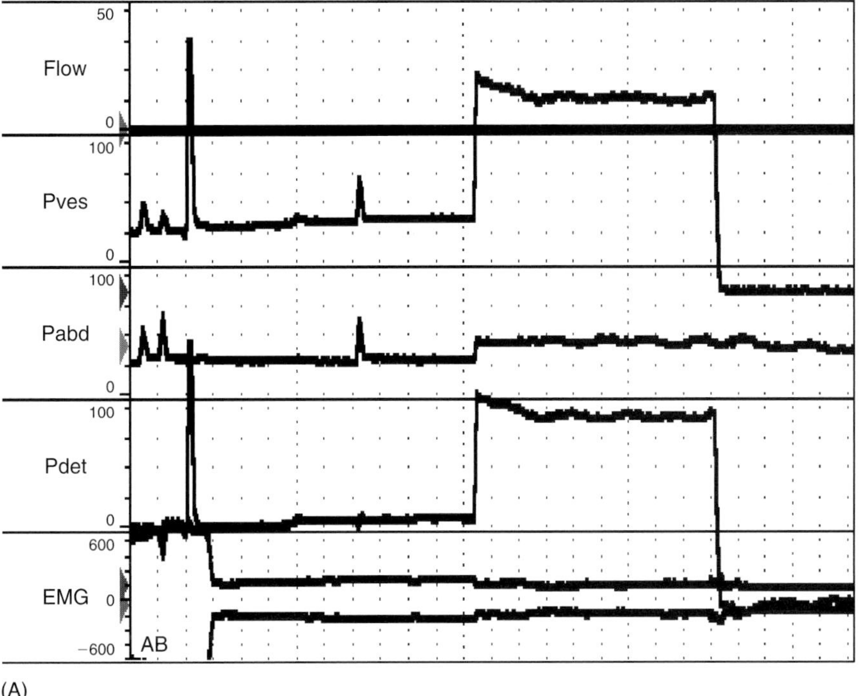

(A)

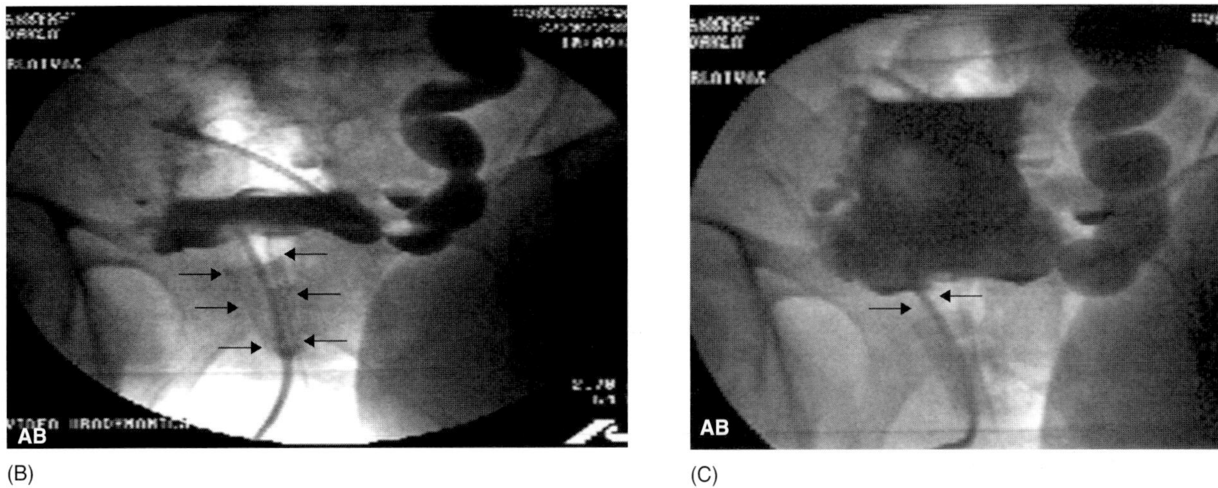

(B) (C)

Fig. 10.18 Grade 5 prostatic obstruction (Schafer grade 6) and type 4 OAB in an 81-year-old man with Parkinson's disease. He developed urinary retention and a prostatic stent was placed, which failed to resolve his urinary retention. Cystoscopy revealed the proximal prostatic urethra and vesical neck to be 'filled' with what appeared to be prolapsing prostatic lobes. (A) Urodynamic tracing. During bladder filling there was an involuntary detrusor contraction at a volume of 70 ml to a detrusor pressure of 123 cmH_2O. He perceived the contraction as pain, but was unable to contract his sphincter or abort the detrusor contraction. Q_{max} = 0.5 ml/s, Pdet@Q_{max} = 108 cmH_2O, Pdetmax = 123 cmH_2O, voided volume = 10 ml, and PVR = 60 ml. (B) X-ray exposed during early bladder filling shows the faint outline of a prostatic urethral stent (arrows) and obvious vesicoureteral reflux into a markedly dilated left ureter. (C) Radiograph exposed at Q_{max} shows no contrast in the urethra. Note that the proximal margin of the stent (arrows) is about 1 cm distal to the bladder neck. At cystoscopy the tissue proximal to the stent appeared to be protruding prostatic lobes causing obstruction. *Comment*: Renal ultrasound showed a normal right kidney, a normal left upper renal pole, and left lower pole hydronephrosis. This almost assuredly is due to a congenital duplication of the left collecting system, despite the fact that a duplication was not seen at cystoscopy. One would expect that with such severe vesicoureteral reflux and a high pressure bladder that he would be at high risk for urosepsis, but, in fact, has never even had a clinical urinary tract infection. He underwent TUR of the obstructing proximal prostatic tissue. Two years thereafter, he was voiding with neither difficulty, incontinence nor urinary infection!

Bladder Outlet Obstruction and Impaired Detrusor Contractility in Women

11

Introduction

Bladder outlet obstruction in women, once thought to be extremely rare, has a reported incidence of 6–23% in patients with persistent lower urinary tract symptoms [1–3]. The etiology of urethral obstruction is depicted in Table 11.1. The incidence of impaired contractility has not been well studied, but in our experience, it is at least as common as urethral obstruction.

Table 11.1 Etiology of urethral obstruction*.

• Prior surgery	14–30%
• Prolapse	28–29%
• Stricture	15%
• Primary bladder neck obstruction	10–16%
• DESD	6%
• Acquired voiding dysfunction	6–33%
• Urethral diverticulum	4%

*From Refs. [1,2]

Diagnosis

The symptoms of bladder outlet obstruction in women are non-specific including storage symptoms (urinary frequency, urgency, and urge incontinence) and voiding symptoms (difficulty starting micturition, hesitancy, weak stream, dysuria, and post-void dribbling). Although it is widely agreed that detrusor pressure uroflow studies are necessary to make the diagnosis of urethral obstruction and to distinguish it from impaired detrusor contractility, there is no consensus on specific urodynamic criteria. In a generic sense, urethral obstruction is characterized by a detrusor contraction of adequate magnitude and duration and a low uroflow. Impaired detrusor contractility is characterized by a weak detrusor contraction and a low uroflow. Empirically, urethral obstruction has been defined as Pdet@$Q_{max} > 20\,cmH_2O$ and $Q_{max} < 12\,ml/s$ and impaired detrusor contractility as Pdet@$Q_{max} < 20\,cmH_2O$ and $Q_{max} < 12\,ml/s$. (Note that the cutoff for Pdet@Q_{max} in men is $40\,cmH_2O$. Nitti et al. [1] proposed that urethral obstruction be defined as "radiographic evidence of obstruction between the bladder neck and the distal urethra in the presence of a sustained detrusor contraction." According to this definition, there is no specific urodynamic criteria, but they observed that obstructed women had lower Q_{max}, higher Pdet@Q_{max}, and higher post-void residual (PVR) (Fig. 11.1).

Chassagne et al. [4] and subsequently Lemack and Zimmern [5] , utilizing various combinations of Pdet@Q_{max}/Q_{max} and using ROC curves, concluded that the best fit of sensitivity (91.5% and 73.6%, respectively), was attained with a cutoff value of Pdet@$Q_{max} = 21\,cmH_2O$ and $Q_{max} = 11\,cmH_2O$.

Blaivas and Groutz [2] devised a bladder outlet obstruction nomogram for women based on cutoff values of Pdet@Q_{max} > 20 cmH_2O and a free (unintubated) Q_{max} < 12 ml/s (Fig. 11.2).

Urethral obstruction may be anatomic or functional (Table 11.2). The two most common known causes of urethral obstruction are genital prolapse (Figs. 11.6 and 11.7) and complications after antiincontinence operations (Figs. 11.8–11.11). Much less commonly, urethral obstruction may be due to urethral diverticulum (Fig. 11.12), urethral stricture (Figs. 11.13–11.15), genital atrophy (Fig. 11.16), or tumor. Functional obstructions include primary vesical neck obstruction (Fig. 11.17), detrusor sphincter dyssynergia due to spinal neurologic lesions (Fig. 11.18), and acquired or learned voiding dysfunction also called dysfunctional voiding (Fig. 11.19). In this latter condition, the patient is unable to fully relax the urethral sphincter during micturition.

Table 11.2 Classification of urethral obstruction.

Anatomic urethral obstruction
Compression
Post-surgical
Prolapse
Urethral diverticulum
Tumor
Urethral stricture
Post-surgical
Traumatic
Atrophy
Functional urethral obstruction
Primary vesical neck
Neurogenic (DESD)
Acquired behavior

The symptoms of impaired detrusor contractility are non-specific and comprise the same spectrum as those associated with urethral obstruction. From a urodynamic standpoint, the hallmark of the diagnosis is a low flow and low detrusor pressure as discussed above (Figs. 11.20 and 11.21). In most instances, the cause of impaired detrusor contractility is not apparent. It is postulated that it is caused by an overdistension injury or longstanding urethral obstruction. Pharmacologic agents, including anticholinergics and tricyclic antidepressants are reversible causes of impaired detrusor contractility. Psychologic causes have been postulated, but not well documented. Neurogenic causes are well known and include lower motor neuron lesions from spinal cord injury, myelodysplasia, multiple sclerosis, spinal stenosis, and herniated disks. In addition, radical pelvic surgery (radical hysterectomy and abdominal perineal resection of the rectum), not infrequently results in damage to the sacral reflex arcs [6,7].

Suggested Reading

1 Nitti VW, Tu LM, Gitlin J. Diagnosing bladder outlet obstruction in women, *J Urol*, 161: 1535, 1999.

2 Blaivas JG, Groutz A. Bladder outlet obstruction nomogram for women with lower urinary tract symptomatology, *Neurourol Urodynam*, 19: 553–554, 2000.

3 Groutz A, Blaivas JG, Chaikin DC. Bladder outlet obstruction in women: definition and characteristics, *Neurourol Urodynam*, 19(3): 213–220, 2000.

4 Chassagne S, Bernier PA, Haab F, Roehrborn CG, Reisch JS, Zimmern PE. Proposed cutoff values to define bladder outlet obstruction in women, *Urology*, 51: 408–411, 1998.

5 Lemack GE, Zimern PE. Pressure flow analysis may aid in identifying women with outflow obstruction, *J Urol*, 163, 1823–1828, 2000.

6 Alsever JD. Lumbosacral plexopathy after gynecologic surgery: case report and review of the literature, *Am J Obstet Gynecol*, 174(6): 1769–1777; discussion 1777–1778, 1996.

7 Sekido N, Kawai K, Akaza H. Lower urinary tract dysfunction as persistent complication of radical hysterectomy, *Int J Urol*, 4(3): 259–264, 1997.

8 Axelrod SL, Blaivas JG. Bladder neck obstruction in women, *J Urol*, 137: 497, 1987.

9 Blaivas JG, Sinha HP, Zayed AAH, Labib KB. Detrusor-external sphincter dyssynergia, *J Urol*, 125: 542–544, 1981.

10 Blaivas JG. The neurophsyiology of micturition: a clinical study of 550 patients, *J Urol*, 127: 958–963, 1982.

11 Blaivas JG, Sinha HP, Zayed AAH, Labib KB. Detrusor-external sphincter dyssynergia: a detailed electromyographic study, *J Urol*, 125: 545–548, 1981.

12 Blaivas JG, Barbalias GA. Characteristics of neural injury after abdominal perineal resection, *J Urol*, 129: 84, 1983.

13 Carr LK, Webster G. Bladder outlet obstruction in women, *Urol Clin N Am*, 23(3): 385–391, 1996.

14 Cherrie RJ, Leach GE, Raz S. Obstructing urethral valve in a woman: a case report, *J Urol*, 129: 1051, 1983.
15 Cormier L, Ferchaud J, Galas JM, Guillemin F, Mangin P. Diagnosis of female bladder outlet obstruction and relevance of the parameter area under the curve of detrusor pressure during voiding: preliminary results, *J Urol*, 167(5): 2083–2087, 2002.
16 Defreitas GA, Zimmern PE, Lemack GE, Shariat SF. Refining diagnosis of anatomic female bladder outlet obstruction: comparison of pressure-flow study parameters in clinically obstructed women with those of normal controls, *Urology*, 64(4): 675–679; discussion 679–681, 2004.
17 Diokno AC, Hollander JB, Bennett CJ. Bladder neck obstruction in women: a real entity, *J Urol*, 132: 294, 1984.
18 Griffiths D. Detrusor contractility – order out of chaos, *Scand J Urol Nephrol*, Suppl(215): 93–100, 2004.
19 Kuo HC. Urodynamic parameters for the diagnosis of bladder outlet obstruction in women, *Urol Int*, 72(1): 46–51, 2004.
20 Massolt ET, Groen J, Vierhout ME. Application of the Blaivas–Groutz bladder outlet obstruction nomogram in women with urinary incontinence, *Neurourol Urodynam*, 24(3): 237–242, 2005.
21 Massey JA, Abrams PH. Obstructed voiding in the female, *Br J Urol*, 61: 36, 1988.
22 McGuire EJ, Letson W, Wang S. Transvaginal urethrolysis after obstructive urethral suspension procedures, *J Urol*, 142: 1037, 1989.
23 Nitti VW, Raz S. Obstruction following anti-incontinence procedures: diagnosis and treatment with transvaginal urethrolysis, *J Urol*, 152: 93, 1994.
24 Patel R, Nitti V. Bladder outlet obstruction in women: prevalence, recognition, and management, *Curr Urol Rep*, 2(5): 379–387, 2001 (review).
25 Tan TL, Bergmann MA, Griffiths D, Resnick NM. Stop test or pressure-flow study? Measuring detrusor contractility in older females, *Neurourol Urodynam*, 23(3): 184–189, 2004.
26 Tan TL, Bergmann MA, Griffiths D, Resnick NM. Which stop test is best? Measuring detrusor contractility in older females, *J Urol*, 169(3): 1023–1027, 2003.
27 Webster GD, Kreder KJ. Voiding dysfunction following cystourethropexy: its evaluation and management, *J Urol*, 144: 670, 1990.

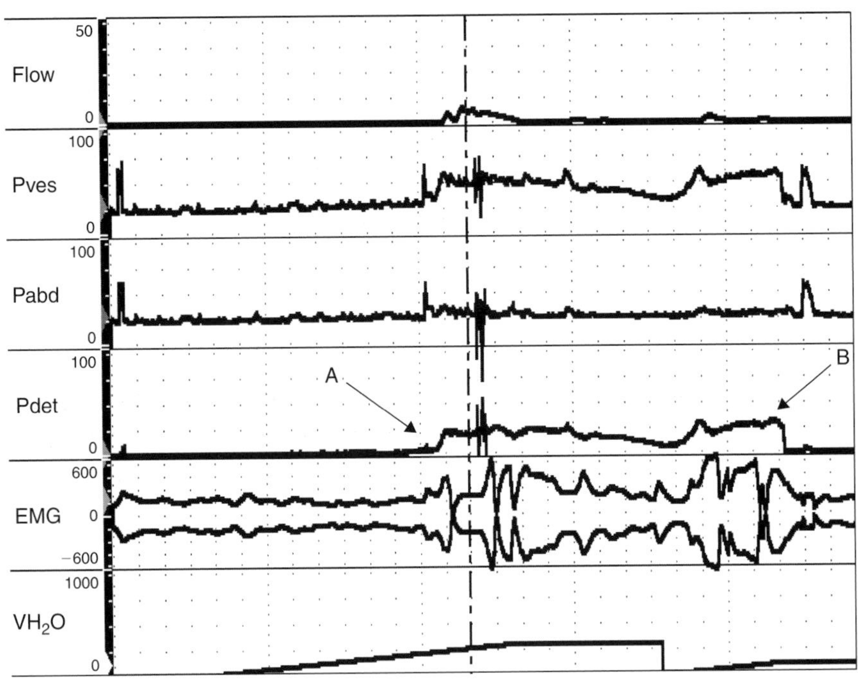

Fig. 11.1 Urethral obstruction according to Dr. Nitti.
(A) Urodynamic study. There is a sustained detrusor contraction (between the arrows A and B) and low flow. Q_{max} = 7.7 ml/s, Pdet@ Q_{max} = 19.5 cmH_2O (vertical dotted line), and Pdetmax = 32 cmH_2O. Despite the apparent sporadic increases in EMG activity, there were no obvious urethral contractions seen at fluoroscopy.

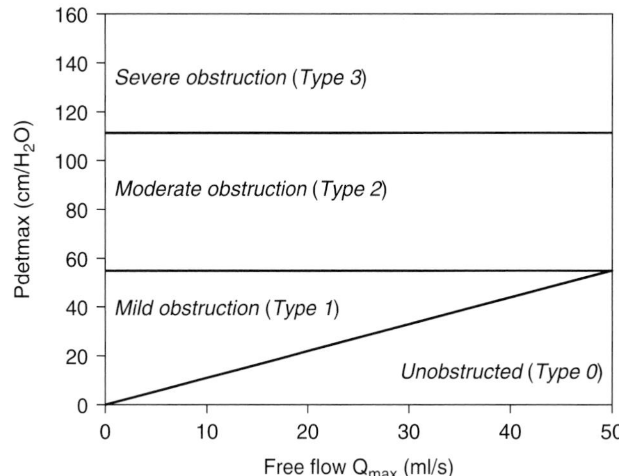

Fig. 11.2 The Blaivas–Groutz nomogram divides women into four groups.

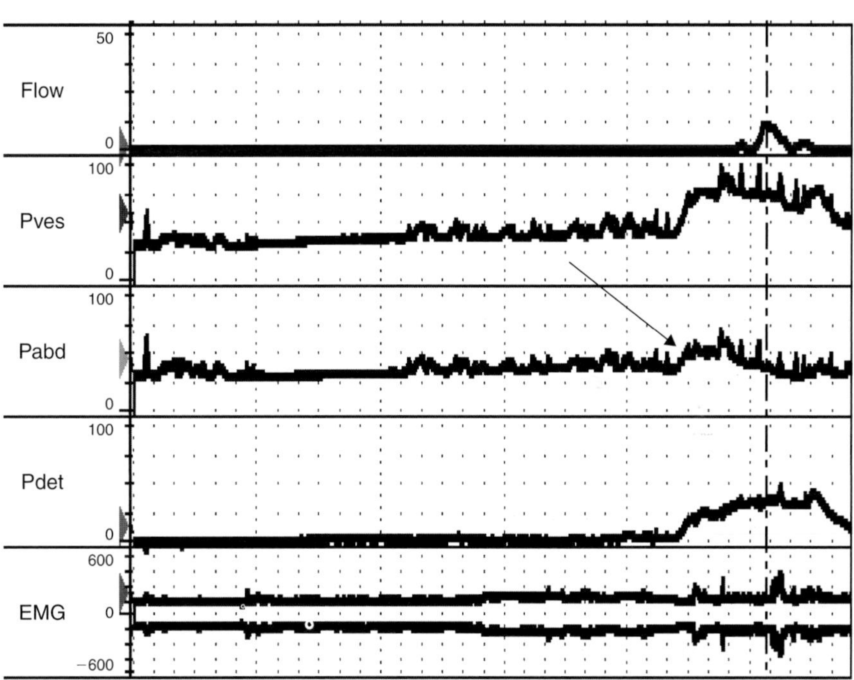

Fig. 11.3 Grade 1 urethral obstruction due to pelvic organ prolapse. The patient is a 70-year-old diabetic woman with procidentia. She complains of severe stress and urge incontinence.

Urodynamic tracing. She initiates micturition by abdominal straining (arrow), but then stops straining and flow increases. Pdet@Q_{max} = 38 cmH_2O and Q_{max} = 12 ml/s (vertical dotted line). This corresponds to grade 1 urethral obstruction.

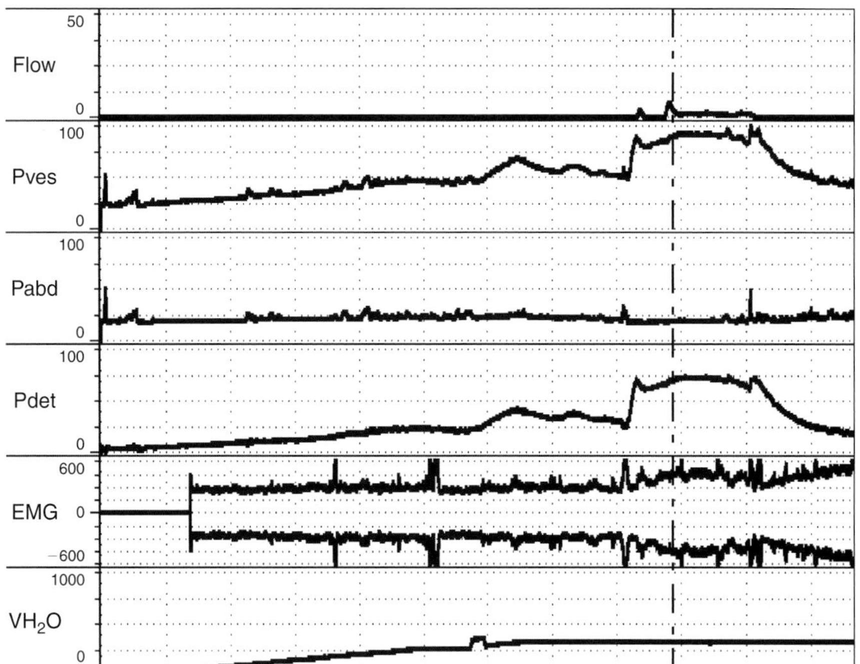

Fig. 11.4 Grade 2 urethral obstruction due to urethral stricture in a 36-year-old woman after pelvic fracture.

Urodynamic tracing. There is a sustained detrusor contraction. Pdet@Q_{max} = 80 cmH_2O and Q_{max} = 5 ml/s (vertical dotted line). This corresponds to grade 2 urethral obstruction on the Blaivas–Groutz nomogram.

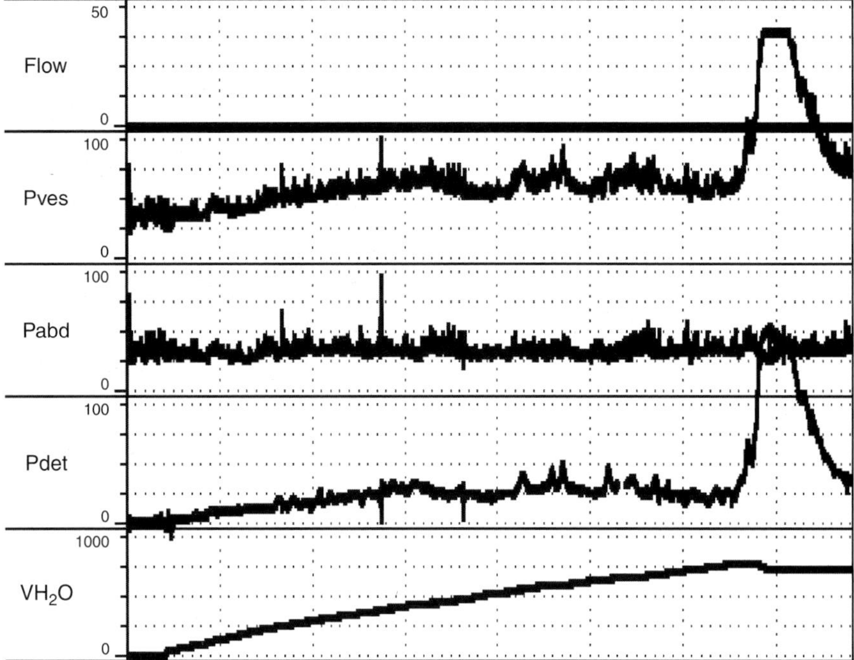

Fig. 11.5 Grade 3 urethral obstruction (primary bladder neck obstruction) in a 52-year-old woman who was asymptomatic, but found to have a distended abdomen due to PVR urine over 1 l.

Urodynamic tracing. There is a sustained voluntary detrusor contraction to 155 cmH_2O and a flow so low that it did not activate the flowmeter. This corresponds to a grade 3 obstruction.

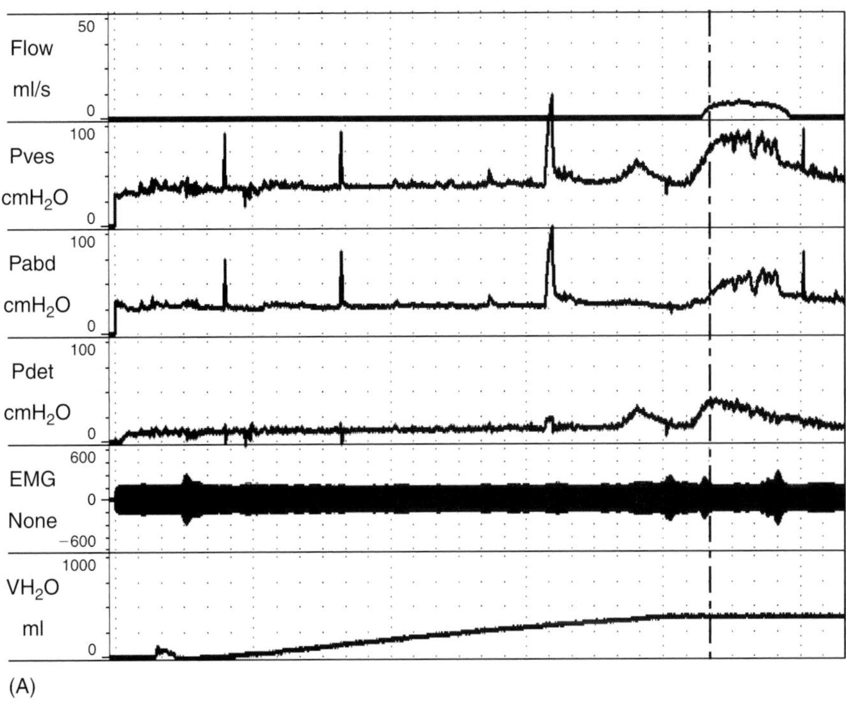

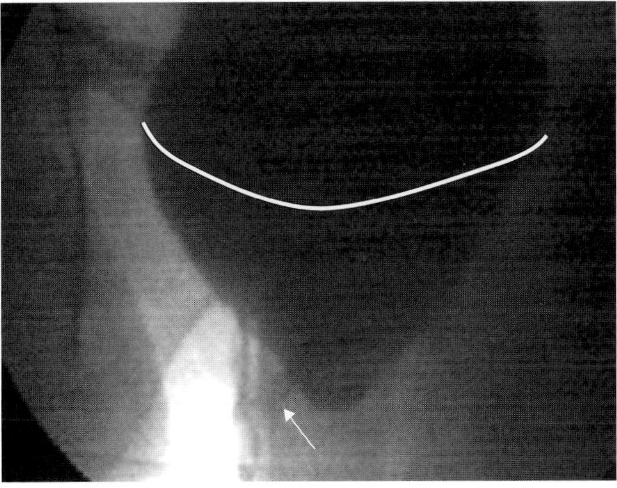

Fig. 11.6 Grade 1 urethral obstruction due to pelvic organ prolapse. The patient is a 68-year-old woman. During voiding there is grade 1 obstruction according to the Blaivas–Groutz nom ogram.

(A) Urodynamic tracing. Q_{max} = 8 ml/s, Pdet@Q_{max} = 36 cmH_2O (vertical dashed line), Pdetmax = 42 cmH_2O, voided volume = 376 ml, and PVR = 13 ml.

(B) X-ray obtained during voiding shows the urethra barely visible (arrow). The white line indicates the lower border of the symphysis pubis.

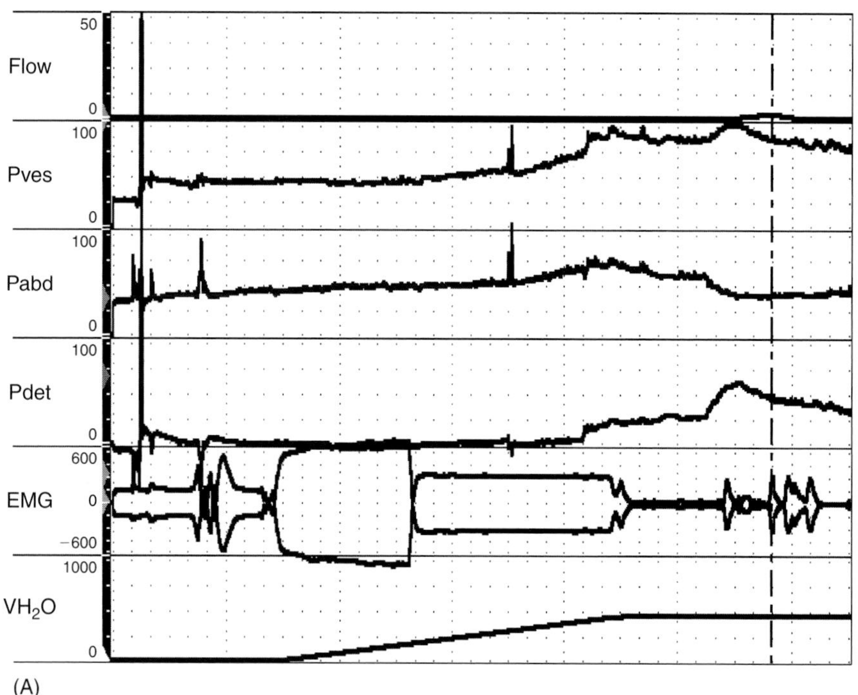

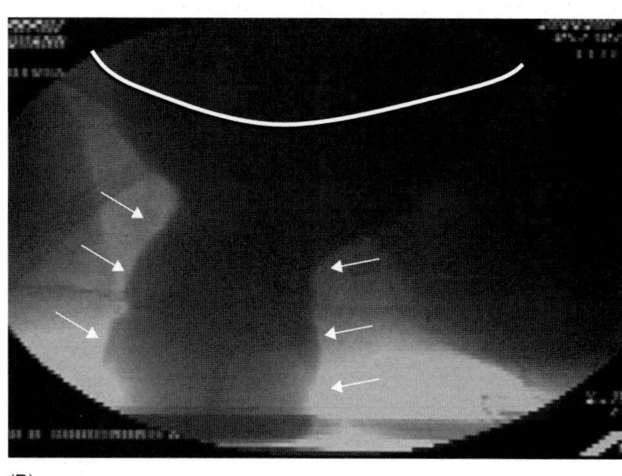

Fig. 11.7 Grade 2 urethral obstruction due to grade 4 cystocele in a 73-year-old woman with procidentia. (A) Urodynamic tracing. Q_{max} = 2.2 ml/s, Pdet@ Q_{max} = 54 cmH_2O (vertical dashed line), voided volume = 28 ml, and PVR = 402 ml.
(B) X-ray shows a grade 4 cystocele. The white line indicates the lower border of the symphysis pubis. The urethra is obscured by the cystocele (arrows).

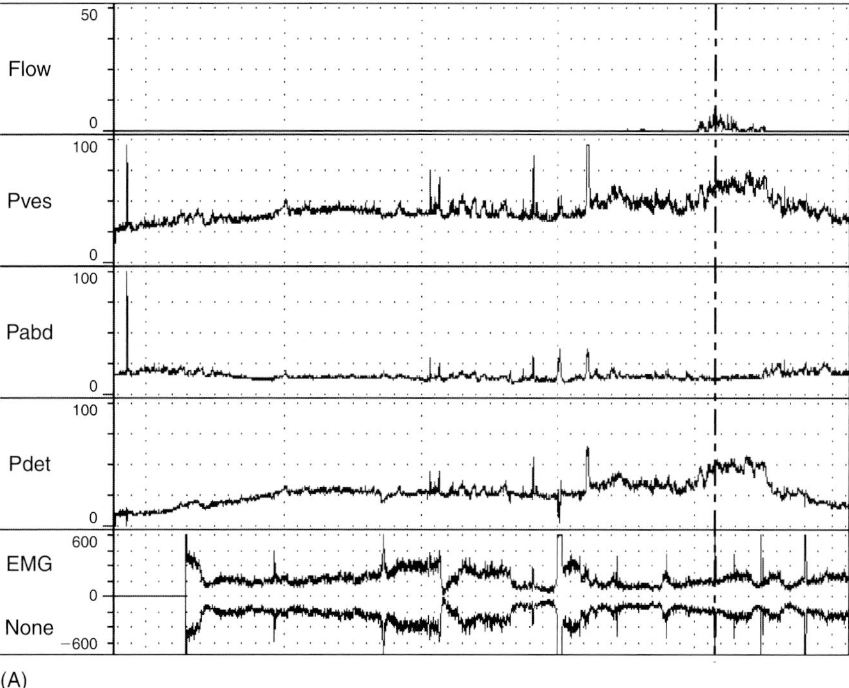

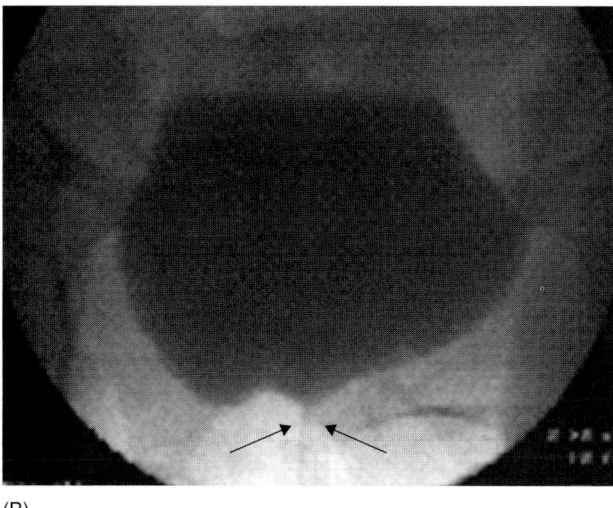

Fig. 11.8 Grade 1 urethral obstruction 5 years status post autologous fascial pubovaginal sling.
(A) Urodynamic tracing. Pdet@Q_{max} = 50 cmH_2O and Q_{max} = 6 ml/s (vertical dashed line). This corresponds to a grade 1 urethral obstruction on the Blaivas–Groutz nomogram.
(B) X-ray exposed at Q_{max} shows a narrow urethra just distal to the vesical neck (arrows).

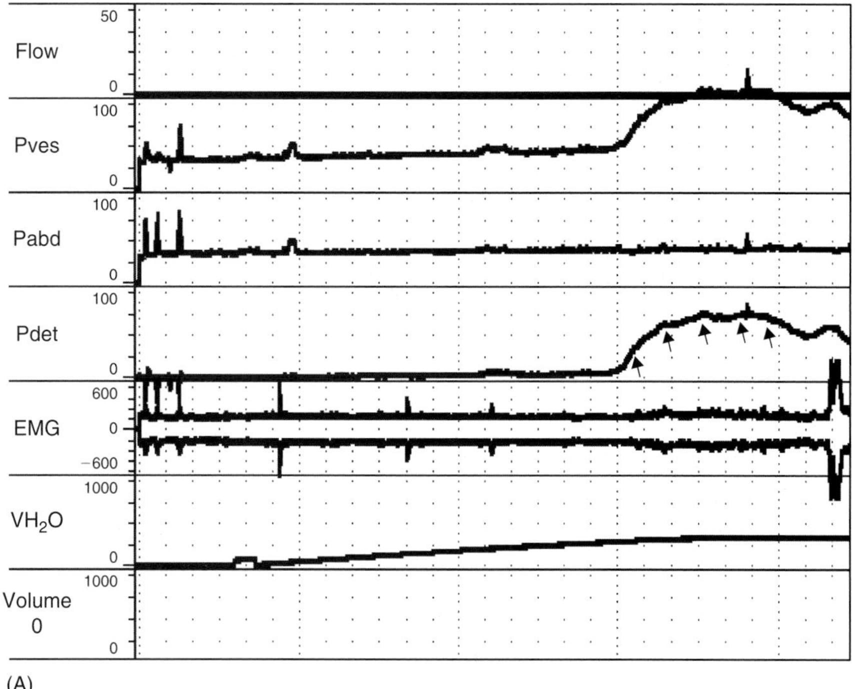

(A)

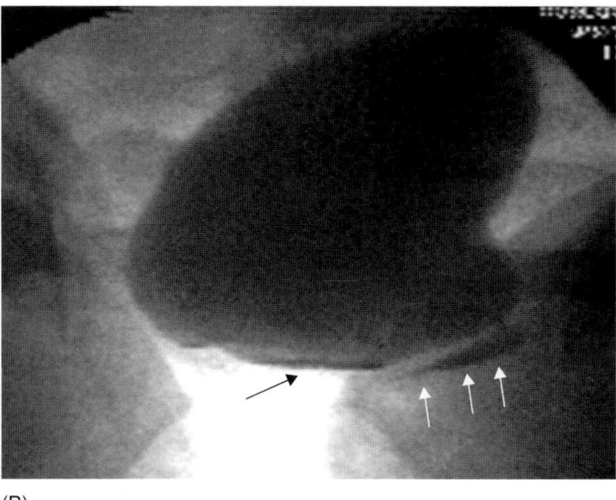

(B)

Fig. 11.9 Urethral obstruction due to autologous fascial pubovaginal sling. (A) Urodynamic tracing. There is a sustained detrusor contraction to over 75 cmH_2O (arrows) and no flow. This corresponds to a grade 2 urethral obstruction on the Blaivas–Groutz nomogram. (B) X-ray exposed at Pdetmax shows complete obstruction of the urethra at the bladder neck (black arrow), presumably from a prior sling operation. Note the left vesicoureteral reflux (white arrows).

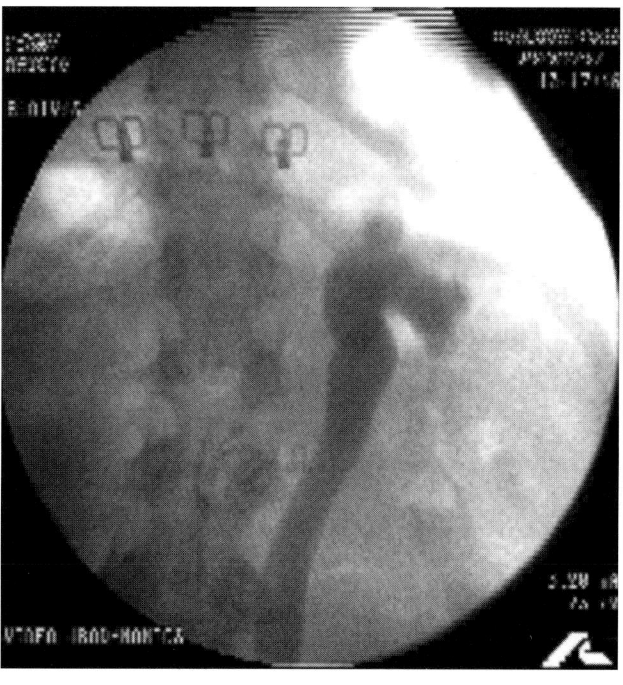

(C)

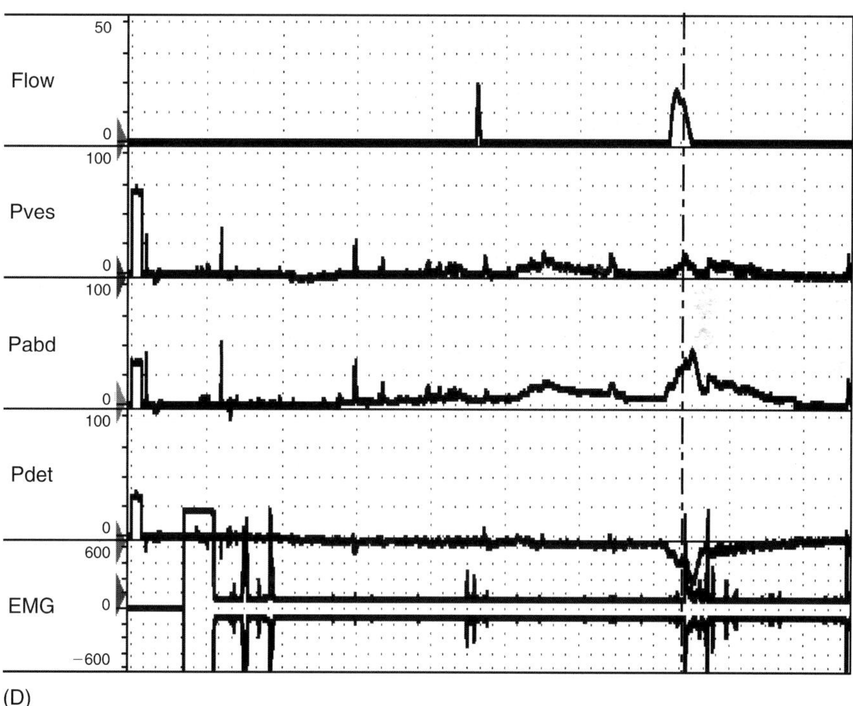

(D)

Fig. 11.9 (continued) (C) The vesicoureteral reflux extends into the left kidney and distends the collecting system (grade 3). (D) Urodynamic tracing for 2 years status post sling incision and left ureteroneocystostomy. She voids normally with a $Q_{max} = 24$ ml/s and a bell shaped curve (vertical line). On the flow tracing there is an artifact that cannot be readily explained, but may be due to unintentional movement of the flowmeter.

Detrusor pressure during uroflow had a negative value of 50 cmH_2O. This is not possible and reflects an artifact due to subtraction of Pabd from Pves. Part of the explanation is the pressure transducers were not properly calibrated. Note that when she coughed, Pabd rose to 52 cmH_2O, but pves only rose to 36 cm. So when during uroflow, pabd rose to almost 50 cm, pdet should fall below zero just because of the calibration error. The likeliest explanation is that she was straining during voiding, raising Pabd, and the vesical pressure was not recording well because of an air bubble or leak. However, the vesical tracing appears to be recording well before and after uroflow and the electronic subtraction everywhere else on the tracing was working pretty well. Further, on visual inspection of the patient during voiding, there was no visible straining. Another possible explanation is that she had a rectal contraction during voiding.

Nevertheless, since she voided with a Pves = 18 cmH_2O and a $Q_{max} = 24$ ml/s, we conclude that her obstruction has been relieved.

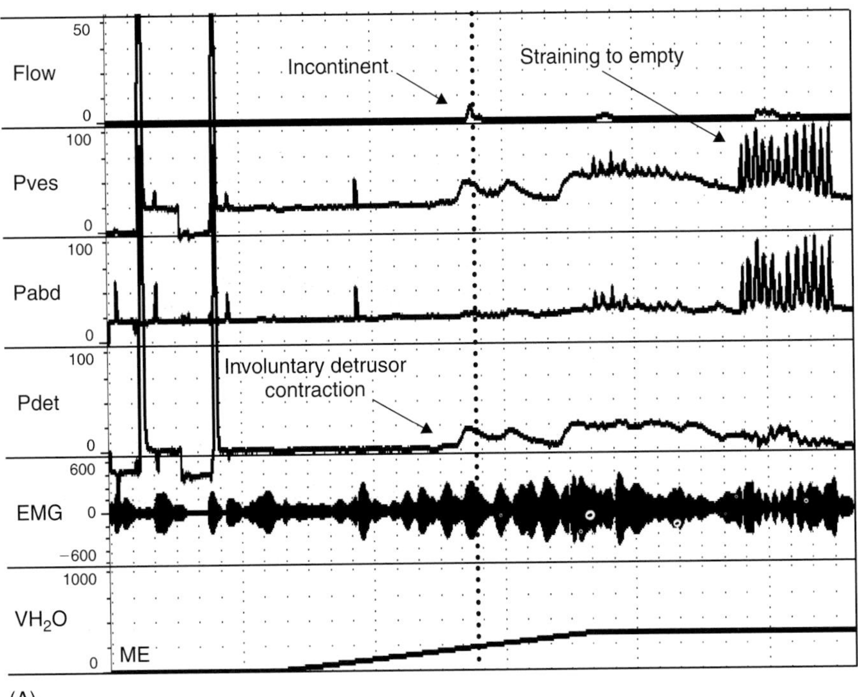

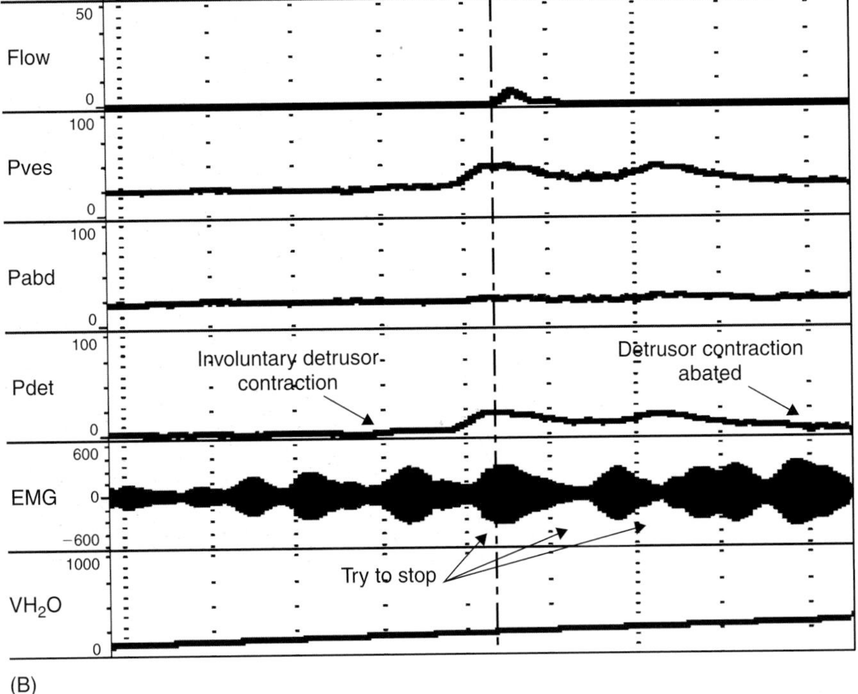

Fig. 11.10 Distal urethral obstruction (grade 1) and type 3 OAB in a 55-year-old woman who developed de novo urge incontinence after undergoing a synthetic sling (TVT). (A) Video-urodynamic study. 150 ml FSF (first sensation of bladder filling) = 176 ml, 1st urge = 190 ml, and severe urge = 210 ml. There was an involuntary detrusor contraction at a volume of 229 ml. She perceived the contraction as urge and was incontinent. She had another involuntary detrusor contraction shortly thereafter, was again incontinent, but still had a large amount in her bladder and then tried to empty by straining. Q_{max} = 7 ml (vertical dotted line), Pdet@Q_{max} = 22 cmH_2O, Pdetmax = 25 cmH_2O, voided volume = 68 ml, and PVR = 290 ml. Uroflow just prior to the urodynamic study: Q_{max} = 7 ml/s, voided volume = 49 ml, and PVR = 150 ml. (B) Magnified view of the first involuntary detrusor contraction. She perceived the contraction as urge and was incontinent. During the detrusor contraction, she was asked to try to stop voiding and she contracted her sphincter, aborted the stream, and the detrusor contraction abated.

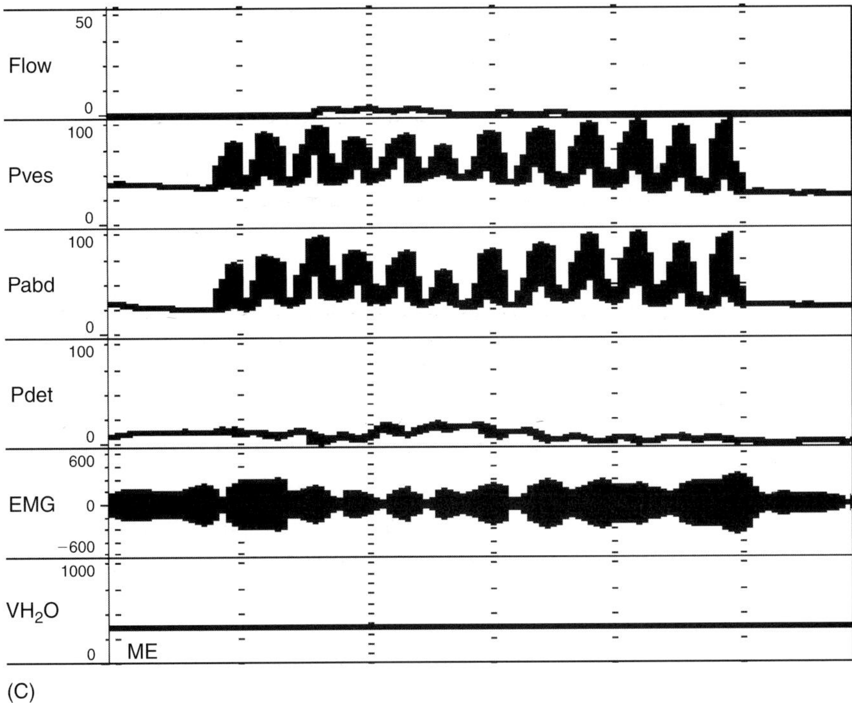

(C)

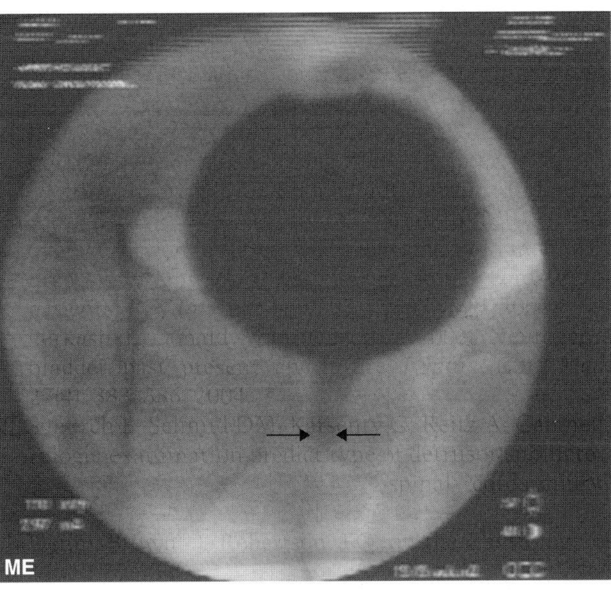

(D)

Fig. 11.10 (continued) (C) Magnified view of her attempt to voluntarily void shows that straining does not appreciably increase her flow. (D) X-ray obtained at Q_{max} (dashed vertical line on Fig. 11.10(A) and (B)) shows a narrowing in the distal urethra consistent with urethral obstruction (arrows). These findings are consistent with obstruction from the synthetic sling or an acquired voiding dysfunction. Comment: She underwent sling incision and her overactive bladder symptoms completely subsided, suggesting that it was mechanical obstruction by the sling that cause the symptoms. She did develop mild sphincteric incontinence, not an acquired voiding dysfunction.

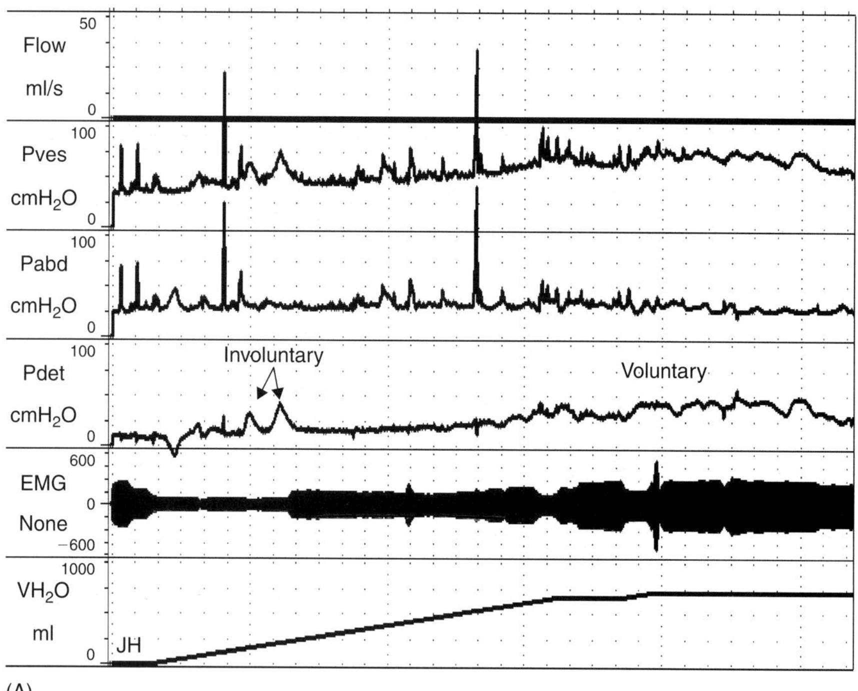

(A)

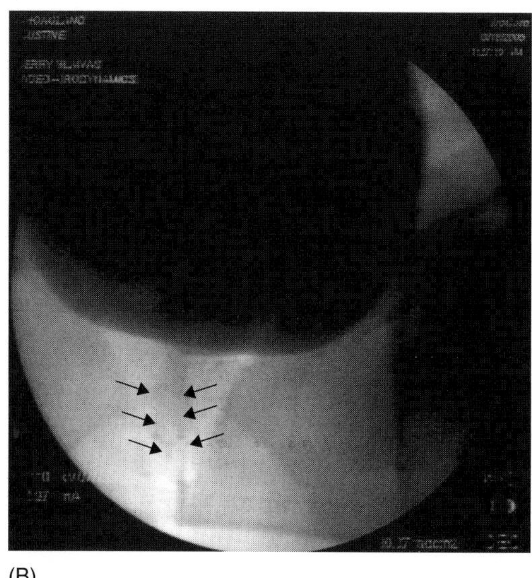

(B)

Fig. 11.11 Proximal urethral obstruction (grade 1) and detrusor overactivity in a 45-year-old woman after multiple synthetic sling surgeries. (A) Urodynamic tracing. During bladder filling there were involuntary detrusor contractions beginning at a volume of 166 ml. She had a voluntary detrusor contraction to 58 cmH_2O. None of the contractions resulted in voiding. (B) X-ray obtained at Q_{max} shows the faint visualization of the urethra (arrows) with a narrowed proximal segment consistent with urethral obstruction from one of the slings.

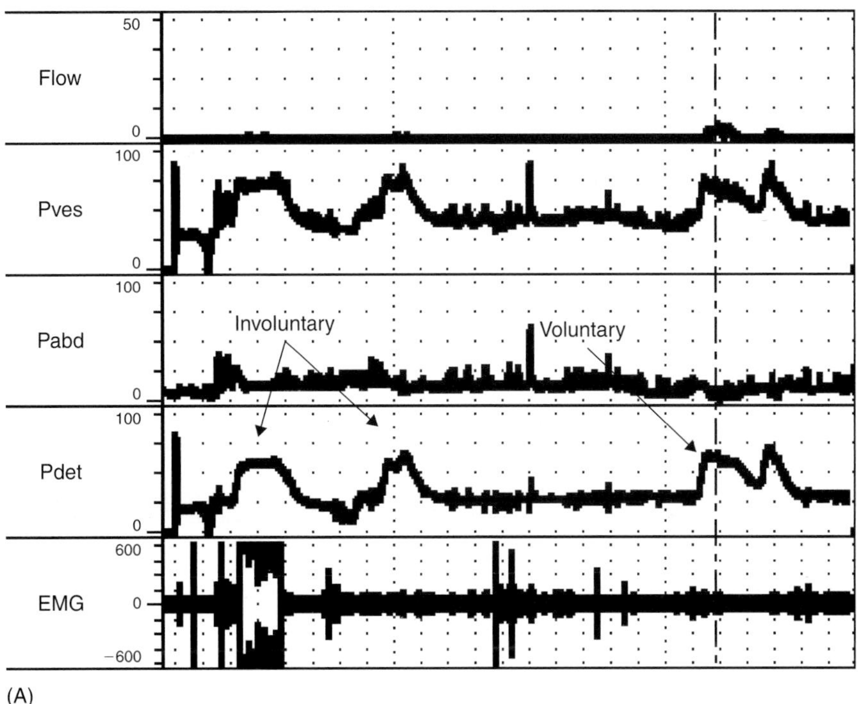

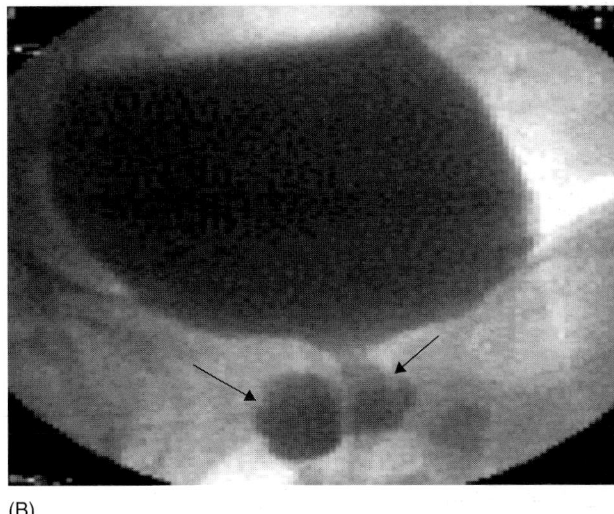

Fig. 11.12 Urethral obstruction due to urethral diverticulum in a 64-year-old woman who had undergone repeated urethral dilations over a 20-year period because of recurring urinary tract infections. (A) Urodynamic tracing. During bladder filling, there are involuntary detrusor contractions that result in incontinence. She finally voids voluntarily. Pdetmax@Q_{max} = 68 cmH_2O, and Q_{max} = 5 ml/s (vertical dashed line). This correlates with grade 2 obstruction on the Blaivas–Groutz nomogram.
(B) X-ray exposed at Q_{max} shows a large, multilocular urethral diverticulum (arrows) causing distal urethral obstruction.

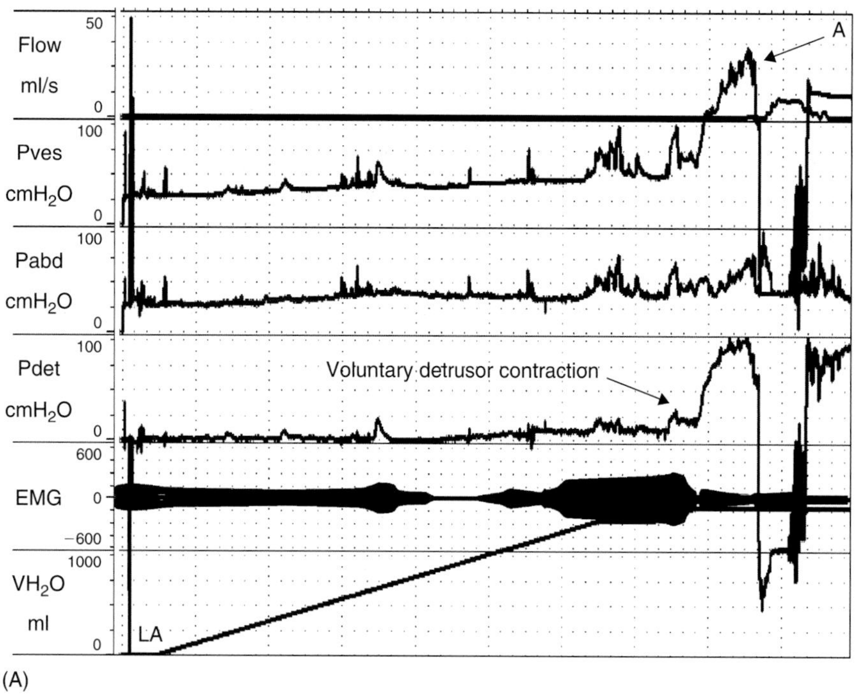

(A)

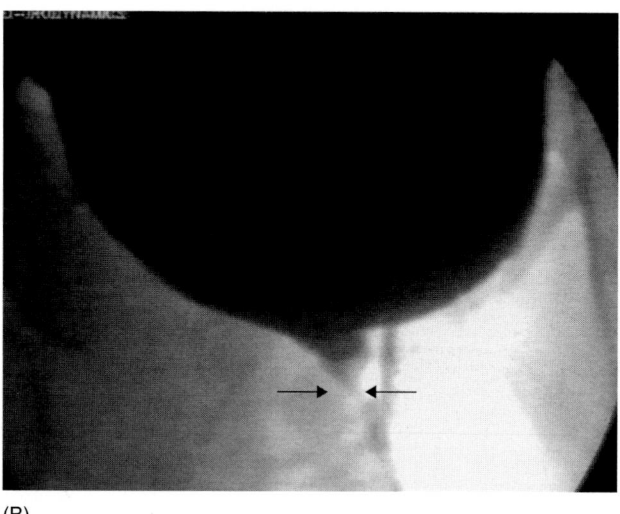

(B)

Fig. 11.13 Urethral obstruction due to urethral stricture of unknown etiology. The patient is a 41-year-old woman with a 3-year history of gradually increasing urinary frequency, urgency, and nocturia. Attempt at cystoscopy was aborted because of inability to pass a 17F cystoscope due to what appeared to be a stricture at the juncture of the middle and distal third of the urethra. (A) Urodynamic tracing. There is a voluntary detrusor contraction to 179 cmH_2O and a Q_{max} = 10 ml/s corresponding to a grade 3 urethral obstruction on the Blaivas–Groutz nomogram. In the midst of the detrusor contraction she began to void the catheter out (arrow A), but it was re-inserted. When the catheter came out, vesical pressure was no longer measured and this caused an artifactual negative pressure registration on the detrusor channel since detrusor pressure is determined by electronic subtraction of abdominal pressure from vesical pressure. (B) X-ray obtained at Q_{max} shows an obstruction at the junction of the middle and distal third of the urethra (arrows).

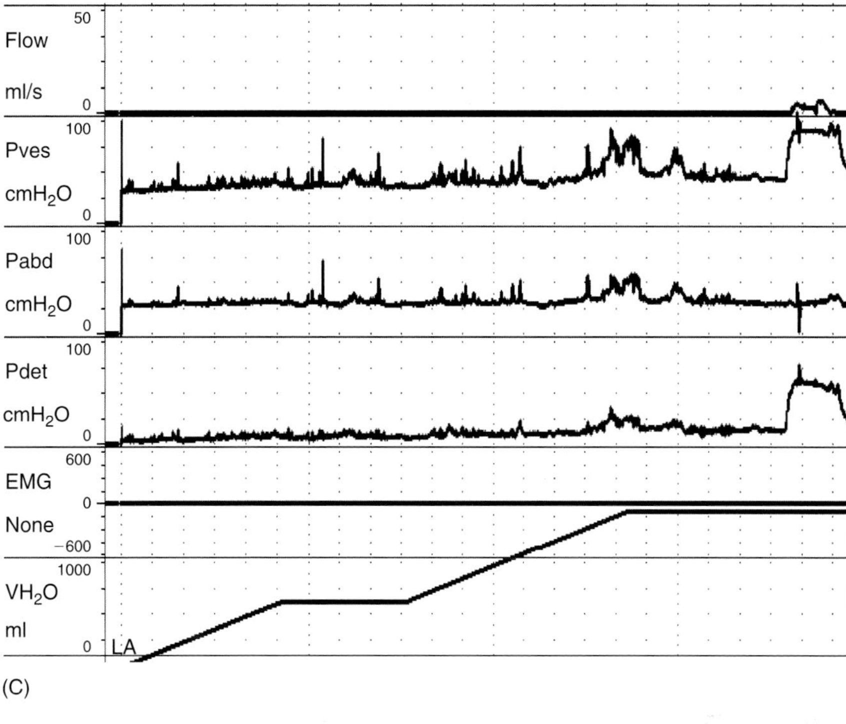

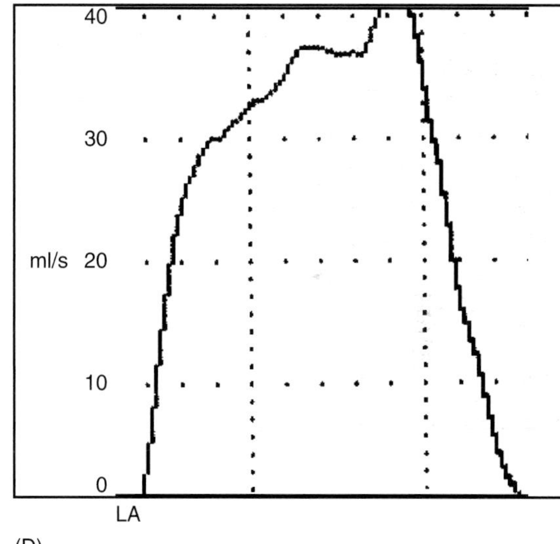

Fig. 11.13 (continued) (C) Urodynamic tracing 3 weeks status post urethroplasty. At a bladder volume of 1,400 ml she had a voluntary detrusor contraction. Pdet@Q_{max} = 70 cmH_2O and Q_{max} = 7 ml/s suggesting urethral obstruction, but she voided normally after removing the urethral catheter. She voided again immediately with a normal bell shaped curve and Q_{max} = 45 ml/s. This computes to a borderline grade 1 obstruction on the Blaivas–Groutz nomogram. (D) Unintubated uroflow 1-year post-operatively. Q_{max} = 42 ml/s, voided volume = 604 ml, and PVR = 0 ml.

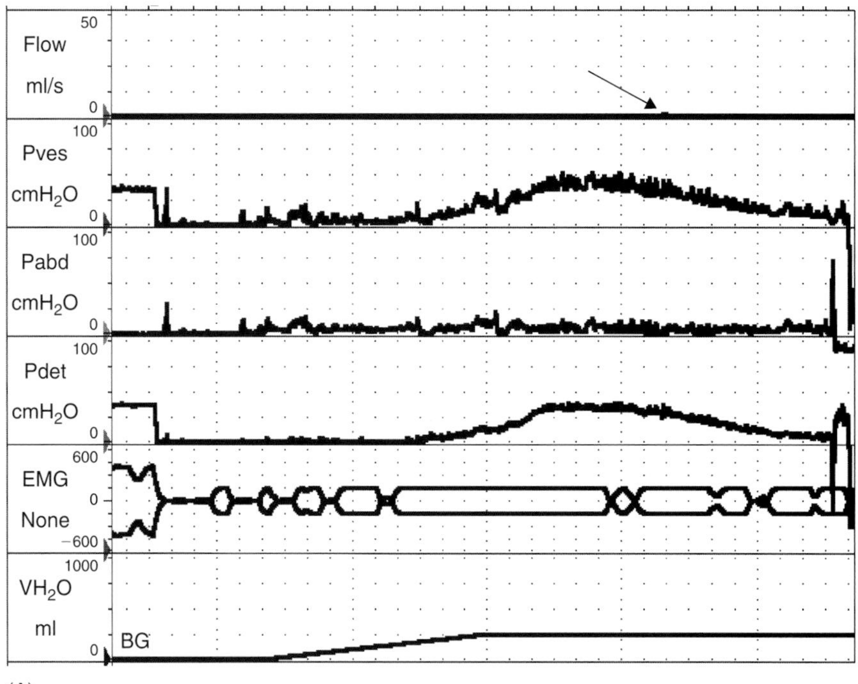

(A)

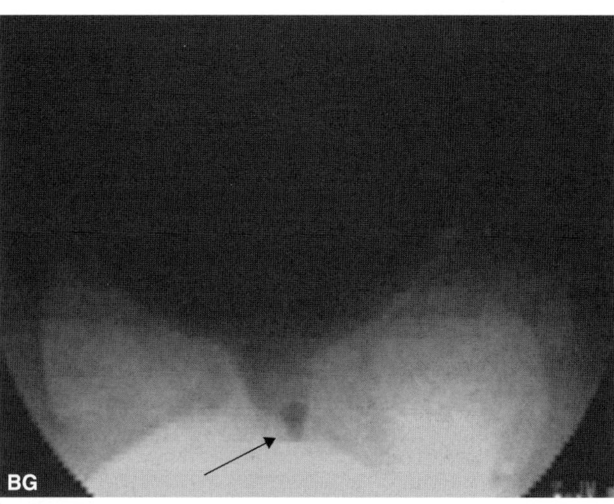

(B)

Fig. 11.14 Urethral stricture status post excision of urethral caruncle. This is an 82-year-old woman referred because of urinary retention following excision of a urethral caruncle. She failed three voiding trials and is currently being managed with an indwelling Foley catheter. (A) Urodynamic tracing. There is a sustained detrusor contraction to about 50 cmH_2O and a Q_{max} = 1 ml/s (arrow). This corresponds to a grade 2 obstruction on the Blaivas–Groutz nomogram. (B) X-ray exposed during voiding at Q_{max} (arrow) shows the obstruction to be at the distal urethra.

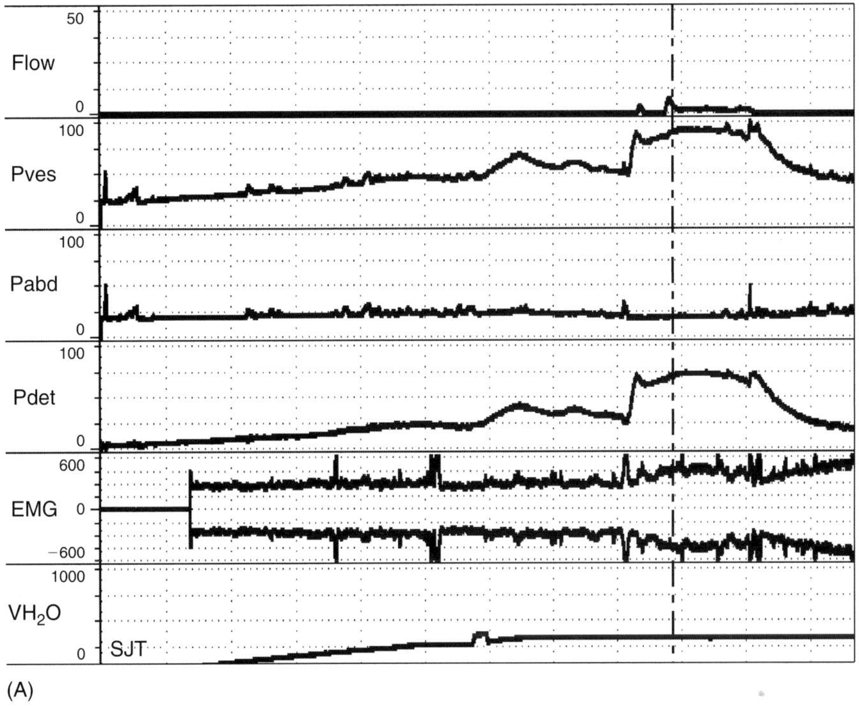

(A)

(B)

Fig. 11.15 Anatomic obstruction due to urethral stricture in a 36-year-old woman after pelvic fracture. (A) Urodynamic tracing. There is a sustained detrusor contraction: Pdet@Q_{max} = 80 cmH_2O and Q_{max} = 5 ml/s (vertical dashed line). This corresponds to grade 2 urethral obstruction on the Blaivas–Groutz nomogram. (B) X-ray obtained at Q_{max} shows distal urethral obstruction (arrows).

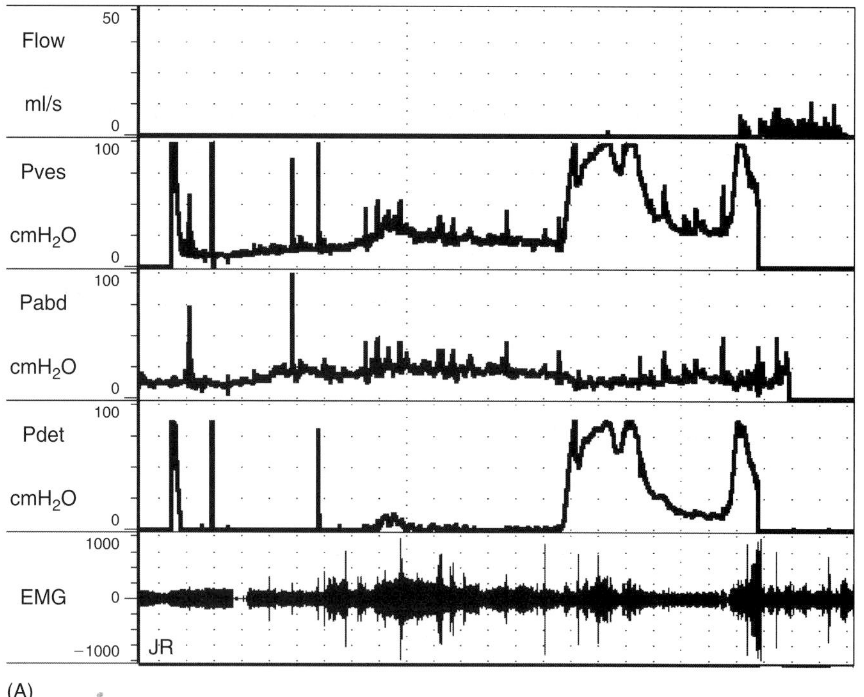

(A)

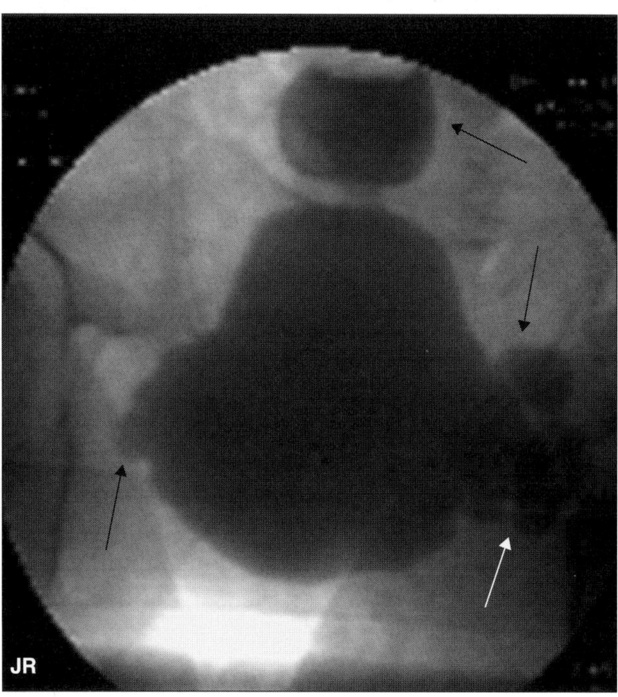

(B)

Fig. 11.16 Urethral obstruction (probably due to atrophic vaginitis). The patient is a 75-year-old woman with a long history of urinary frequency and a single episode of urinary retention treated with a temporary Foley catheter. On examination there was severe genital atrophy and cystoscopy showed the urethra to be concentrically scarred and narrowed and had to be dilated in order to introduce the 17F cystoscope. (A) Urodynamic tracing. Both of the detrusor contractions are voluntary, but the flow is very low. During the second detrusor contraction, the catheter was removed to see if flow would improve, but there was still severe obstruction that correlated with a grade 2 obstruction on the Blaivas–Groutz nomogram. Pdet@ Q_{max} = 88 cmH_2O and Q_{max} = 7 ml/s. After removal of the catheter she continued to void with an interrupted stream and a Q_{max} = 10 cmH_2O. (B). X-ray exposed during flow. No contrast is seen in the urethra suggesting the bladder neck as the site of obstruction. The bladder is markedly trabeculated and there are multiple diverticula (arrows).

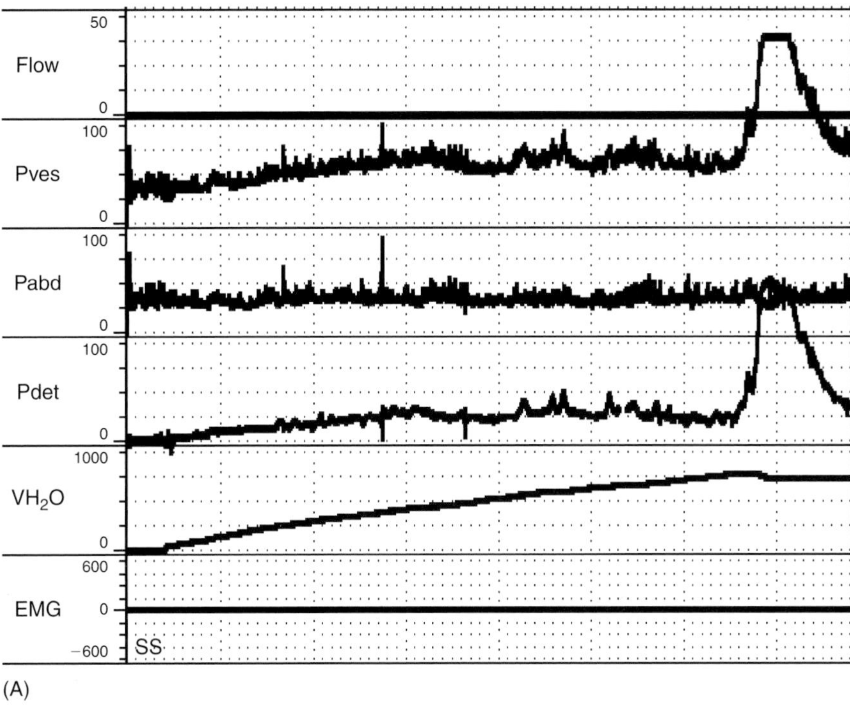

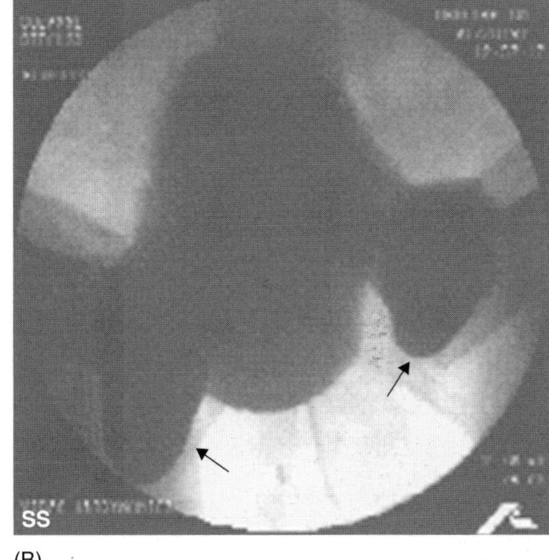

Fig. 11.17 Grade 3 urethral obstruction (primary bladder neck obstruction) in a 52-year-old woman who was asymptomatic, but found to have a distended abdomen associated with PVR urine over 1l. (A) Urodynamic tracing. There is a sustained voluntary detrusor contraction to 155 cmH_2O and a flow so low that it did not activate the flowmeter. This corresponds to a grade 3 obstruction. The EMG channel was not recorded. (B) X-ray obtained during Pdetmax shows no contrast in the urethra (vesical neck obstruction) and two large bladder diverticula (arrows).

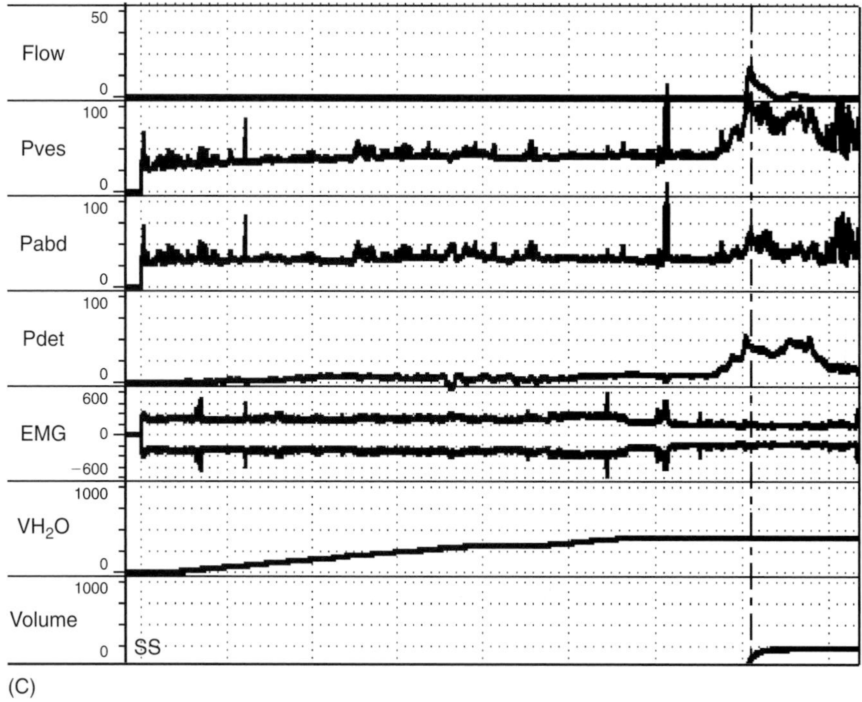

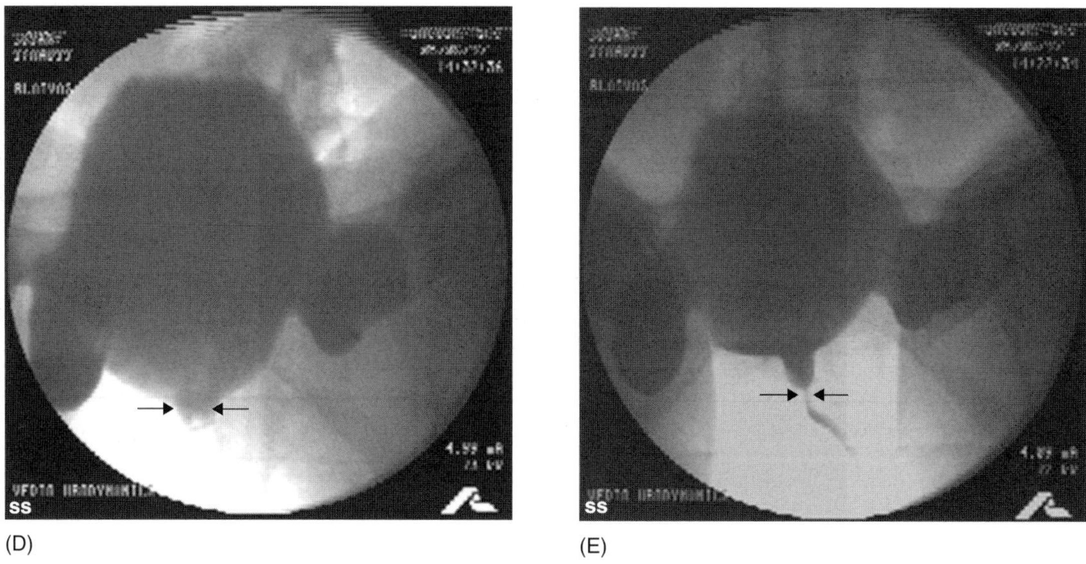

Fig. 11.17 (continued) (C) Urodynamic tracing obtained 6 months status post transurethral incision and resection of bladder neck. She voided with a voluntary detrusor contraction (Pdet@Q_{max} = 37 cmH_2O and Q_{max} = 18 ml/s). This is consistent with mild (grade 1) urethral obstruction, a marked improvement from her pre-operative status. (D) X-ray obtained at bladder capacity shows an open vesical neck at rest (arrows). (E) X-ray obtained during voiding shows a narrowed distal urethra.

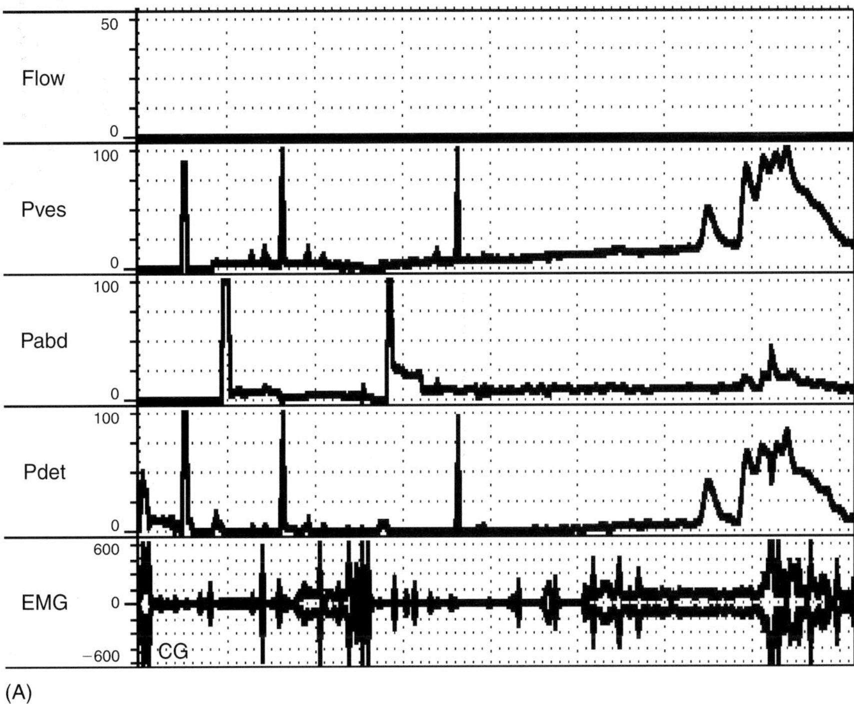

Fig. 11.18 Detrusor external sphincter dyssynergia and bladder neck obstruction in a 17-year-old paraplegic woman. (A) Urodynamic tracing. At a bladder volume of 125 ml, there is a sustained involuntary detrusor contraction (Pdetmax = 90 cmH_2O). During the detrusor contraction, there is a marked increase in EMG activity consistent with a diagnosis of DESD. However, the increased EMG activity occurs long after the onset of the detrusor contraction. This is not typical. Usually, in DESD the increased EMG activity occurs before or synchronous with the detrusor contraction. The current EMG findings may be artifactual due to the use of surface EMG electrodes instead of needle electrodes.
(B) X-ray exposed at Pdetmax shows no contrast at all in the urethra. The likeliest cause is synchronous bladder neck obstruction and DESD. It is possible, albeit unproven, that in this patient the striated urethral musculature extends all the way to the vesical neck.

Note the irregular contour of the bladder base consistent with a trabeculated bladder.

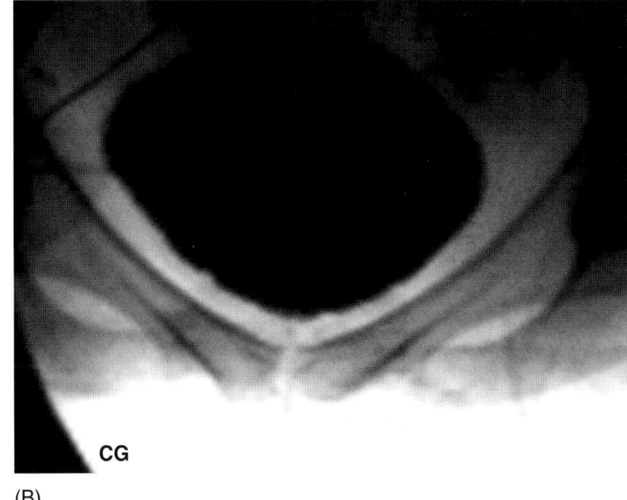

(B)

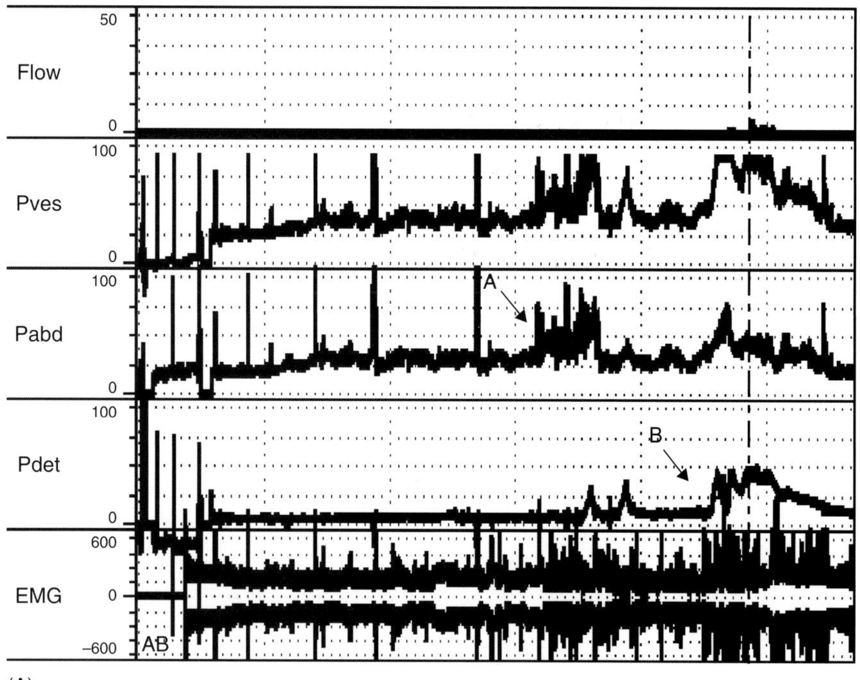

(A)

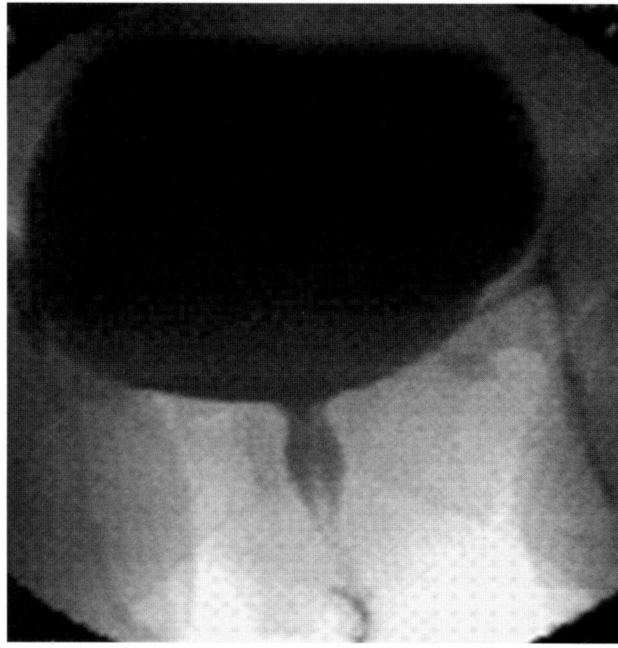

(B)

Fig. 11.19 Acquired voiding dysfunction in a 65-year-old woman. She complained of difficulty voiding and a "start/stop" voiding pattern. (A) Urodynamic tracing. During bladder filling there are multiple, sporadic increases in EMG activity. At the arrow A, she tries to void, strains and finally has two low magnitude detrusor contractions accompanied by further increases in EMG activity and no voiding (this is more easily seen in real time; the current tracing is compressed owing to page spacing limitations). She finally develops a sustained detrusor contraction (arrow B), but is still unable to relax her sphincter and she voids with an interrupted stream, obstructed by her own sphincter contraction. Pdet@Q_{max} = 50 cmH_2O and Q_{max} = 6 ml/s (vertical dashed line), consistent with grade 2 urethral obstruction on the Blaivas–Groutz nomogram. (B) X-ray obtained at Q_{max} (vertical dashed line) shows a wide open proximal two-thirds of the urethra and barely discernible visualization of the distal third. Without synchronous pressure/flow data, the appearance of this urethra would be considered normal.

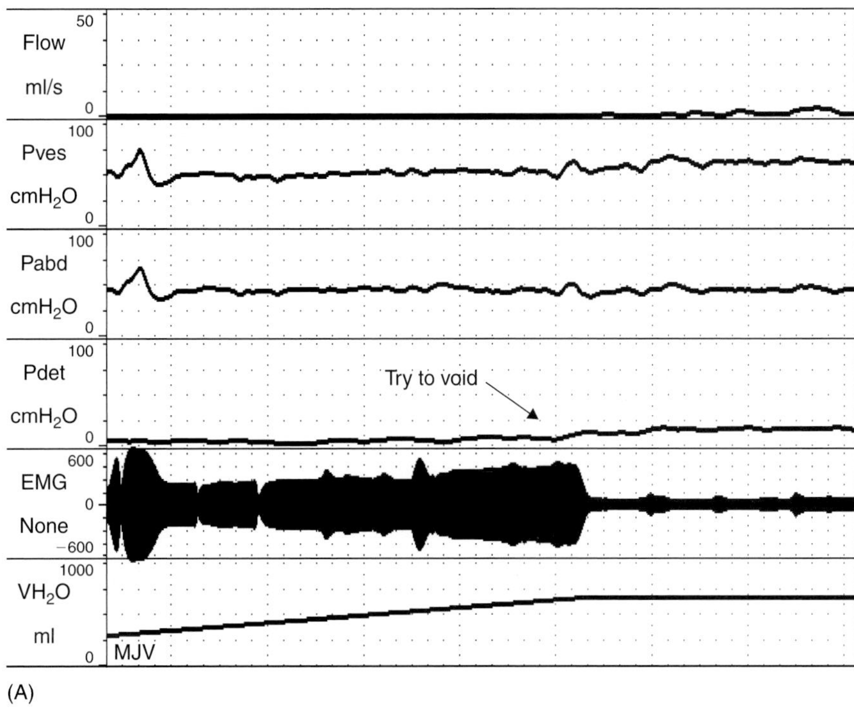

(A)

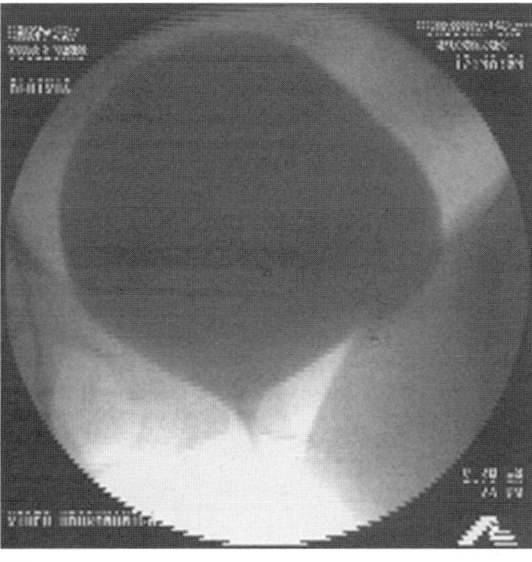

(B)

Fig. 11.20 Impaired detrusor contractility and type 1 OAB in a 77-year-old woman. Her chief complaint is urge incontinence just as she reaches the toilet. (A) Urodynamic study. FSF = 311 ml, 1st urge = 431 ml, and severe urge = 600 ml. There were no involuntary detrusor contractions. Bladder capacity was 665 ml. Q_{max} = 4 ml/s, Pdet@Q_{max} = 15 cmH_2O, Pdetmax = 17 cmH_2O, voided volume = 111 ml, PVR = 495 ml, and PVR prior to urodynamic study = 0 ml. (B) X-ray obtained during voiding at Q_{max}.

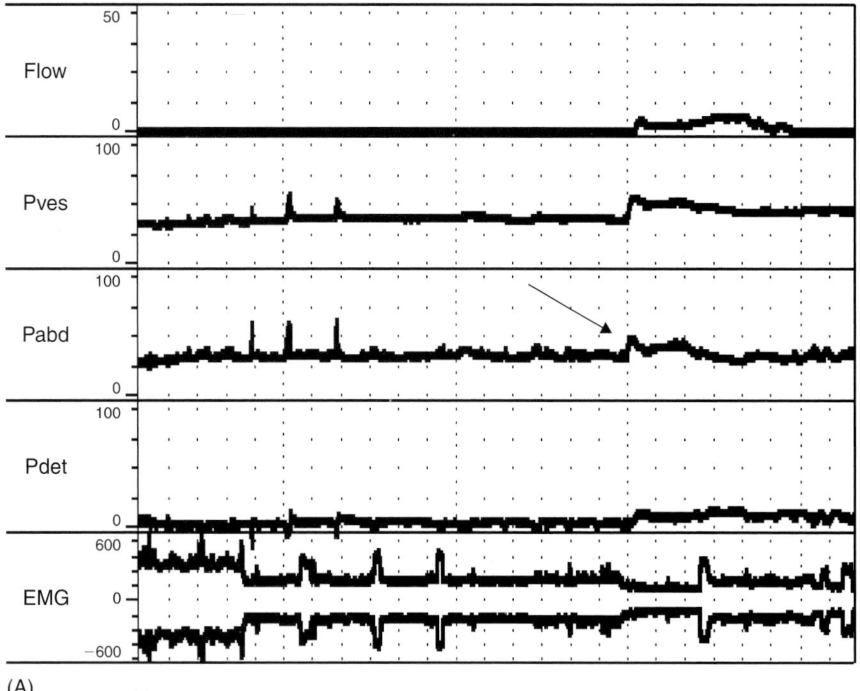

(A)

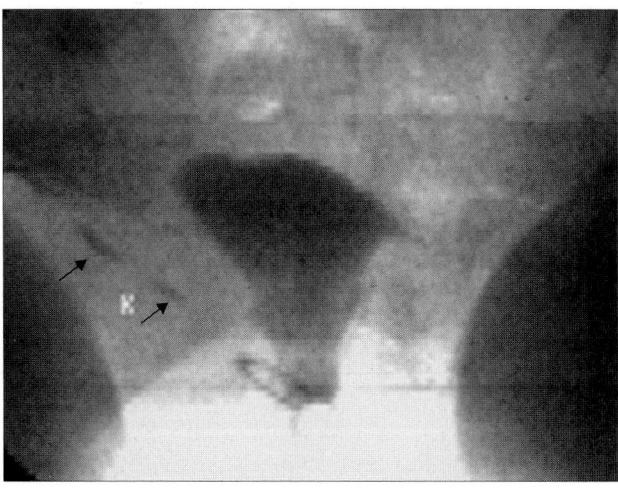

(B)

Fig. 11.21 Impaired detrusor contractility in a 31-year-old woman with recurrent stress incontinence after a vaginal wall sling. (A) Urodynamic tracing. At a bladder volume of 305 ml, she strains to initiate micturition (arrow) and then generates a voluntary detrusor contraction showing impaired detrusor contractility. (Q_{max} = 7.1 ml/s, Pdet@ Q_{max} = 14.2 cmH_2O, Pdetmax = 15 cmH_2O, voided volume = 305 ml, and PVR = 0 ml.) (B) X-ray obtained at Q_{max} shows a wide open urethra, but the view is not obliqued enough to show details. She also has grade 1 right vesicoureteral reflux (arrows).

12 Neurogenic Bladder: The Effect of Neurologic Lesions on Micturition

Micturition is normally accomplished by activation of the micturition reflex (see chapter 2, Normal micturition). The micturition reflex is integrated and modulated at numerous sites throughout the central nervous system including the pontine mesencephalic reticular formation (pontine micturition center), parasympathetic and somatic components of the sacral spinal cord (the sacral micturition center), and the thoracolumbar sympathetics [1–4].

Neurologic lesions above the pons usually leave the "micturition reflex" intact and, when they affect voiding at all, generally result in loss of voluntary control. In these patients micturition is physiologically normal (there is a coordinated relaxation of the sphincter during detrusor contraction, but the patient has simply lost the ability to either initiate or prevent voiding) [4,5]. There is great variability in the degree of the patient's awareness, control, and concern about micturition. Some patients have either no awareness or concern and simply void involuntarily (Fig. 12.1). This pattern is also called type 4 overactive bladder (OAB) [6] (see chapter 9, overactive bladder).

Some patients with suprapontine neurologic lesions can sense the impending onset of an involuntary detrusor contraction and are able to voluntarily contract the sphincter and abort the detrusor contraction before it starts. This pattern is called type 2 OAB (Fig. 12.2). Such a patient usually complains of urgency, but not urge incontinence. Others are aware of the involuntary detrusor contraction and can contract the striated sphincter, but this does not abort the detrusor contraction and incontinence ensues. This pattern is called type 3 OAB (Fig. 12.3). In addition to urinary urgency, these patients also complain of urge incontinence.

Some patients with supraspinal neurologic lesions have both involuntary detrusor contractions and impaired detrusor contractility (Fig. 12.4). Others have detrusor areflexia or an acontractile detrusor (Fig. 12.5), but the neurophysiologic pathways responsible for this have not been well described. Sometimes it is difficult to distinguish between low bladder compliance, involuntary detrusor contractions, and/or detrusor areflexia (Fig. 12.6).

Interruption of the neural pathways connecting the "pontine micturition center" to the "sacral micturition center" usually results in detrusor-external sphincter dyssynergia (DESD) or other manifestations of poor coordination of the micturition reflex such as weak, poorly sustained detrusor contractions [4,7,8]. DESD is characterized by involuntary contractions of the striated musculature of the urethral sphincter during an involuntary detrusor contraction. It is seen exclusively in patients with neurologic lesions between the brain stem (pontine micturition center) and the sacral spinal cord (sacral micturition center). These include traumatic spinal cord injury, multiple sclerosis, myelodysplasia, and other forms of transverse myelitis.

There are three main types of DESD. In type I there is a concomitant increase in both detrusor pressure and EMG activity (Fig. 12.7). At the peak of the detrusor contraction, the sphincter suddenly relaxes and unobstructed voiding occurs. Type II DESD is characterized by sporadic contractions of the external urethral sphincter throughout the detrusor contraction (Fig. 12.8). In type III DESD there is a crescendo–decrescendo pattern of sphincter contraction which results in urethral obstruction throughout the entire detrusor contraction (Fig. 12.9).

The diagnosis of DESD should be suspected in any patient with a neurologic lesion involving the spinal cord. Conversely, in patients without such a lesion, this diagnosis should be viewed with skepticism. In neurologically normal patients, a presumed diagnosis of DESD is almost always due to an acquired disorder of micturition characterized by a contraction of the striated sphincter in a conscious or subconscious attempt to abort micturition. The correct diagnosis is best attained by videourodynamic evaluation with EMG monitoring. In DESD the onset of the detrusor contraction is preceded by an increase in sphincter EMG activity. In learned voiding dysfunction the sphincter EMG activity diminishes just prior to the contraction, then sporadically increases as the patient contracts and relaxes the sphincter (identical to Fig. 12.3). If EMG is unavailable, the characteristics of the urethral contractions seen at fluoroscopy often provide enough information for a definitive diagnosis.

Sacral neurologic lesions have a variable effect on micturition depending on the extent to which the neurologic injury affects the parasympathetic, sympathetic, and somatic systems. In complete parasympathetic lesions the bladder is areflexic and the patient is in urinary retention (similar to Fig. 12.5). In many cases, there is also low bladder compliance. When, in addition to a parasympathetic lesion, there is also a sympathetic one, the proximal urethra loses its sphincteric function. Clinically, this results in incomplete bladder emptying (due to the acontractile detrusor) and sphincteric incontinence (due to the non-functioning proximal urethra) (Fig. 12.10) [9–12].

Somatic neurologic lesions affect pudendal afferents and efferents. In addition to loss of perineal and peri-anal sensation, these lesions abolish the bulbocavernosus reflex and impair the ability to voluntarily contract the urethral and anal sphincters. Herniated disks, diabetic neuropathy, multiple sclerosis, and spinal cord cause sacral neurologic lesions tumors. They are also commonly encountered after extensive pelvic surgery such as abdominoperineal resection of the rectum and radical hysterectomy [9–12].

In addition to documenting the effect that the neurologic abnormality has on micturition, videourodynamic evaluation is also important for detecting urologic risk factors that require either active treatment or aggressive followup to prevent complications such as hydronephrosis, vesicoureteral reflux, urolithiasis, urosepsis, and renal failure. Urologic risk factors include detrusor-external sphincter dyssynergia, low bladder compliance, and sustained high magnitude detrusor contractions. For patients who experience autonomic dysreflexia, the relationship between the signs and symptoms (sweating, headache, hypertension, bradycardia) and bladder filling, detrusor contraction, sphincter contraction, or vesicoureteral reflux is noted.

Suggested Reading

1 Bradley WE, Conway CJ, Bladder Representation in the Pontine–Masencephalic Reticular Formation, Exp. Neurol, 1966, 16:237.
2 Bradley WW, Timm, GE, Scott, FB, Innervation of the Detrusor Muscle and Urethra, Urol. Clin NA, 1:30,1974.
3 De Groat WC, Nervous Control of the Urinary Bladder in the cat.
4 Blaivas JG. The neurophysiology of micturition: a clinical study of 550 patients, *J Urol*, 127: 958, 1982.
5 Khan Z, Starer P, Yang WC, Bhola A, Analysis of voiding disorders in patients with cerebrovascular accidents, *Urology*, 1990, 32:256.
6 Flisser AJ, Walmsely K, Blaivas JG. Urodynamic classification of patients with symptoms of overactive bladder, *J Urol*, 169(2): 529–534, 2003.
7 McGuire EJ, Brady S. Detrusor–sphincter dyssynergia. *J Urol*, 121: 774, 1979.
8 Blaivas JG, Sinha HP, Zayed AAH, Labib KB. Detrusor-external sphincter dyssynergia, *J Urol*, 125: 541, 1981.
9 McGuire EJ. Urodynamic evaluation after abdominal–perineal resection and lumbar intervertebral disc herniation, *Urology*, 6: 63, 1975.
10 Norlen L. Influence of the sympathetic nervous system on the lower urinary tract and clinical implications, *Neurourol Urodynam*, 1: 125, 1982.
11 Blaivas JG, Barbalias GA. Characteristics of neural injury after abdominal perineal resection of the rectum, *J Urol*, 129: 84, 1983.
12 Yalla SV, Andriole G. Vesicourethral dysfunction following pelvic visceral ablative surgery, *J Urol*, 132: 503, 1984.
13 Dangas N, Parashou E, Lymberi M, Kehayas P. Responses of renal function to elevated intravesical pressure, *Br J Urol*, 72: 539–543, 1993.
14 Ersoz M, Tunc H, Akyuz M, Ozel S. Bladder storage and emptying disorder frequencies in hemorrhagic and ischemic stroke patients with bladder dysfunction, *Cerebrovasc Dis*, 20(5): 395–399, 2005.
15 Hansen RB, Biering-Sorensen F, Kristensen JK. Bladder emptying over a period of 10–45 years after a traumatic spinal cord injury, *SpinalCord*, 42(11): 631–637, 2004.
16 Kaplan SA, Chancellor MB, Blaivas JG. Bladder and sphincter behavior in patients with spinal cord lesions, *J Urol*, 46: 113–117, 1991.
17 Morrison JFB. Bladder control: role of the higher levels of central nervous system. In Torrens M, Morrison JFB (eds) *The Physiology of the Lower Urinary Tract*, London, UK: Springer–Verlag, 1987, Chapter 8.
18 Ockrim J, Laniado ME, Khoubehi B, Renzetti R, Finazzi Agro E, Carter SS, Tubaro A. Variability of detrusor overactivity on repeated filling cystometry in men with urge symptoms: comparison with spinal cord injury patients, *BJU International*, 95(4): 587– 590, 2005.
19 Perkash I. Donald Munro Lecture 2003. Neurogenic bladder: past, present, and future, *J Spinal Cord Med*, 27(4): 383–386, 2004.
20 Schurch B, Schmid DM, Karsenty G, Reitz A. Can neurologic examination predict type of detrusor sphincter-dyssynergia in patients with spinal cord injury? *Urology*, 65(2): 243–246, 2005.
21 Denny-Brown D, Robertson, EG, on the Physiology of Micturition, Brain, 1933, 56:149.
22 Kuru M. Nervous Control of Micturition, Physiol Rev. 1965, 45:425.
23 Langworthy OR, Kolb LG, Lewis LG, Physiology of Micturition, Baltimore, The williams and Wilkins Co, 1940.
24 Torrens, M, Morrison, JFB (eds), The Physiology of the Lower Urinary Tract, Berlin, Springer-Verlag, 1987.

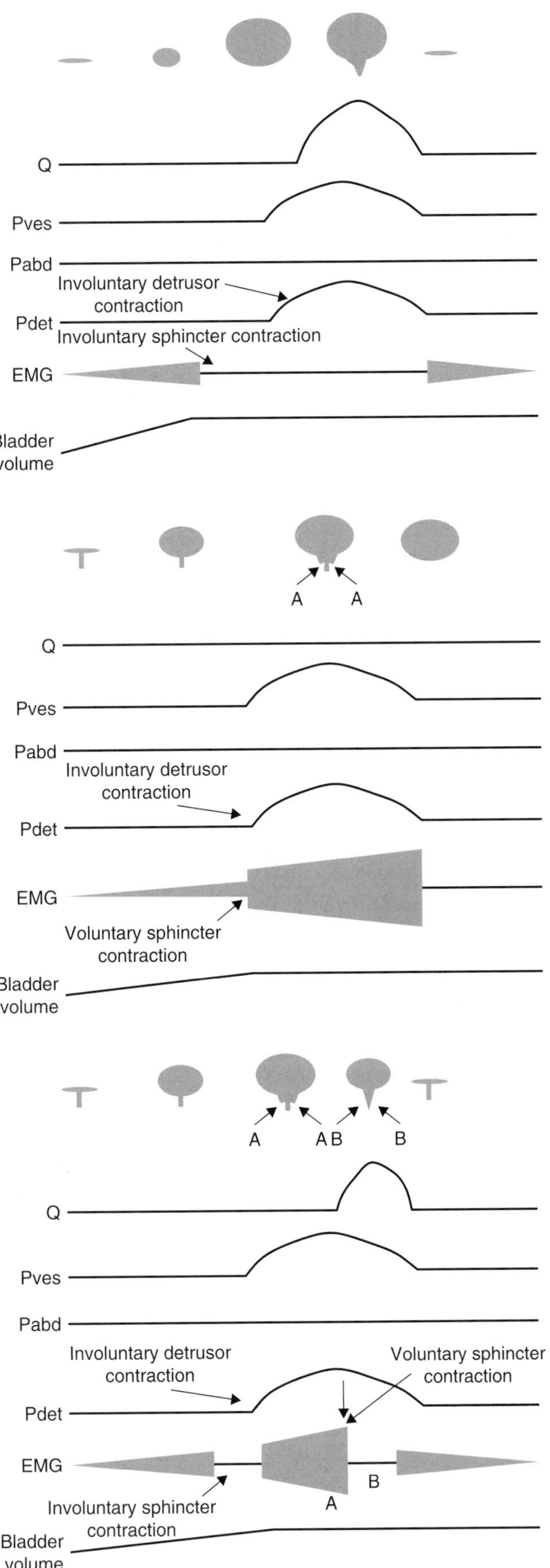

Fig. 12.1 Detrusor hyperreflexia (type 4 OAB) due to neurologic lesions above the brain stem that leaves the pontine micturition center intact. This results in a normal micturition reflex that the patient cannot completely control. In this example, the patient has no awareness of the involuntary detrusor contraction and simply voids "normally," but without control. The urodynamic tracing is identical to a normal micturition reflex.

Fig. 12.2 Detrusor hyperreflexia (type 2 OAB). In this example, the impending onset of an involuntary detrusor contraction is sensed by the patient who immediately contracts the striated sphincter. This is manifest as increased EMG activity. At this point, the urethra is dilated in its proximal extent with obstruction in the distal third by the sphincter contraction (arrows "A"). Through a reflex mechanism, the detrusor contraction is aborted and continence maintained (no flow, flat Q tracing).

Fig. 12.3 Detrusor hyperreflexia (type 3 OAB). An involuntary detrusor contraction is heralded by a sudden and complete relaxation of the sphincter EMG. As soon as the patient senses the detrusor contraction, he contracts his sphincter (increased EMG activity) in an attempt to prevent incontinence. At this point, the urethra is dilated in its proximal urethra with obstruction in the distal third by the sphincter contraction (arrows A), momentarily maintaining continence. Once the sphincter fatigues, the urethra opens and incontinence ensues (arrows B).

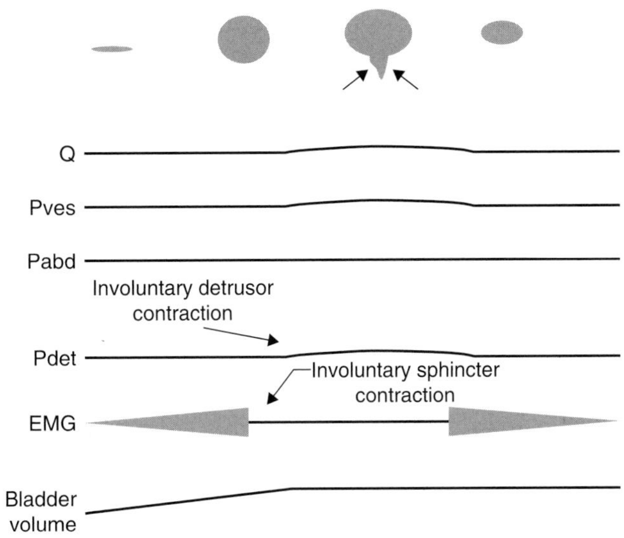

Q
Pves
Pabd
Involuntary detrusor contraction
Pdet
Involuntary sphincter contraction
EMG
Bladder volume

Fig. 12.4 Detrusor hyperreflexia and impaired detrusor contractility. An involuntary detrusor contraction is heralded by a sudden and complete relaxation of the sphincter EMG, but the detrusor contraction is barely discernible as a subtle rise in detrusor pressure. Uroflow is low, but the urethra opens normally (arrows). The patient does not empty completely.

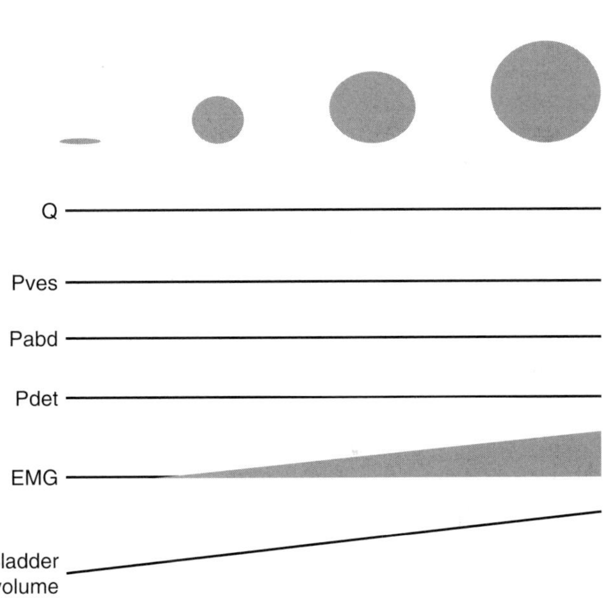

Fig. 12.5 Detrusor areflexia. Despite the bladder filling to a large volume, there is no detrusor contraction at all and the urethra remains closed.

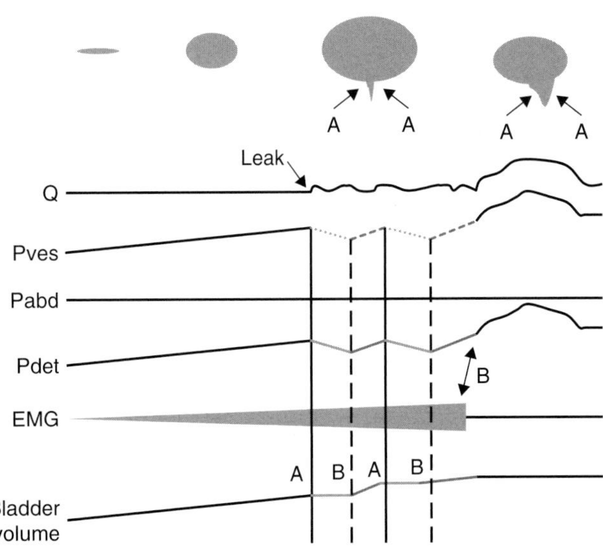

Fig. 12.6 Low bladder compliance versus involuntary detrusor contraction. During bladder filling there is a gradual rise in detrusor pressure and the patient begins to void/leak with a low flow rate. Is this a detrusor contraction or low bladder compliance? There are two clues that this is low compliance. Firstly, each time the bladder infusion is stopped (vertical solid lines) detrusor pressure falls, and when bladder infusion is started again (vertical dashed line) detrusor pressure rises. Secondly, the rise in detrusor pressure is unassociated with any EMG changes. At the end of bladder filling, there is complete relaxation of the striated sphincter (EMG silence) heralding the onset of an involuntary detrusor contraction (arrow B). The detrusor pressure continues to rise after bladder filling has stopped confirming that detrusor contraction and not low bladder compliance causes the pressure rise.

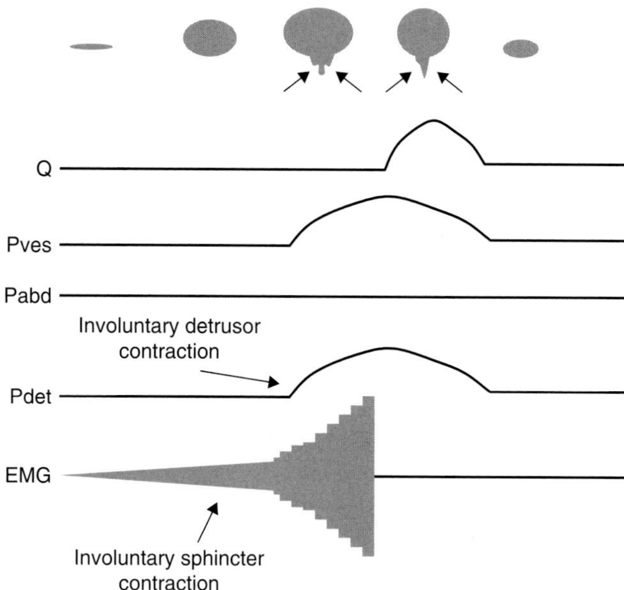

Fig. 12.7 Type 1 DESD: The involuntary sphincter contraction, precedes the involuntary detrusor contraction. At the peak of the detrusor contraction, there is a sudden and complete relaxation of the striated sphincter (EMG silence) and (unobstructed) voiding ensues. During the first half of the detrusor contraction, there is the classic appearance of DESD – a dilated proximal urethra and narrowed distal urethra associated with increased EMG activity and an involuntary detrusor contraction.

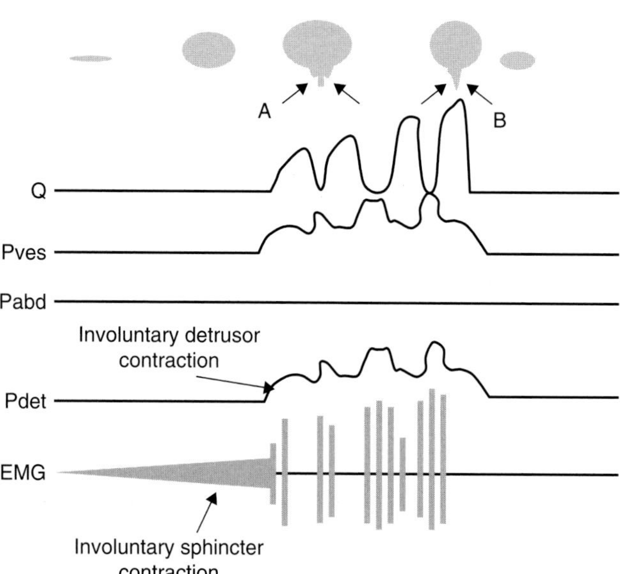

Fig. 12.8 Type 2 DESD: There are sporadic involuntary sphincter contractions throughout the involuntary detrusor contraction. During the sphincter contractions, the patient is obstructed by his own sphincter (A); during sphincter relaxation, voiding is unobstructed (B).

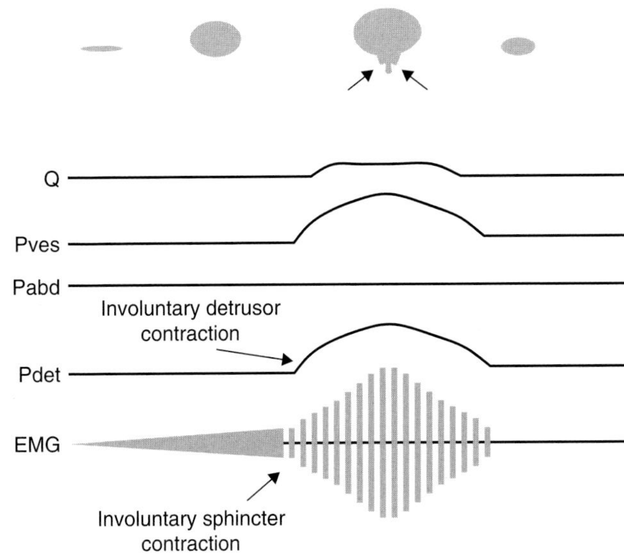

Fig. 12.9 Type 3 DESD: The involuntary sphincter contraction precedes the involuntary detrusor contraction. There is a crescendo–decrescendo pattern in EMG activity and voiding is obstructed throughout.

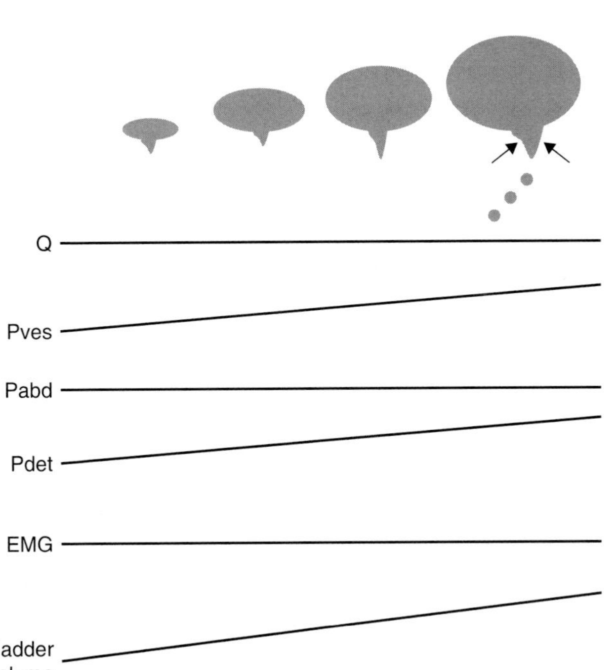

Fig. 12.10 Detrusor areflexia, low bladder compliance, and open bladder neck due to parasympathetic and sympathetic injury. During bladder filling there is a gradual rise in detrusor pressure and the patient begins to void/leak with a flow rate too low to activate the flowmeter.

13 Cerebral Vascular Accident, Parkinson's Disease and Other Supra Spinal Neurologic Disorders

Cerebrovascular accident (CVA) has been estimated to afflict 83–160 per 100,000 populations annually and is the third most common cause of disability in the United States. Arterial occlusion, hemorrhage, and congenital malformation are the most common etiologies. Arteriosclerotic vascular disease is frequently associated with hypertension and diabetes. Intracranial hemorrhage is usually due to rupture of aneurysms located at the base of the brain. Many patients after CVA suffer from lower urinary tract symptoms and urodynamic abnormalities. During the first month after stroke, incontinence is very common, with a reported incidence as high as 70%. However, it is usually transient, and in many patients it is due, at least in part, to immobility and dependency subsequent to paralysis and cognitive disorders.

Detrusor hyperreflexia is the most common urodynamic abnormality after CVA and is thought to be the result of a release of the spinal micturition reflexes from cerebral inhibitory centers (Fig. 13.1). Detrusor-external sphincter dyssynergia (DESD) is not seen after stroke, but some patients have voluntary sphincter contractions during involuntary detrusor contractions (type 3 overactive bladder (OAB), formerly termed pseudo-dyssynergia) (Fig. 13.2). This should not be misinterpreted as DESD as it is a conscious or subconscious attempt to suppress involuntary micturition. Some patients have detrusor hyperreflexia and impaired detrusor contractility (Fig. 13.3). Others have detrusor hyperreflexia and low bladder compliance (Fig. 13.4). Of course, detrusor hyperreflexia after stroke may be associated with pre-morbid conditions such as prostatic obstruction and sphincteric incontinence, not pictured here. Prostatic obstruction and stroke pose a difficult therapeutic dilemma. Inexplicably, as many as 25% of patients develop urinary retention due to detrusor areflexia in the immediate period after stroke, but this usually subsides over time.

Borrie and associates studied 151 patients with CVA in a 1-year period. Seventeen percent had pre-existing urinary incontinence. At 1, 4, and 12 weeks post-stroke, 60%, 42%, and 29% of the survivors, respectively, were incontinent. Cystometry was performed in those with moderate or severe urinary incontinence and involuntary detrusor contractions were present in 85% of those who had been continent prior to their stroke. Factors associated with urinary incontinence at 4 weeks were moderate or severe motor deficit, impaired mobility, and mental impairment. Badlani and associates reported urodynamic findings in CVA patients.

Detrusor hyperreflexia was present in 46%, areflexia was present in 20%, and the rest were found to have a normal urodynamic evaluation.

Parkinson's disease

Parkinson's disease is one of the most common neurologic entities causing voiding dysfunction. It affects men and women equally, mainly in the sixth and seventh decades of life. The usual clinical findings (tremor, bradykinesia, and muscular rigidity) are thought to be caused by a dopamine deficiency in the substantial nigra. Voiding dysfunction has been reported in 35–75% of patients. Urinary urgency, frequency, and urge incontinence are the predominant symptoms; the remainder generally have obstructive symptoms consisting of hesitancy, incomplete emptying, or urinary retention.

The majority of patients with Parkinson's disease have detrusor hyperreflexia. If the patient senses the involuntary detrusor contraction, he or she may voluntarily contract the sphincter in an attempt at maintaining continence (Fig. 13.5). This voluntary contraction of the external sphincter was termed "pseudo-dyssynergia" in the older literature and type 3 OAB in our current classification system. Another common urodynamic finding is a delay in the relaxation of the external sphincter at the onset of voluntary micturition. This finding, which may mimic DESD, has been termed "sphincter bradykinesia" and is a characteristic of patients with Parkinson's disease who have generalized skeletal muscle rigidity. Sphincter bradykinesia can be seen on fluoroscopy, sphincter electromyography (EMG), or with simultaneous measurement of the urethral pressure at the level of the external urethral sphincter. Prostatic obstruction is not uncommon in men with Parkinson's disease and may be associated with sphincter bradykinesia (Fig. 13.6). It poses the same therapeutic dilemma as discussed above in those with stroke. In the general population, the estimated risk of incontinence after prostatectomy is estimated at approximately 2% or less. However, the risk of incontinence after prostatectomy in a Parkinsonian patient is approximately 20% or more. Post-prostatectomy incontinence in the Parkinsonian is generally not due to iatrogenic injury to the sphincter; rather it is almost always caused by detrusor hyperreflexia.

A less common urodynamic finding in the patient with Parkinson's disease is impaired detrusor contractility (Fig. 13.7). Detrusor areflexia is relatively uncommon in Parkinson's disease and may be the manifestation of widespread neurologic dysfunction, as is seen in multi-system atrophy syndromes of which the Shy–Drager syndrome is most well known to urologists (see Fig. 13.8).

Multi-system atrophy

The term multiple system atrophy has been applied to a number of disease entities, which have a common pathologic expression of neuronal atrophy. The Shy–Drager syndrome is but one manifestation of multiple system atrophy. The variability of the pathologic presentations includes Parkinsonism, cerebellar ataxia, and autonomic failure. Disturbances of continence and micturition and erectile impotence invariably accompany the other neurologic changes in the Shy–Drager syndrome and may be the presenting symptom.

Urethral sphincter EMG, using needle electrodes and oscilloscopic monitoring, is valuable in differentiating between multiple system atrophy and Parkinson's disease. Patients with multiple system atrophy have marked abnormalities of their striated urethral sphincter EMG, while Parkinsonian patients do not. The EMG abnormalities are due to degeneration of Onuf's nucleus that results in denervation of the striated urethral and anal sphincter.

Berger and associates compared the urodynamic findings in 29 patients with Parkinson's disease and nine patients with the Shy–Drager syndrome. All patients with Parkinson's disease exhibited detrusor contractions during the urodynamic study and all had normal filling pressures; 90% had detrusor hyperreflexia. Among the patients with Shy–Drager syndrome, 67% had detrusor areflexia, 33% had detrusor hyperreflexia, and 45% had low bladder compliance (Fig. 13.9). In most patients with Shy–Drager syndrome who had a voiding cystourethrogram, an open bladder neck at rest was also demonstrated, indicating sympathetic denervation. The EMG of the external sphincter showed some form of lower motor neuron lesions in all the Shy–Drager patients and in none of the Parkinson's. In the latter group, the sphincter EMG was normal in 39% and showed involuntary sphincter activity in 61%. A typical urodynamic study in a patient with Shy–Drager syndrome is seen in Figure 13.8.

Other intracranial diseases

Lower urinary tract dysfunction and abnormal urodynamic findings may be associated with intracranial diseases including Huntington's chorea, cerebellar ataxia, cerebral palsy, hereditary ataxias, and cerebral aneurysms. As a general rule, detrusor behavior has been demonstrated to be hyperreflexia with coordinated sphincter function. Discussed below are the urodynamic manifestations of some of the more common intracranial neurologic diseases.

Traumatic brain injury

Traumatic brain injury is the most common form of severe neurologic impairment as a result of trauma. Severe head injuries occur in approximately 50,000–75,000 people per year in the United States. With lesions above the pontine micturition center, especially those involving the frontal lobes, uninhibited detrusor contractions are the most frequent form of bladder dysfunction. Even though incontinence is a major problem, post-void residual urines are rarely elevated. In a few patients with more isolated brain stem injuries who have involvement below the pontine micturition center, detrusor-sphincter dyssynergia may occur.

Dementia

Dementia is a diffuse deterioration in intellectual function manifested principally by memory deficits and changes in conduct. Possible etiologies include "aging", occult head injury, encephalitis, pre-senile dementia (Alzheimer's, Pick's, and Jakob–Creutzfeldt disease), normal pressure or communicating hydrocephalus, and neurosyphilis. The mechanism of neurogenic bladder dysfunction in these diseases has not been identified, in part due to the difficulty in differentiating the possible effects of the underlying organic disease on specific cerebro-cortical areas from depression or inattention to personal hygiene. The most common urodynamic finding is detrusor hyperreflexia.

Mental retardation

Urinary incontinence and nocturnal enuresis are more commonly reported in mentally retarded people than in the normal population. Our knowledge of the cause and characteristic of urinary disorders in the mentally retarded is limited. Hellstrom and associates studied a group of 21 mentally retarded patients with long-standing urinary symptoms. It was possible to perform the urodynamic examination in all cases. Thirteen patients voided during the study. The most common abnormalities were detrusor areflexia in nine patients and detrusor hyperreflexia in eight patients. The findings were essentially normal in four cases.

Comatose patients

Wyndaele studied 135 patients with various degrees of coma, and found involuntary detrusor contractions with complete micturition in 76% of patients when the indwelling catheter was removed. With pharmacologic intervention and intermittent catheterization, the remaining 24% started to urinate within 1 week. Most patients in acute and prolonged coma have spontaneous, involuntary micturition without dyssynergic sphincter.

Suggested Reading

1 Badlani GH, Vohra S, Motola JA. Detrusor behavior in patients with dominant hemispheric strokes. *Neurourol Urodynam*, 10: 119–123, 1991.

2 Berger Y, Blaivas JG, DeLaRocha ER, Salinas J. Urodynamic findings on Parkinson's disease. *J Urol*, 138: 836–838, 1987.

3 Berger Y, Salinas J, Blaivas JG. Urodynamic differentiation of Parkinson's disease and the Shy–Drager syndrome (SD). *Neurourol Urodynam*, 9: 117–121, 1990.

4 Bonney W, Gupta S, Arndt S, Anderson K, Hunter DR. Neu-robiological correlates of bladder dysfunction in schizophrenia. *Neurourol Urodynam*, 12: 347–348, 1993.

5 Borrie MJ, Campbell AJ, Caradoc-Davies TH, Spears GFS. Urinary incontinence after stroke: a prospective study. *Age Aging*, 15: 177–181, 1986.

6 Brocklehurst JC, Andrews K, Richards B, Laycock PF. Incidence and correlates of incontinence in stroke patients. *J Am Geriatric Soc*, 33: 540–542, 1985.

7 Eardley I, Quinn NP, Fowler CJ, et al. The value of urethral sphincter electromyography in the differential diagnosis of Parkinsonism. *Br J Urol*, 64: 360–362, 1989.

8 Flisser AJ, Walmsely K, Blaivas JG. Urodynamic classification of patients with symptoms of overactive bladder. *J Urol,* 169(2): 529–534, 2003.

9 Garrett VE, Scott JA, Costich J, Aubrey DL, Gross J. Bladder emptying assessment in stroke patients. *Arch Phys Med Rehab,* 70: 40–43, 1989.

10 Hellstrom PA, Jarvelin MR, Kontturi MJ, Huttunen NP. Bladder function in the mentally retarded. *Br J Urol,* 66: 475–478, 1990.

11 Khan Z, Starer P, Bhola A. Urinary incontinence in female Parkinson's disease patients. *Urology,* 33: 486–489, 1989.

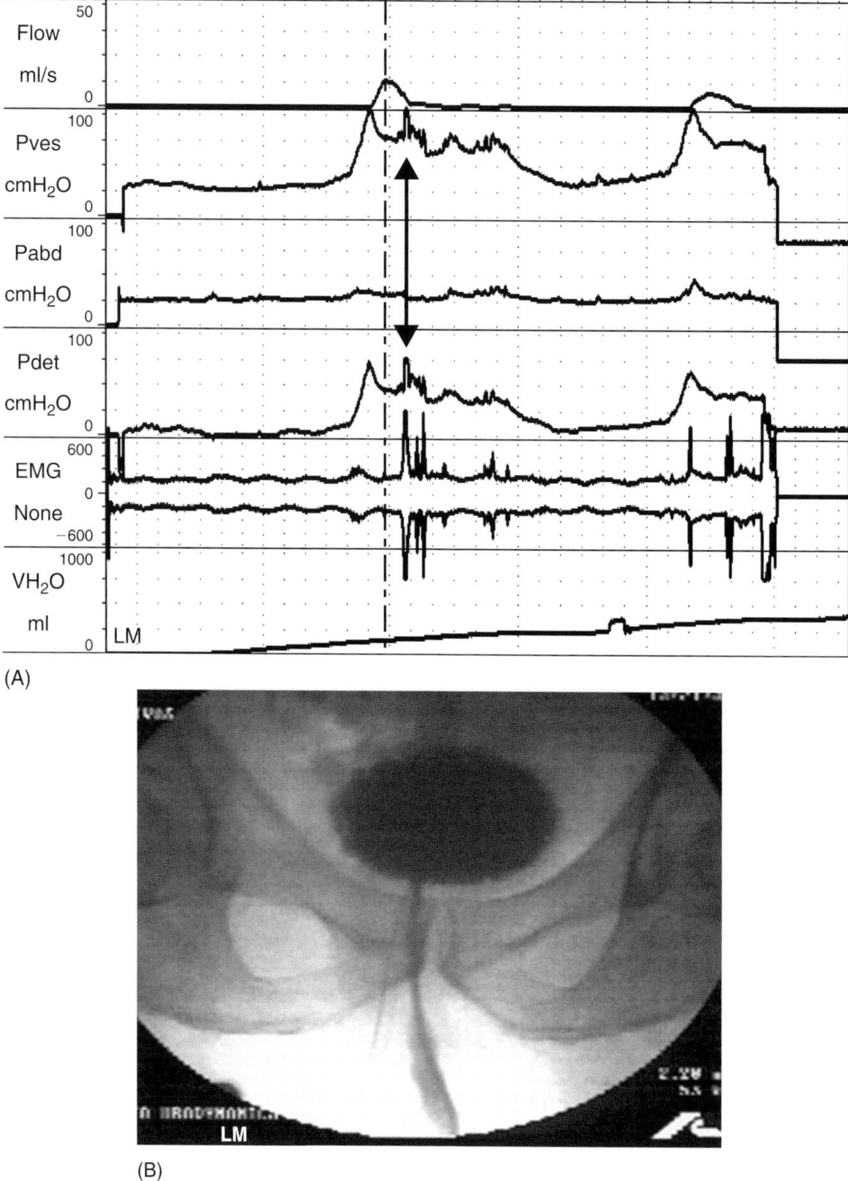

Fig. 13.1 Detrusor hyperreflexia (type 4 detrusor overactivity) due to CVA. LM is a 66-year-old man 3 years after CVA that left him with left hemiparesis and incontinence. (A) Urodynamic tracing. FSF (first sensation of filling) = 155 ml; 1st urge and severe urge = 243 ml. During bladder filling there was a spontaneous involuntary detrusor contraction at a volume of 240 ml. He perceived the contraction as urge, but was not able to contract his sphincter and he voided involuntarily. After the detrusor contraction had almost abated, when the bladder was almost empty, there was an involuntary sphincter contraction that obstructed the urethra and caused a momentary rise in detrusor pressure (arrow). The detrusor contraction continued and the remaining bladder urine was voided with a flow of only about 1 ml/s. Pdet/Q study Q_{max} = 13 ml, Pdet@Q_{max} = 46 cmH_2O (vertical dotted line), and Pdetmax = 77 cmH_2O. This corresponds to a Schafer grade 2 which is not considered to be urethral obstruction. Voided volume = 243 ml and post-void residual = 0 ml. (B) X-ray obtained near the end of micturition shows a normal caliber bulbar urethra. The prostatic urethra seems narrowed, but was wide open on earlier views that are not reproduced here. The bladder has an irregular contour consistent with coarse trabeculations.

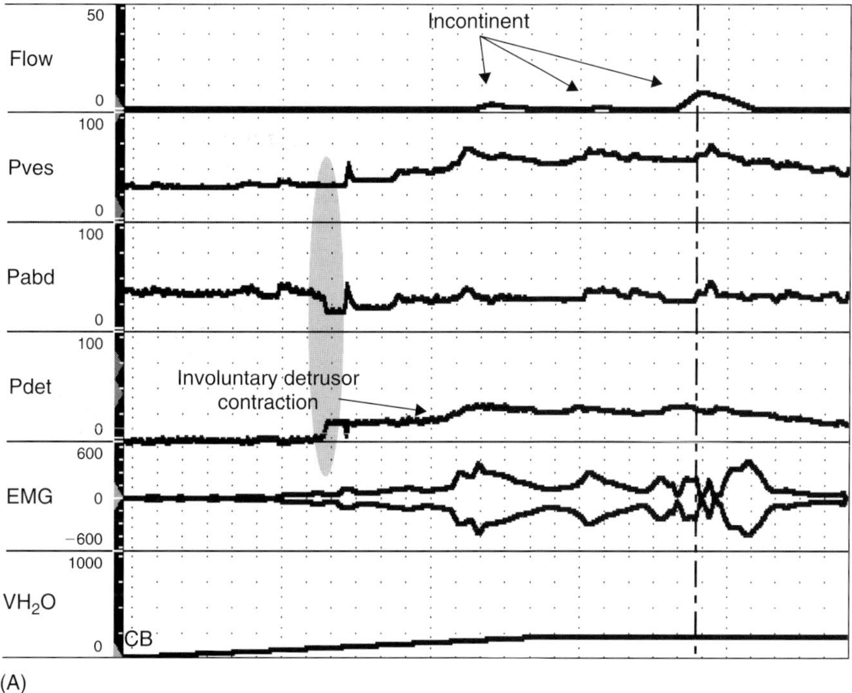

(A)

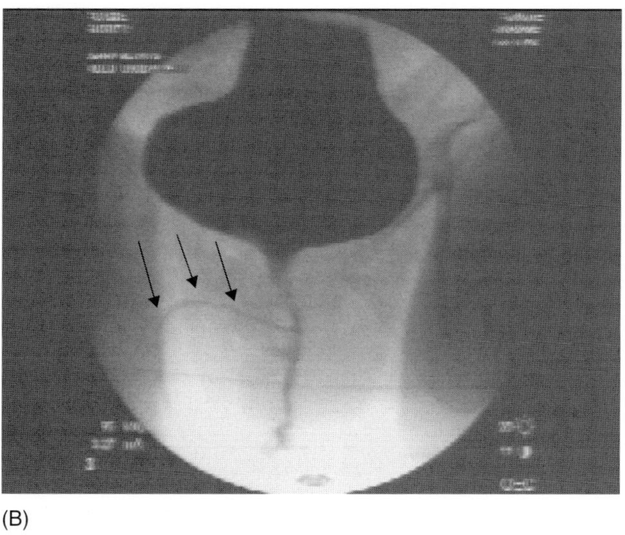

(B)

Fig. 13.2 Detrusor hyperreflexia (type 3 OAB) due to CVA mimicking DESD. CB is a 68-year-old hemiparetic woman due to stroke suffered 2 years earlier. She has no cognitive deficits. Her chief complaint is "I have to go many times during the day but I get there in time; at night, I don't get there in time." A 24-hour voiding diary showed a voided volume = 2,453 ml/15 voids, daytime = 1,403 ml/12 voids, and nighttime = 1,050 ml/3 voids. Maximum voided volume = 330 ml. NPI = 43. She described one urge incontinence episode. Pad test showed 160 g urine loss.

[A] Urodynamic tracing. FSF (first sensation of filling) = 55 ml, 1st urge = 119 ml, and severe urge = 182 ml. At the shaded oval, there is a sudden (artifactual) fall in Pabd that causes a rise in Pdet. There was a spontaneous involuntary detrusor contraction at a volume of 184 ml. She contracted her sphincter repeatedly in an attempt to prevent incontinence, but each time the sphincter fatigued, she voided involuntarily (arrows). Q_{max} = 9 ml/s, Pdet@ Q_{max} = 28 cmH_2O, Pdetmax = 34 cmH_2O, voided volume = 130.4 ml, and post-void residual = 64 ml. (B) X-ray obtained at Q_{max} (vertical dotted line on urodynamic tracing) shows a normal urethra. The arrows point to the urethral catheter. The radiographic contrast seen distal to the bend in the catheter is urine that has been trapped in the vagina.

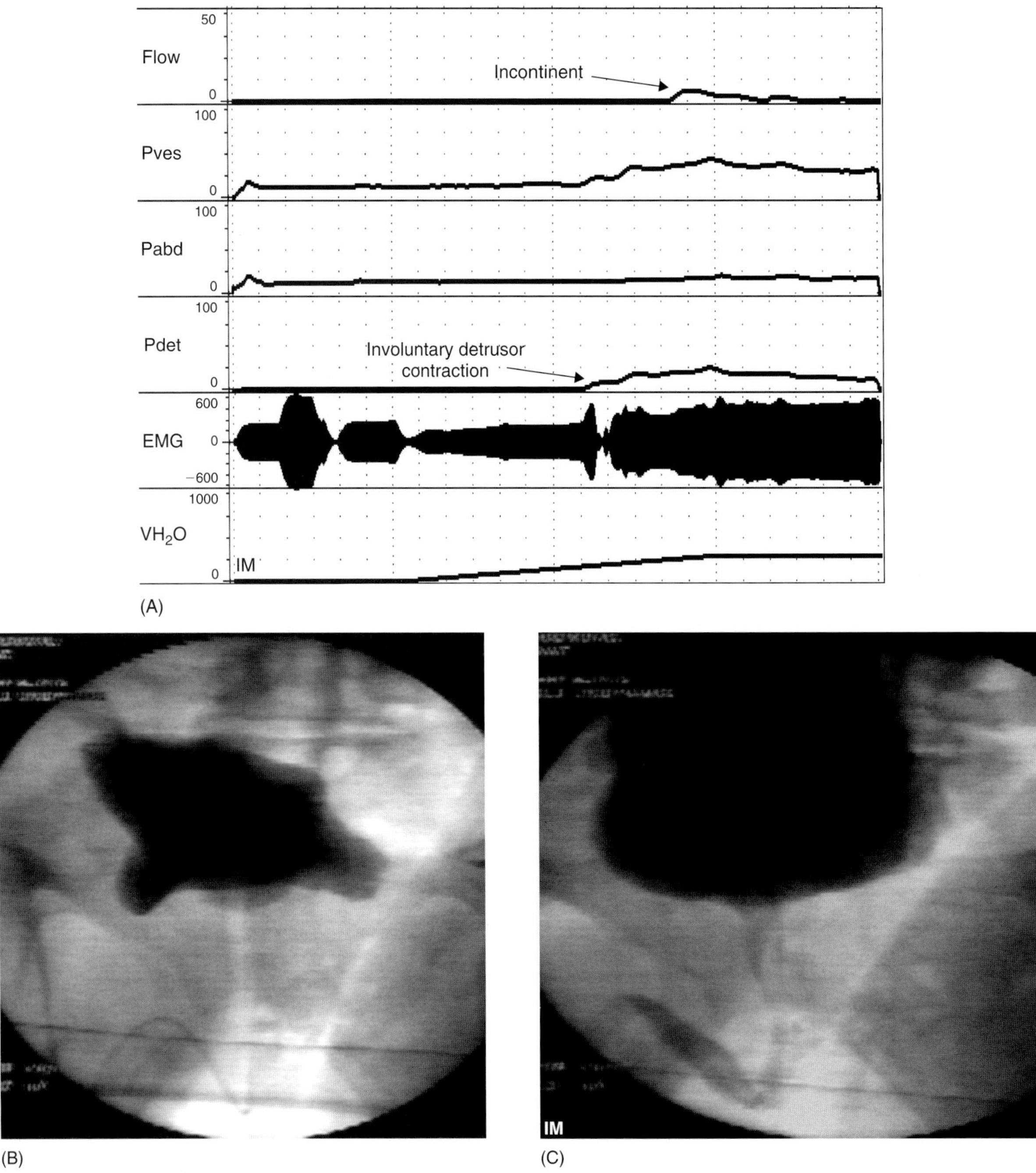

Fig. 13.3 Detrusor hyperreflexia and impaired detrusor contractility associated with CVA. IM is an 82-year-old man who is 4 months status post CVA that resulted in right hemiparesis. There are no cognitive deficits. He complains of urinary frequency, urgency, urge incontinence, and soaks through large pads day and night. (A) Urodynamic study. FSF = 120ml, 1st urge = 228ml, and severe urge = 257ml. At a bladder volume of 269ml there was an involuntary detrusor contraction. He perceived the contraction as urge. He contracted his sphincter and temporarily prevented incontinence, but the detrusor contraction continued and after a short time, he voided involuntarily. Note that there is a disparity between the EMG tracing and pressure flow curves. One would expect that when the EMG becomes silent just after the detrusor contraction occurred, Pdet would fall and voiding ensue. Further, the EMG activity is increased throughout the detrusor contraction, but there appears to be no correlation between the increased EMG activity, uroflow, detrusor pressure, and the radiographic appearance of the urethra. When such a disparity exists, we believe that the EMG is artifact. Q_{max} = 6ml/s, Pdet@Q_{max} = 20cmH_2O, and Pdetmax = 26cmH_2O. According to the Schafer nomogram, this represents a very weak bladder without urethral obstruction. Voided volume = 171ml; PVR = 101ml. (B) X-ray obtained with about 50ml in the bladder. (C) X-ray obtained during voiding at Q_{max} shows poor visualization of the prostatic urethra, but the bulbar and anterior urethra are well seen.

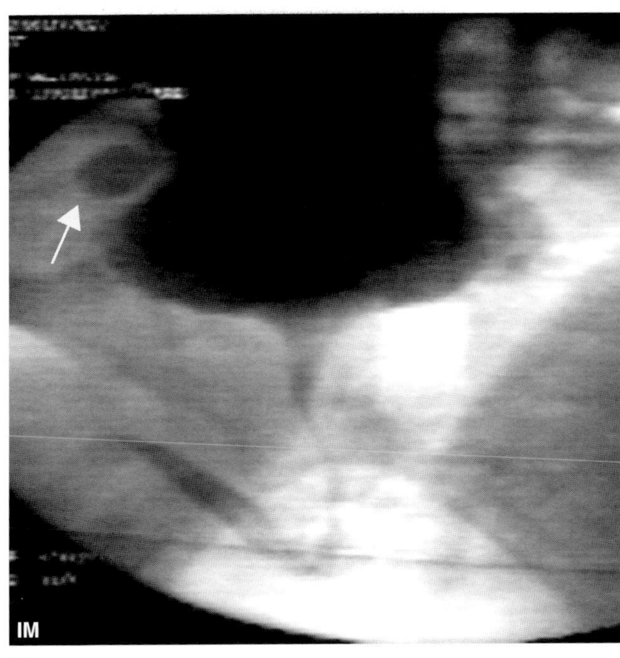

(D)

Fig. 13.3 (continued) (D) X-ray obtained toward the end of micturition. The prostatic urethra is visualized better and a bladder diverticulum is apparent (arrow).

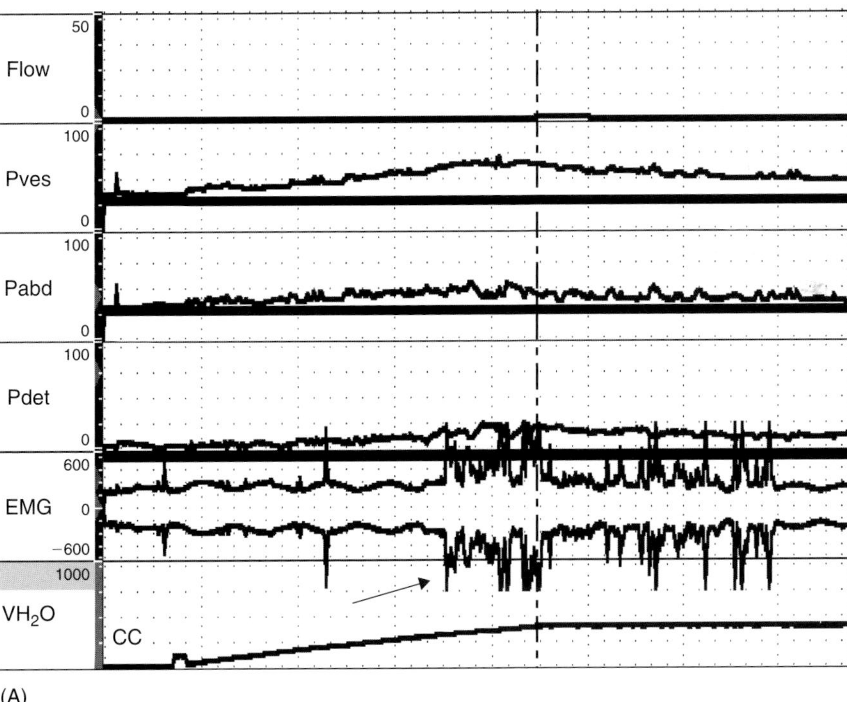

(A)

Fig. 13.4 Detrusor hyperreflexia versus low bladder compliance after CVA. CC is a 79-year-old woman 1 year status post CVA with residual right hemiparesis; 10 years prior she underwent resection of a brain stem meningioma. She complains of urinary frequency, urgency, urge incontinence, and nocturia every hour. (A) Urodynamic tracing. FSF = 291 ml, 1st urge = 334 ml, and severe urge = 402 ml. At the arrow, she contracted her sphincter in an attempt to prevent incontinence, but once she relaxed, she voided involuntarily (vertical dotted line). Once she developed the severe urge, bladder filling was stopped and detrusor pressure declined, but it is not possible to determine from the tracing whether this "voiding" was due to a low magnitude detrusor contraction or low bladder compliance. The vesical and abdominal tracings are difficult to interpret because of multiple rectal contractions. The three black thick horizontal lines on the pressure tracings are intended to visually make it clearer that the gradual rise in vesical pressure is mostly due to increasing detrusor pressure, since there is also a gradual rise in Pabd and also some rectal contractions that make the Pdet tracing difficult to evaluate.

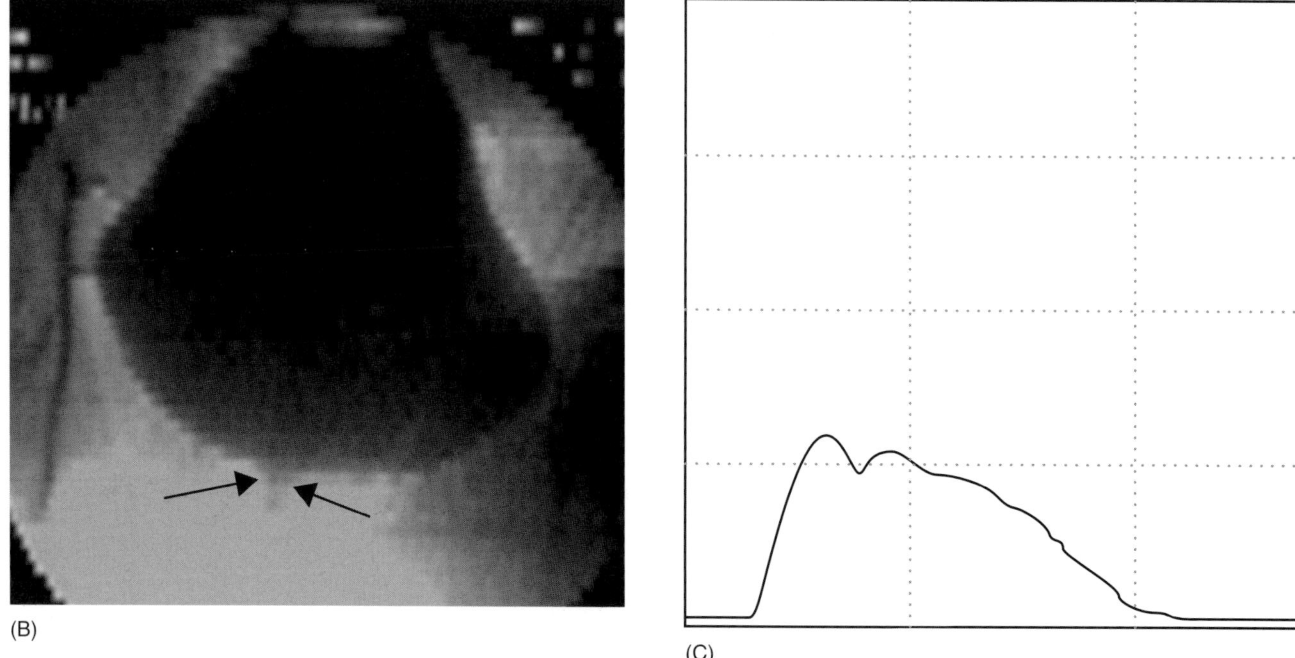

(B)

(C)

Fig. 13.4 (continued) If one considers Pves to approximate Pdet, bladder compliance is low (11 ml/cmH_2O). Unintubated uroflow: Q_{max} = 11 ml/s, voided volume: 127 ml, pattern: descending slope, and PVR = 20 ml. Pressure/flow study: Q_{max} = 7 ml, Pdet@Q_{max} = 7 cmH_2O, Pdetmax = 16 cmH_2O, voided volume = 126 ml, and PVR = 380 ml. (B) X-ray exposed with 350 ml in the bladder, at the arrow on the urodynamic tracing, shows an open vesical neck. (C) Unintubated uroflow immediately after urodynamic study. Q_{max} = 11 ml/s, voided volume = 127 ml, and PVR = 20 ml. **Comment**: This study nicely demonstrates the conundrums that derive when there is a disparity between the clinical and urodynamic findings. CC's history is classic for detrusor hyperreflexia secondary to stroke, but the urodynamic study showed a relatively large capacity bladder, an open bladder neck at rest, and possibly, low bladder compliance, but no involuntary detrusor contractions. These findings suggest a thoracolumbar neurologic lesion. Further, during the urodynamic study, her uroflow was very low and PVR was over 350 ml. After the study, though, she voided with a near normal uroflow and low PVR. To compound things further, her nocturia was proven to be mostly due to nocturnal polyuria. None of these findings explain her OAB symptoms. Treatment comprised behavior modification and late afternoon diuretics for the nocturnal polyuria.

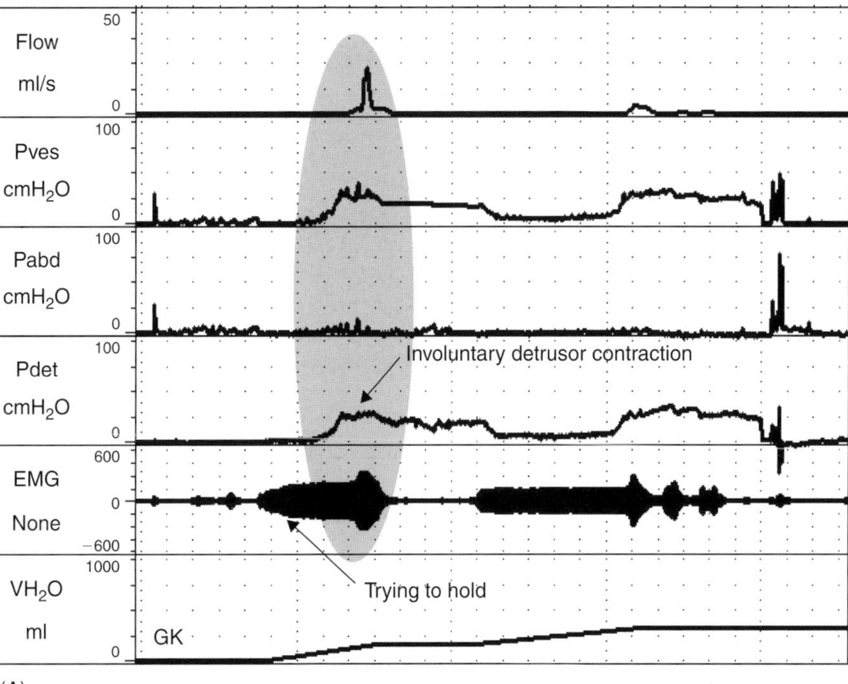

(A)

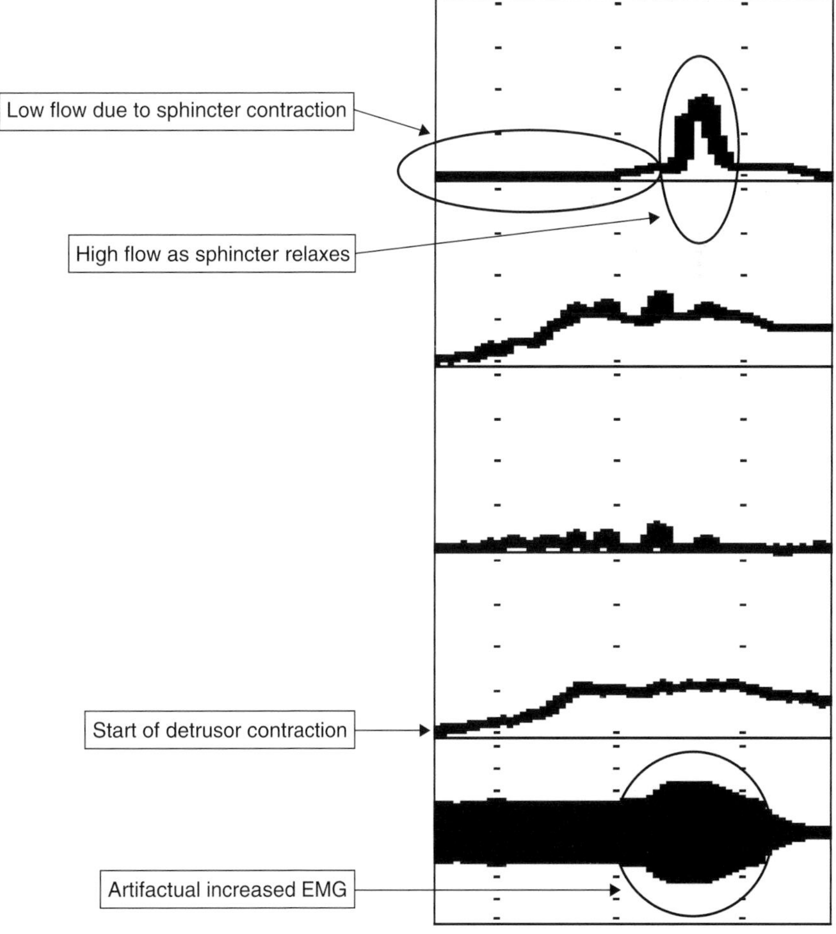

(B)

Fig. 13.5 Detrusor hyperreflexia and "pseudo-dyssynergia" (type 3 OAB) in a woman with Parkinson's disease. GK is a 70-year-old woman: "I wanted to know if I'm a candidate for the tension free vaginal tape (TVT) operation . . . I need something, because I'm always in the bathroom, because I have to go back to urinate . . . I have pressure, most of the time." She voids about 10–12 times a day. "I never really make 2 hours in between, because I feel like I have to go. If I don't go, I can have an accident. I wear a heavy sanitary napkin, which is usually damp; leakage is not one of my main problems, but the urge is, and I think about it all the time." (A) Urodynamic tracing. She perceived an urge to void at about 50 ml and began to contract her sphincter to try to prevent incontinence (arrow). Bladder filling was continued and at a volume of 110 ml she had an involuntary detrusor contraction and voided to completion. Her flow curve begins as a slow rise, then there is a sudden rise in flow, and then a gradual decline again, but throughout this detrusor pressure remains nearly constant. The only explanation for this is a sudden relaxation of her sphincter, yet the EMG activity appears to increase during the increased flow; this must be an artifact (see inset). Later on there is another involuntary detrusor contract and she again contracts her sphincter to try to prevent incontinence but the sphincter contraction is ineffective and she leaks. (B) Enlarged view of the area of interest.

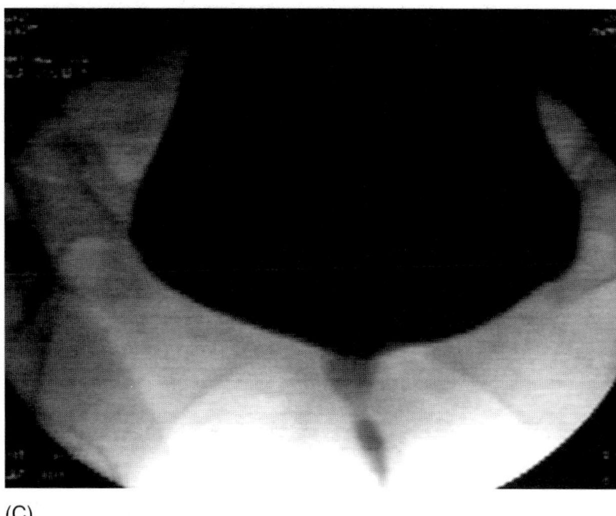

(C)

Fig. 13.5 (continued) (C) X-ray obtained during voiding at Q_{max} (shaded oval in (A)) shows a normal urethra.

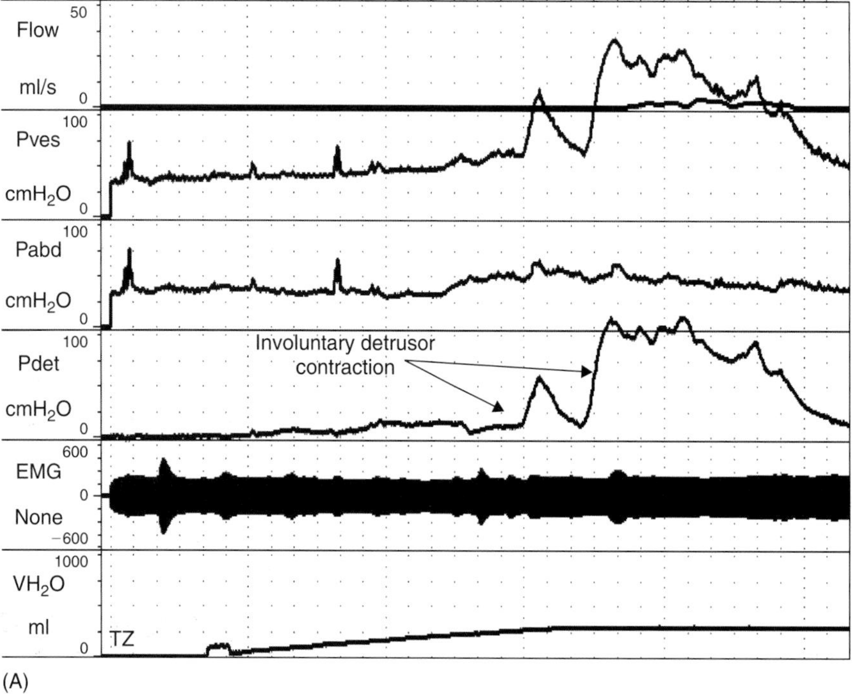

(A)

Fig. 13.6 Sphincter bradykinesia and grade 5 prostatic urethral obstruction in a 65-year-old man with Parkinson's disease. TZ has had Parkinson's disease for about 12 years. He complains of urge incontinence most days (mostly when he's frozen, but he keeps urinary bottles everywhere at home because he won't be able to make it in time). He ordinarily voids more than once an hour during the day and has nocturia about every 1–2 hours at night. He wears absorbent pads most days, and he changes them 2+ times per day and they are wet. His American Urological Association (AUA) symptom score is 20. He's had these symptoms for several years and is treated with tamsulosin and oxybutinin, but doesn't consider symptoms bad enough to require further interventions. (A) Urodynamic tracing. FSF = 177 ml, 1st urge = 194 ml, and severe urge = 277 ml. During bladder filling there was a spontaneous involuntary detrusor contraction at a volume of 277 ml, but little change in EMG activity. This is characteristic of sphincter bradykinesia. Q_{max} = 4.8 ml/s, Pdet@Q_{max} = 95 cmH_2O, Pdetmax = 116 cmH_2O, voided volume = 275 ml, and post-void residual = 30 ml. This corresponds to a Schafer grade 5 urethral obstruction.

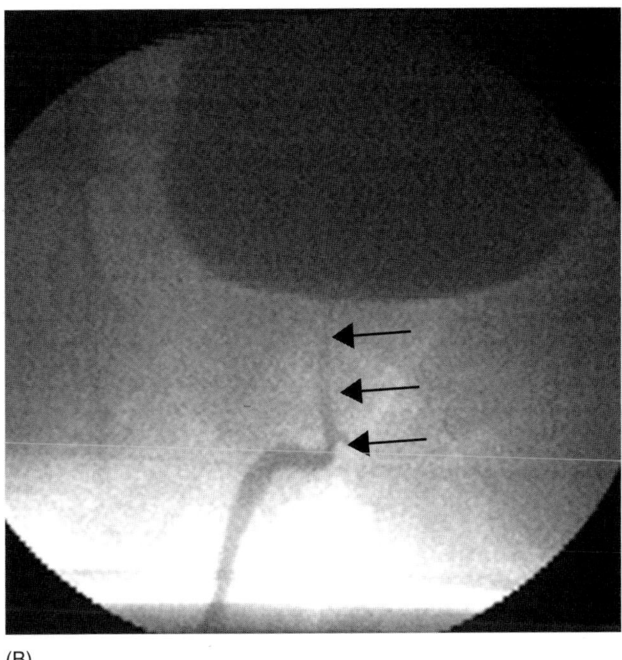

(B)

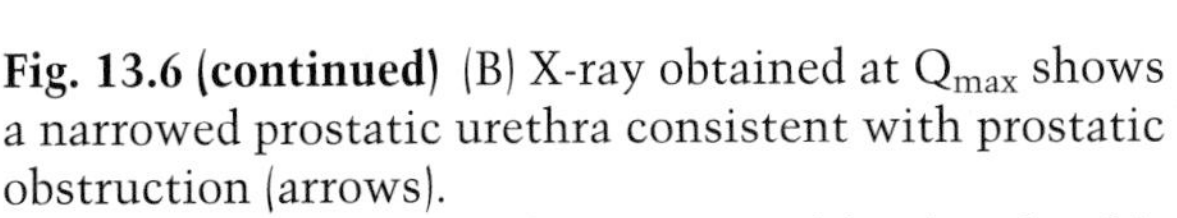

Fig. 13.6 (continued) (B) X-ray obtained at Q_{max} shows a narrowed prostatic urethra consistent with prostatic obstruction (arrows).

Comment: Theoretically, a patient like this should do well after surgery to relieve the prostatic obstruction because he appears to have good voluntary control of his sphincter and can abort the involuntary detrusor contraction and prevent incontinence. In practice, though, the results are not as good in our experience. In many patients there is initial success, but as the Parkinson's disease progresses, they develop urge incontinence due to refractory detrusor overactivity.

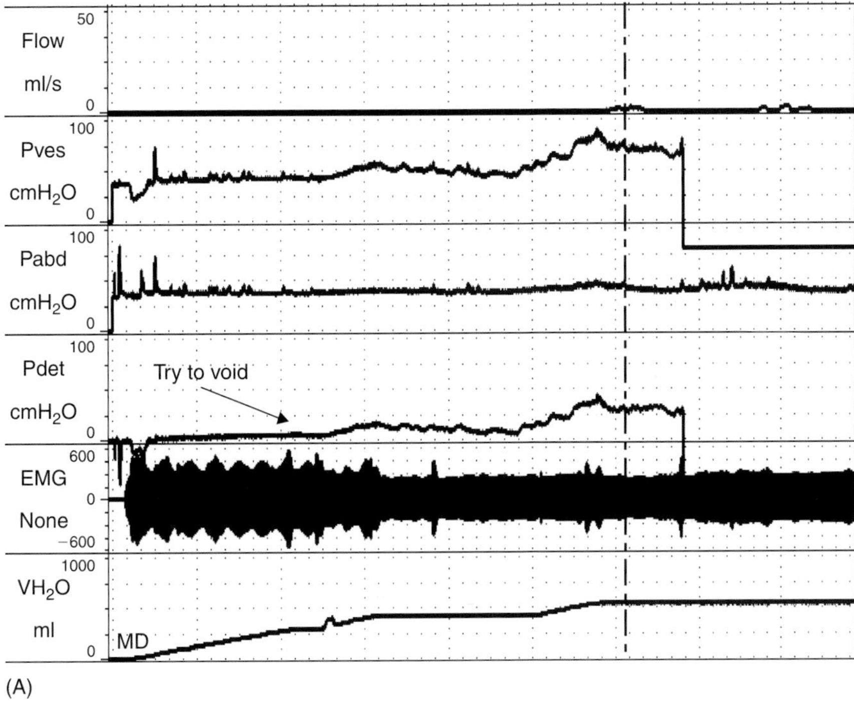

(A)

Fig. 13.7 Impaired detrusor contractility in a 74-year-old man with Parkinson's disease. MD is a 74-year-old man with Parkinson's disease. He underwent transurethral resection of the prostate (TURP) 12 years prior. His chief complaint is feeling of incomplete bladder emptying, weak stream, and hesitancy. He ordinarily voids more than once an hour during the day and has nocturia about every 1–2 hours at night. His American Urological Association (AUA) symptom score is 24. Despite the severity of his symptoms, he did not consider them to be a problem and declined treatment. (A) Urodynamic tracing. FSF = not felt, 1st urge = 106 ml, and severe urge = 265 ml. Bladder capacity was 553 ml. There were no involuntary detrusor contractions. Once he perceived a strong urge to void, he attempted micturition. At first there were sporadic increases in EMG activity, but eventually he appeared to relax his sphincter and had a long, undulating detrusor contraction and eventually voided with a weak flow. Q_{max} = 3 ml/s and Pdet@Q_{max} = 30 cmH_2O (vertical line on urodynamic tracing).

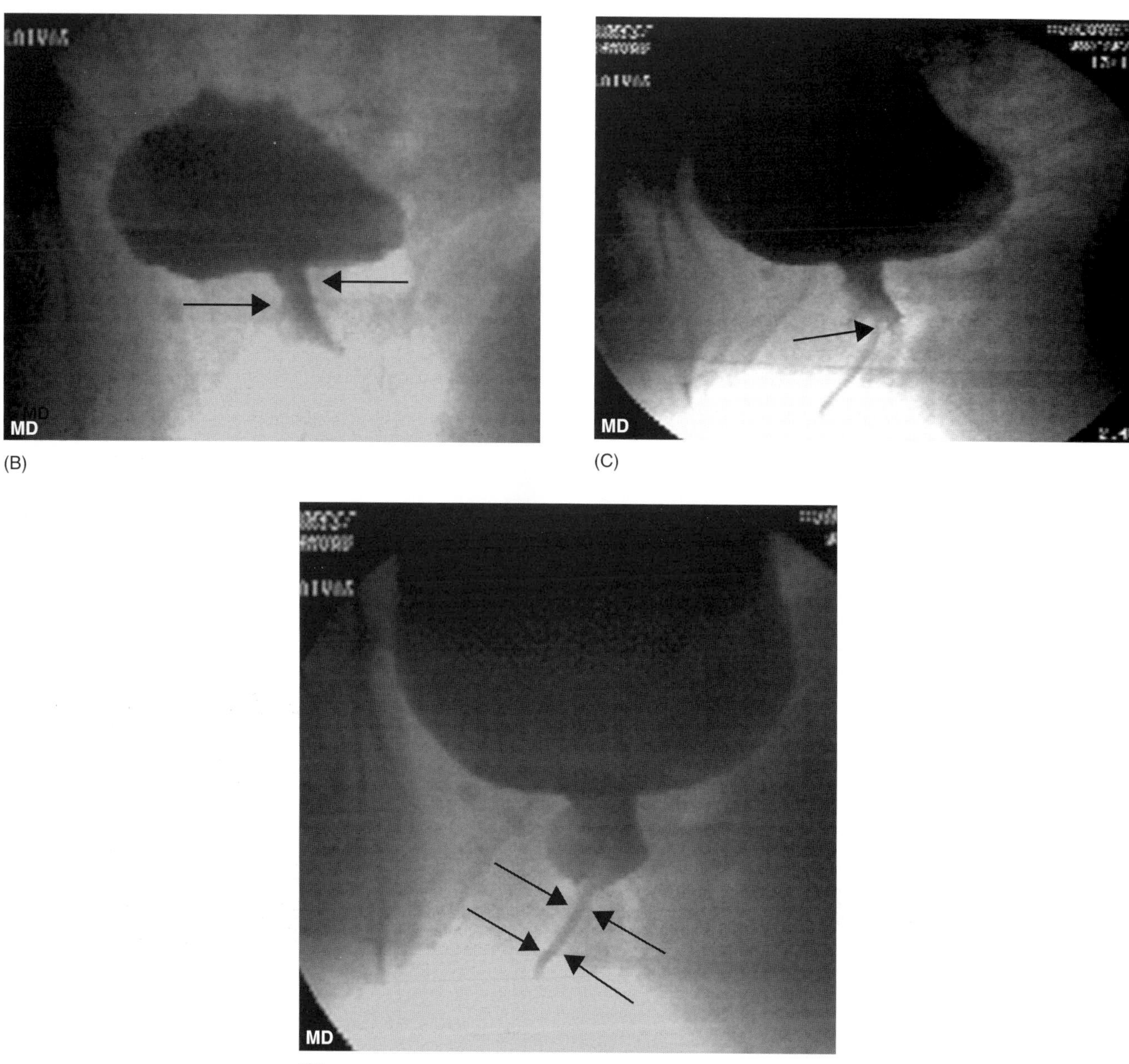

(B) (C) (D)

Fig. 13.7 (continued) This corresponds to a very weak detrusor contraction on the Schafer nomogram. Voided volume = 220 ml and PVR = 325 ml. After removal of the urodynamic catheter, he voided again, also with a very low flow (arrow), but subsequently an unintubated uroflow showed: Q_{max} = 10 ml/s, voided volume = 148 ml, pattern: prolonged, and PVR = 0 ml. (B) X-ray exposed with 50 ml in the bladder shows a TURP defect (contrast in the entire prostatic urethra) (arrows). (C) With further bladder filling, contrast is seen all the way down to the verumontanum (arrow). (D) X-ray exposed at Q_{max} (vertical dotted line on urodynamic tracing) shows a dilated prostatic urethra and a narrowed membranous and bulbar urethra (arrows). In the setting of impaired detrusor contractility, it is not possible to determine whether this represents urethral obstruction, unless a micturitional pressure profile is done. From a radiologic view, this is the classic appearance of DESD.

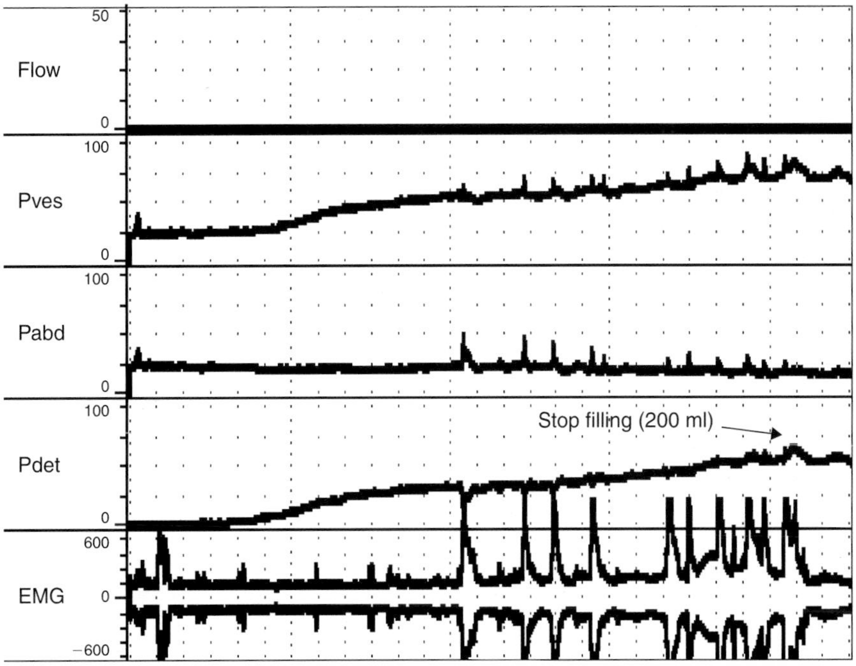

Fig. 13.8 Typical urodynamic study in Shy–Drager syndrome showing detrusor areflexia, low bladder compliance, and open bladder neck at rest. A Urodynamic tracing. During bladder filling, there is a steep rise in detrusor pressure and when filling is stopped, Pdet falls showing that this due to low bladder compliance and not a detrusor contraction. The sporadic bursts of EMG activity are movement artifacts as each burst is accompanied by an increase in Pabd and Pves.

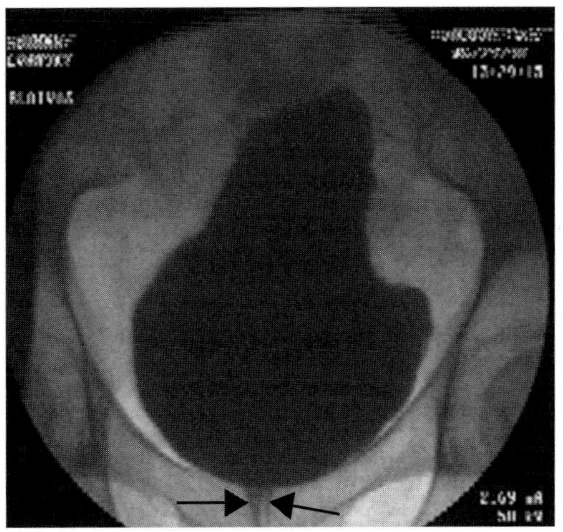

Fig. 13.9 X-ray shows an open bladder neck with 175 ml at the bladder (arrows).

Spinal Cord Injury, Multiple Sclerosis, and Diabetes Mellitus

14

Despite the logic that would dictate otherwise, the correlation between the anatomic pattern of neurologic pathology and underlying pathophysiology is too unreliable to permit diagnosis and treatment of neurogenic bladder without urodynamic testing [1,2]. Urodynamic patterns in neurogenic bladder have been described in Chapter 12, Neurogenic Bladder. Herein, we discuss three specific neurologic disorders, all of which can result in similar urodynamic abnormalities.

Spinal cord injury

Spinal cord injury (SCI) has a prevalence of 2.3/100,000 populations in the USA. Historically, urologic complications were the main cause of death, but with modern treatment of SCI, life expectancy is nearly normal. The recognition that high detrusor pressures are the major cause of urologic complications is a key reason for the improved survival. Life-long urologic surveillance is a central component to the care of the SCI patient.

The clinical course of SCI begins with spinal shock, which is followed by a recovery phase, and a final phase during which there are no further neurologic changes.

Spinal shock

Immediately after SCI, there is usually a period of spinal shock during which there is a flaccid paralysis and absence of reflex activity below the level of the lesion with the single exception of the bulbocavernosus reflex which usually remains intact. The duration of spinal shock is very variable. In most instances, reflex detrusor activity reappears after 2–12 weeks, but in some cases it may not return for as long as 6–12 months. During the period of spinal shock the bladder is areflexic and the patient develops urinary retention. Urodynamic evaluation is generally not necessary at this stage and optimal management is intermittent catheterization.

Recovery stage

The recovery stage is heralded by the return of reflex activity. Although the level of the neurologic lesion cannot predict the pathophysiology with certainty, most patients after cervical and/or thoracic injury develop detrusor hyperreflexia and most of these have detrusor–external sphincter dyssynergia (DESD). The pattern after lumbar injuries is quite variable, but most patients after sacral injuries develop detrusor areflexia. Occasionally patients with cervical or thoracic lesions develop detrusor areflexia. Some of these patients have occult secondary lower motor neuron lesions, but in others the cause is never found. Urodynamic studies are useful at this stage, particularly if high detrusor pressures are found as that may influence treatment.

Stable phase

Once there is no longer any sign of any neurologic recovery, a fairly stable urodynamic pattern ensues. However, even at this stage, over time a number of other conditions may emerge which require specific treatment depending upon the underlying cause. It is for this reason that a lifetime of urologic surveillance is necessary. For example, patients with detrusor areflexia may over the course of time, develop low bladder compliance and those with DESD may develop secondary bladder neck or prostatic obstruction. Treatment is dependent upon an accurate urodynamic assessment. Of particular importance is uncovering urodynamic risk factors, which, without proper treatment, lead to significant upper tract complications including hydronephrosis, vesicoureteral reflux, stones, infection and, ultimately, renal failure. These risk factors include low bladder compliance, DESD, and severe bladder outlet obstruction.

The most common urodynamic finding in suprasacral SCI is DESD (Figs. 14.1–14.3). In thoracolumbar lesions, the effect on micturition is variable (Figs. 14.4 and 14.5).

Autonomic dysreflexia

Autonomic dysreflexia is an exaggerated sympathetic neural response to afferent stimulation that is unique to patients with spinal injury above the level of the level of sympathetic outflow (approximately T6). The symptoms include headache, sweating, flushing, sudden and severe hypertension, and reflex bradycardia. Bladder or bowel distension is the most common precipitating event but a number of other noxious stimuli may precipitate the condition including urinary tract infection, bladder stones, bedsores, ingrown toenails, osteomyelitis, and even micturition itself (particularly in patients with bladder neck obstruction). Any of these conditions may cause sympathetic discharges, which causes reflex vasoconstriction. This results in systemic hypertension. The carotid body senses the rise in blood pressure and reflex vagal discharge causes vasodilation and bradycardia as part of the normal homeostatic mechanism to lower blood pressure. However, if the neural signal cannot traverse the SCI, vasoconstriction persists below the level of the neurologic lesion and the hypertension persists because compensatory this mechanisms are ineffective. Vasodilation above the level of the lesion results in profuse sweating, flushing, and "goose bumps." Immediate treatment is necessary to remove the noxious stimulus.

Most patients with autonomic dysreflexia know exactly what triggers it and they usually develop a prodrome several minutes to several seconds before the onset of clinical symptoms. Moreover, the symptoms usually subside within seconds to minutes after removing the precipitating cause (in this instance it is usually the full bladder that causes symptoms; emptying the bladder results in cessation of the dysreflexia). Thus, it is possible in most instances to complete the urodynamic investigation without subjecting the patient to severe symptoms. Patients whose injury is at or above T6 level and those with a history of autonomic dysreflexia should have their blood pressure monitored during lower urinary tract instrumentation. Emergency medication should be available if autonomic dysreflexia persists after emptying the bladder and removing the catheters such as nifedipine 10mg sublingually, chlorpromazine 1mg IV, and phentolamine 5mg IV may be needed to abort a life-threatening autonomic dysreflexia episode. If during bladder filling or manipulation the patient complains of dysreflexia symptoms and the blood pressure is dangerously high, the bladder should be emptied immediately. If the patient does not state that the symptoms are subsiding within about 30–60 seconds, the catheters should be removed and if there is still no response, one of the above medications should be administered. If emptying the bladder is effective, it is possible to resume the urodynamic study at a slow filling rate, monitoring the patient carefully.

Multiple sclerosis

Multiple sclerosis is caused by focal inflammatory and demyelinating lesions scattered throughout the nervous system. This leads to a wide variety of neurologic signs and symptoms. The incidence is approximately 10 new cases per 100,000 people between the ages of 20 and 50 years in the USA, but there are wide regional variations. MS is more common in women than men and usually begins between the second and fifth decade of life. In approximately 60% of the patients, the disease is manifest by exacerbations and remissions. The clinical course is described as acute, progressive, chronic, and benign.

Some type of bladder dysfunction is seen in nearly all patients during the course of their disease. As with the other conditions in this chapter, there is generally a rather poor correlation between the patient's urologic symptoms, neurologic abnormalities, and urodynamic findings. Even patients without overt urologic symptoms can have underlying urologic pathology.

Both voiding symptoms and urodynamic findings may change over the course of time. Wheeler and coworkers noted that 55% of patients had different urodynamic findings after repeat examination. Blaivas and associates found 15% of patients had markedly different urodynamic findings upon repeat studies. The most important conditions which predispose patients with MS to grave urologic complications are: (1) detrusor-external sphincter dyssynergia in men; (2) low bladder compliance and high detrusor filling pressure (>40 cmH_2O); and (3) presence of an indwelling catheter.

The most common urodynamic pattern in MS is detrusor hyperreflexia, which occurs in 50–99% of patients (Fig. 14.6). In up to 50% of patients with detrusor hyperreflexia DESD is also documented (Figs. 14.7–14.9). Detrusor areflexia and/or impaired detrusor contractility, is seen in 20–30% of cases (Fig. 14.10). Unfortunately, while straining increases intraabdominal and intravesical pressure, many patients are unable to relax the external sphincter and this causes a functional obstruction which results in incomplete voiding or complete urinary retention.

Diabetic neurogenic bladder

The prevalence of diabetes mellitus is estimated to be 1–2% of the population of the USA, or 1,000–2,000 per 100,000 populations. Autonomic neuropathy is common and it has been proposed that such neuropathy is a major cause of lower urinary tract symptoms (LUTS). However, coexisting urologic conditions, such as benign prostatic hyperplasia (BPH), overactive bladder (OAB), and stress incontinence may also cause symptoms.

Diabetic cystopathy is characterized by decreased bladder sensation that leads to increasing intervoiding intervals which, in turn, causes increased bladder capacity. The bladder eventually becomes overstretched causing impaired detrusor contractility, culminating in detrusor areflexia, and incomplete bladder emptying (Fig 14.11). It is thought that the primary pathologic process causing the neuropathy is a metabolic derangement of the Schwann cell that results in segmental demyelinization and impairment of nerve conduction.

For many years, it was thought that diabetic cystopathy was the most common finding in patients with diabetes mellitus [3,4]. In Frimodt-Moller's study, 25–50% of unselected patients with diabetes mellitus had evidence of diabetic cystopathy and in routine urodynamic studies of unselected diabetic patients, diabetic cystopathy has been reported to occur in 27–85%, but our study does not support that data.

However, other studies have shown detrusor overactivity to be much more common. In one study, of 182 patients with diabetes mellitus who underwent urodynamic study because of LUTS, 55% had detrusor overactivity, 23% had impaired detrusor contractility, 11% had indeterminate findings, 10% had detrusor areflexia, and 1% was normal. Bladder outlet obstruction occurred in 36%, all of who were men [2]. Figure 14.12 depicts a type 1 diabetic man with detrusor hyperreflexia and prostatic urethral obstruction.

Suggested Reading

1 AMIS ES Jr, BLAIVAS Jg: Neurogenic Bladder Simplified. RAD Clin. N. America 29(3):571–80, 1991.

2 Kaplan SA, Chancellor MB and Blaivas Jg: Bladder and Sphincter behavior in patients with spinal cord lesions. J. Urol 146(1):113–7, 1991.

3 Frimodt-Moller C. Diabetic cystopathy. I. A clinical study on the frequency of bladder dysfunction in diabetics, *Dan Med Bull*, 23: 267, 1976.

4 Frimodt-Moller C, Oleson KP. Diabetic cystopathy. IV. Micturition cystourethrography compared with urodynamic investigation, *Dan Med Bull*, 23: 291, 1976.

5 Anderson RU. Urodynamic patterns after acute spinal cord injury: association with bladder trabeculation in male patients, *J Urol*, 129: 777, 1983.

6 Arnold EP, Fukui J, Anthony A, Utley WLF. Bladder function following spinal cord injury: a urodynamic analysis of the outcome, *Br J Urol*, 56: 172, 1984.

7 Blaivas JG, Barbalias GA. Detrusor external sphincter dyssynergia in men with multiple sclerosis: an ominous urologic condition, *J Urol*, 131: 94, 1984.

8 Blaivas JG. The neurophysiology of micturition: a clinical study of 550 patients, *J Urol*, 127: 958, 1982.

9 DiBlasio C, Weiss JP, Blaivas JG, Tash JA, Gerboc J. Diabetes and LUTS: dispelling the myth, *J Urol*, 169 (4, Suppl): 374, 2003.

10 Hackler RH, Hall NM, Zampieri TA. Bladder hypocompliance in the spinal cord injury population, *J Urol*, 141: 1390, 1989.

11 Kaplan SA, Chancellor MB, Blaivas JG. Bladder and sphincter behavior in patients with spinal cord lesions, *J Urol*, 146: 113, 1991.

12 Killorin W, Gray M, Bennett JK, et al. The value of urodynamic and bladder management in predicting upper urinary tract complications in male spinal cord injury patients, *Paraplegia*, 30: 427–430, 1992.

13 Light JK, Faganel J, Beric A. Detrusor areflexia in suprasacral spinal cord injuries, *J Urol*, 134: 295, 1985.

14 McGuire EJ, Woodside JR, Borden TA, et al. Prognostic value of urodynamic testing in myelodysplasic patients, *J Urol*, 126: 205–209, 1981.

15 McGuire EJ, Noll F, Maynard F. A pressure management system for the neurogenic bladder after spinal cord injury, *Neurourol Urodynam*, 10: 223, 1991.

16 McGuire EJ, Savastano JA. Urodynamics and management of the neuropathic bladder in spinal cord injury patients, *J Am Paraplegia Soc*, 8: 28–32, 1985.

17 Ruutu M. Cystometrographic patterns in predicting bladder function after spinal cord injury, *Paraplegia*, 23: 243, 1985.

18 Weld KJ, Graney MJ, Dmochowski RR. Differences in bladder compliance with time and associations of bladder management with compliance in spinal cord injured patients, *J Urol*, 163(4): 1228–1233, 2000.

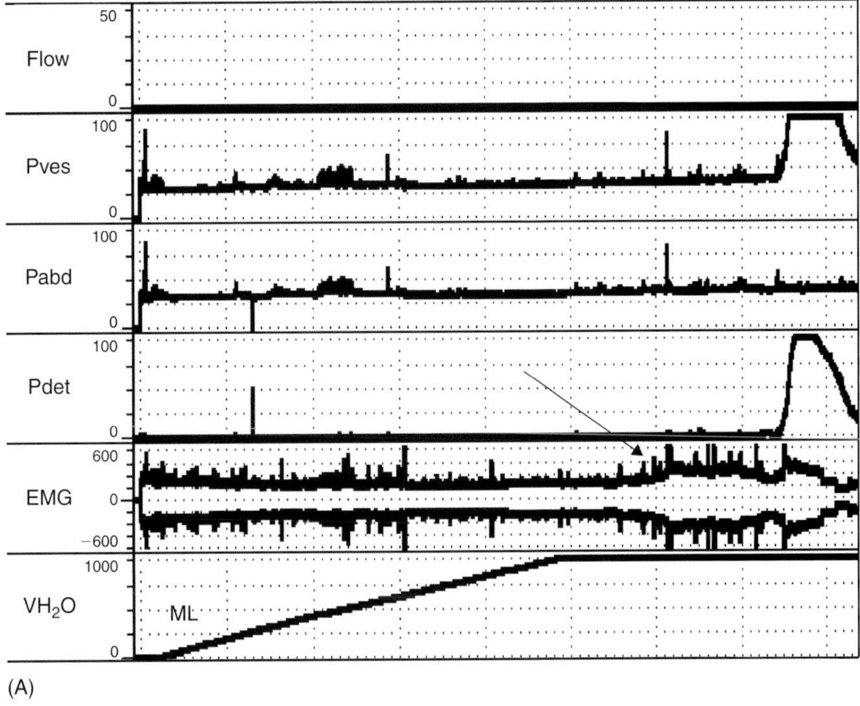

(A)

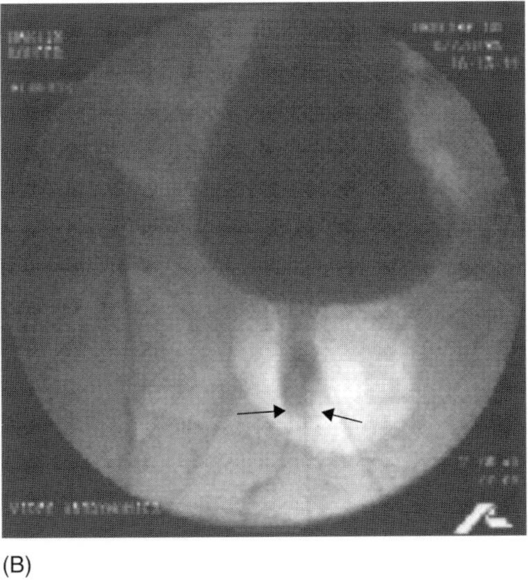

(B)

Fig. 14.1 (A) DESD. This is a classic urodynamic tracing of DESD – an involuntary contraction of the striated sphincter that precedes and continues throughout the involuntary detrusor contraction. The increased electromyography (EMG) activity (arrow), that proxies for the sphincter contraction, begins long before the onset of the involuntary detrusor contraction. The flat line at the peak of the Pves and Pdet tracings is caused by a preset computer cutoff than can be switched on or off. Actual Pdetmax=115 cmH_2O. The bladder volume at which the detrusor contraction occurred in this patient (1,000 ml) is unusual. Most patients with DESD have a much smaller bladder capacity. (B) X-ray obtained at Pdetmax shows the classic picture of DESD – complete obstruction at the membranous urethra (arrows) and a trabeculated bladder, described as a "Christmas tree" shaped bladder.

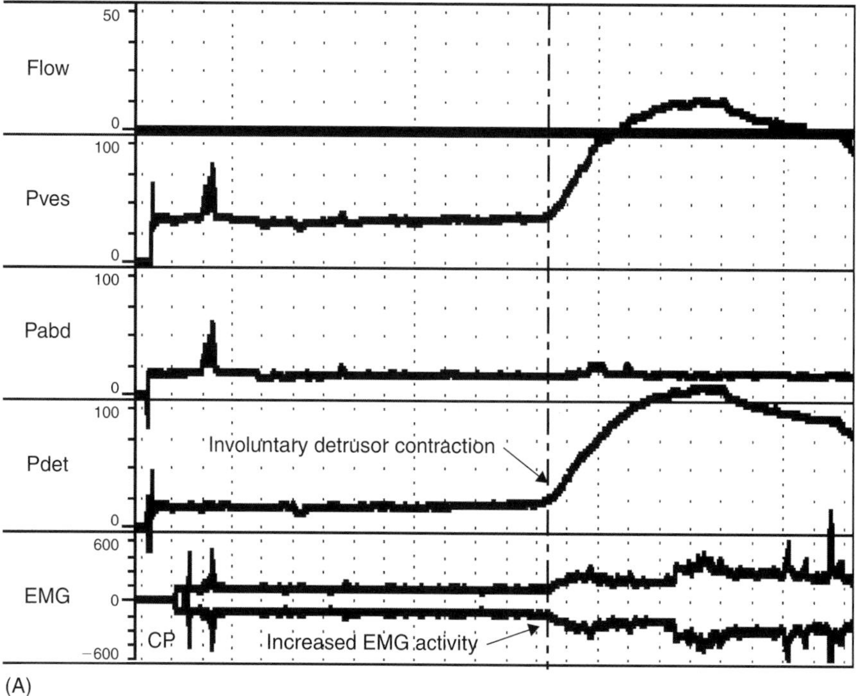

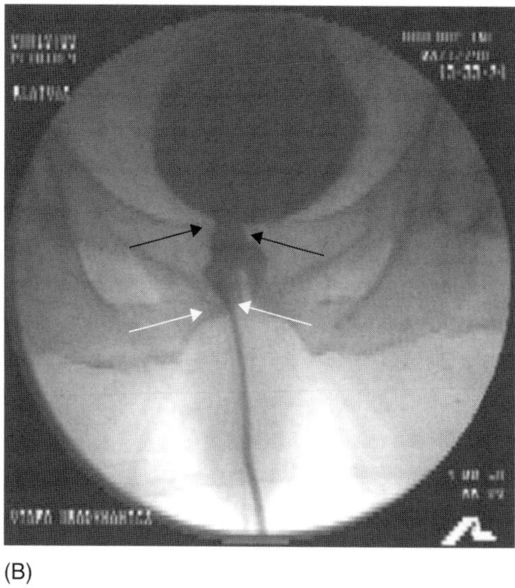

Fig. 14.2 DESD and mild bladder neck obstruction. CP is a 67-year-old male paraplegic caused by an arteriovenous malformation at T6. (A) Urodynamic tracing. Note that the increase in EMG activity occurs just prior to the onset of the detrusor contraction. (B) The prostatic urethra is dilated and completely obstructed at the membranous urethra by the involuntary sphincter contraction (white arrows). In addition, though, there is narrowing of the bladder neck and proximal urethra (black arrows) suggestive of secondary bladder neck or prostatic obstruction.

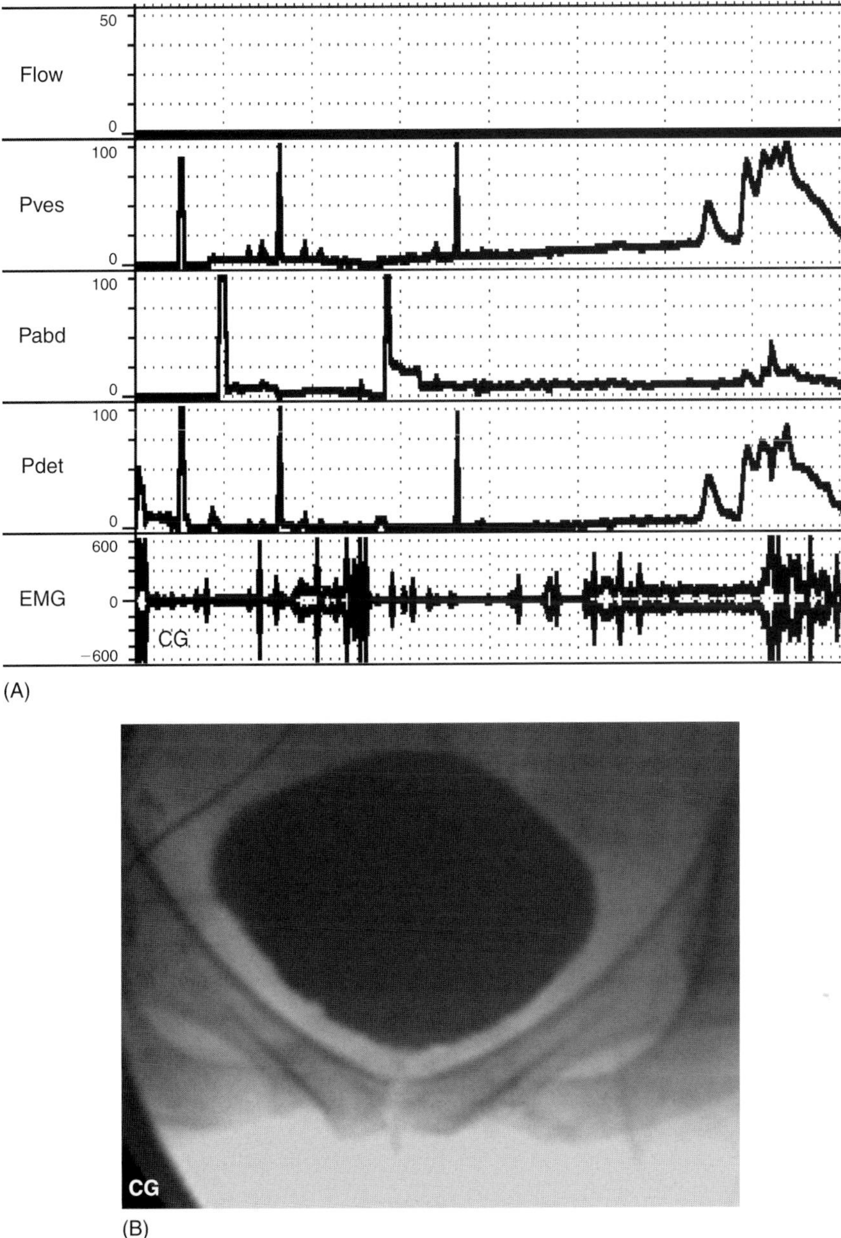

Fig. 14.3 DESD and bladder neck obstruction in a 17-year-old paraplegic woman due to a traumatic incomplete T7 SCI suffered in a motor vehicle accident 4 years earlier. She had been treated with intermittent self-catheterization but had incontinence refractory to anticholinergics. (A) Urodynamic tracing. At a bladder volume of 125 ml, there is a sustained involuntary detrusor contraction (Pdetmax = 90 cmH_2O). During the detrusor contraction, there is a marked increase in EMG activity consistent with a diagnosis of DESD. However, the increased EMG activity occurs long after the onset of the detrusor contraction. This is not typical. Usually, in DESD, the increased EMG activity occurs before or synchronous with the detrusor contraction. This may be an artifact when surface EMG electrodes are used instead of needle electrodes. There are three types of DESD associated with increasingly complete neurologic lesions. Type 1 is where the EMG is active for the first part of the involuntary detrusor contraction, then quiets after reaching peak detrusor pressure. In type 2 DESD, there is sporadic EMG activity throughout the detrusor contraction. In type 3 DESD, the EMG is continuously active (in a crescendo–decrescendo pattern) throughout the contraction, constituting the most dangerous variety of DESD associated with the highest detrusor pressures. (B) X-ray exposed at Pdetmax shows no contrast at all in the urethra. The likeliest cause is synchronous bladder neck obstruction and DESD. It is possible, albeit unproven, that in this patient the striated urethral musculature extends all the way to the vesical neck.

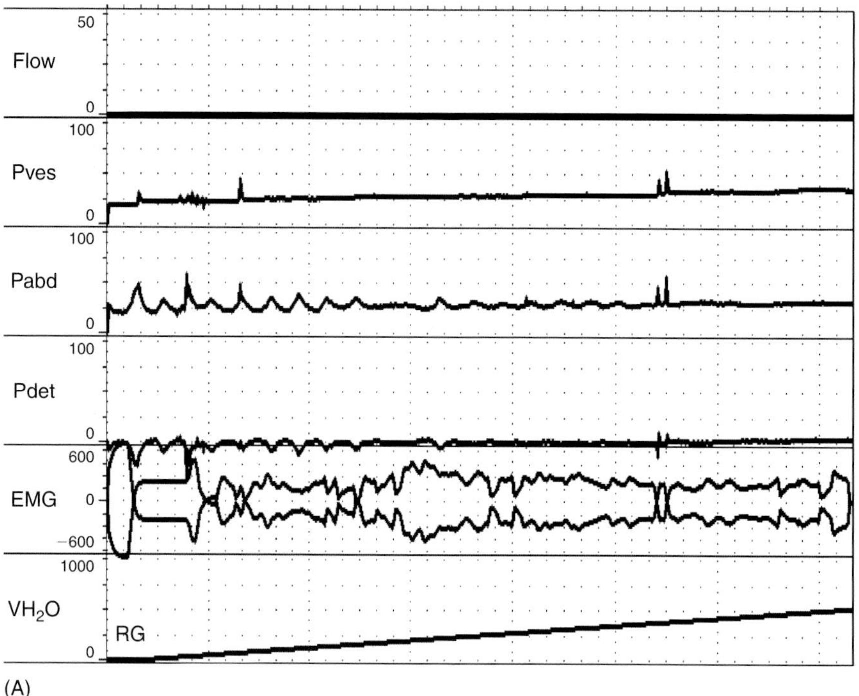

(A)

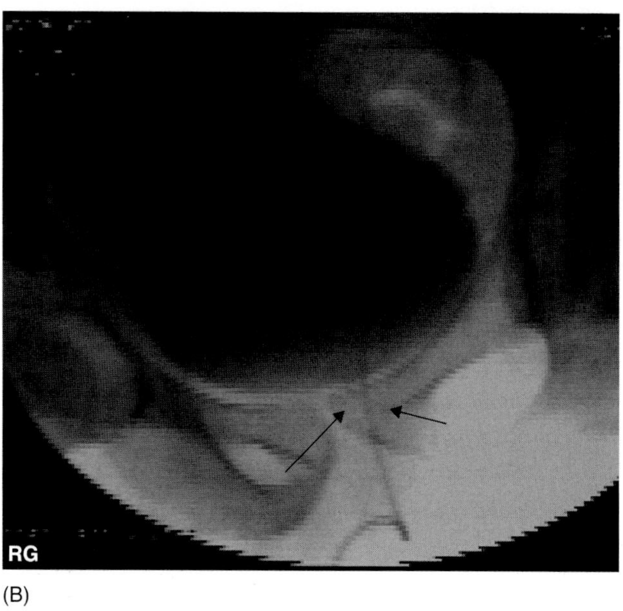

(B)

Fig. 14.4 Detrusor areflexia in a 22-year-old paraplegic man. He sustained a T12 (level) incomplete SCI in an auto-accident 6 years previously. He was initially treated with intermittent self-catheterization, but discontinued it about 4 years ago when he began to void (only by straining). On examination, anal sphincter tone and control are absent and the bulbocavernosus reflex is absent, but perianal sensation is intact. (A) Urodynamic tracing. FSF (first sensation of filling)=431 ml, first and severe urge=518 ml. He was asked to void but was unable to generate a detrusor contraction. (B) X-ray obtained at bladder capacity shows a closed vesical neck (arrows).

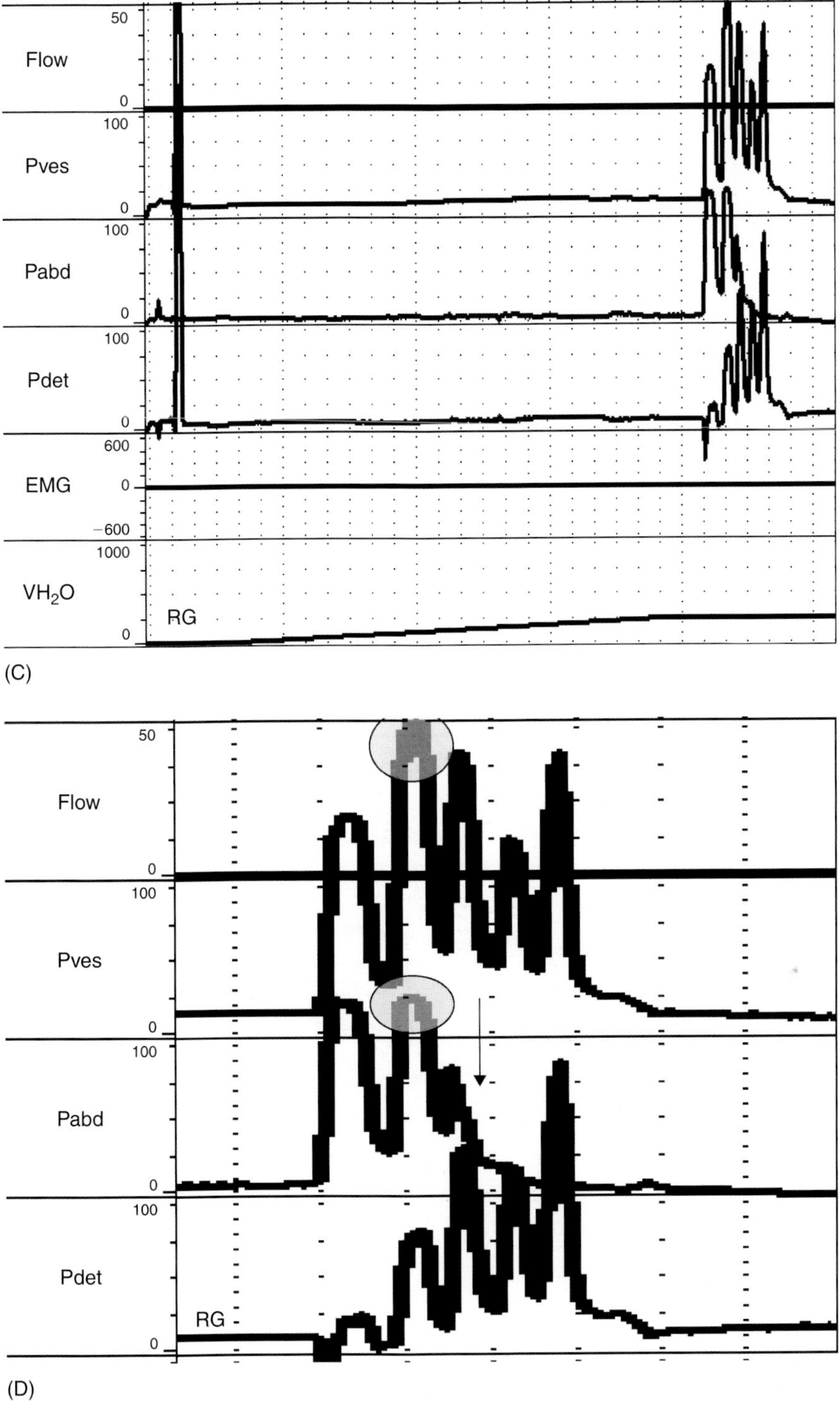

Fig. 14.4 (continued) (C) Repeat urodynamic tracing 1 year later again shows an areflexic bladder, but this time he is asked to void in his usual fashion and he strains to vesical pressures of nearly 200 cmH_2O. He voided with a strong stream, but uroflow was not measured as he was supine. During voiding there are artifactual increases in Pdet (see Fig. 14.4(D)). The EMG tracing was not used in this study. (D) The artifactual rise in detrusor pressure is likely due to a phenomenon called damping, presumably due to tiny air bubbles in the Pabd tubing or transducer. The net effect is that the spikes of pressure are not fully recorded. This is evident in the shaded ovals that show a flattened appearance in the Pabd tracing compared to the spikes in the Pves tracing. The net effect is that the Pabd pressure is artifactually lower than Pves resulting in an artifactual increase in Pdet. At the arrow, the Pabd catheter begins to slip out of the rectum. Once this happens, Pabd is no longer recorded and Pdet is (artifactually) equal to Pves.

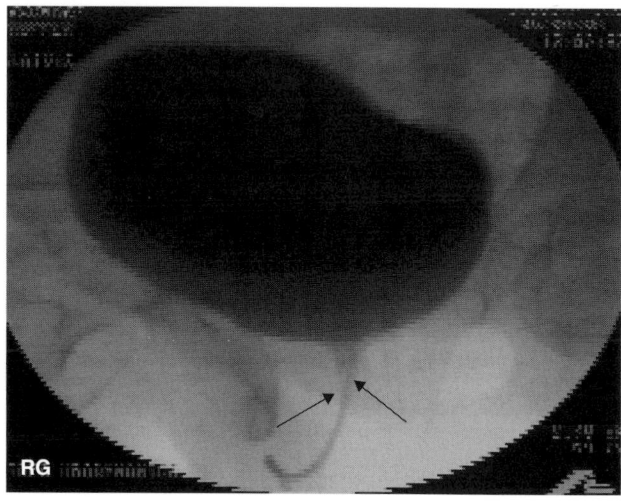

(E)

Fig. 14.4 (continued) (E) During voiding, the bladder neck opens (arrows).

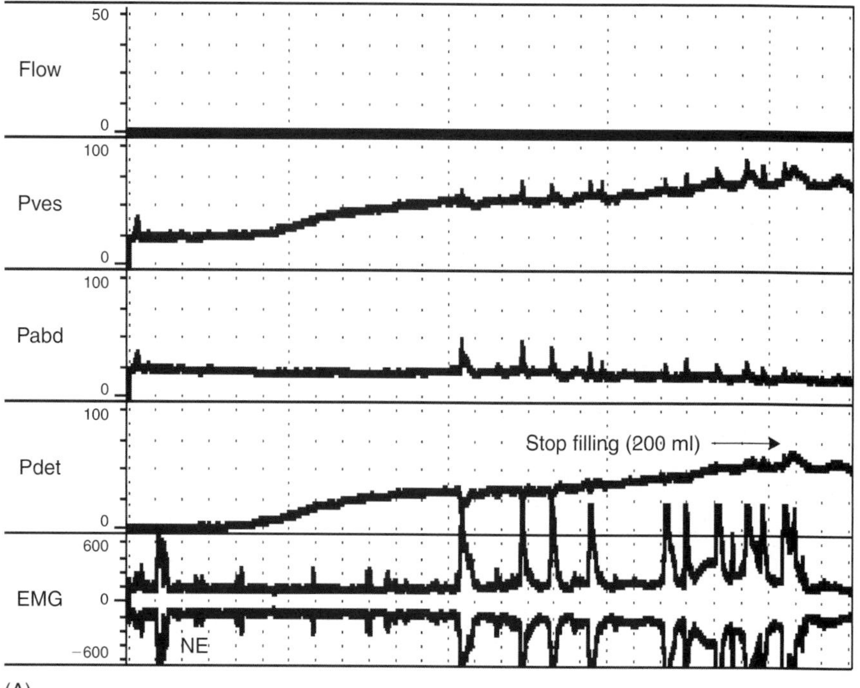

(A)

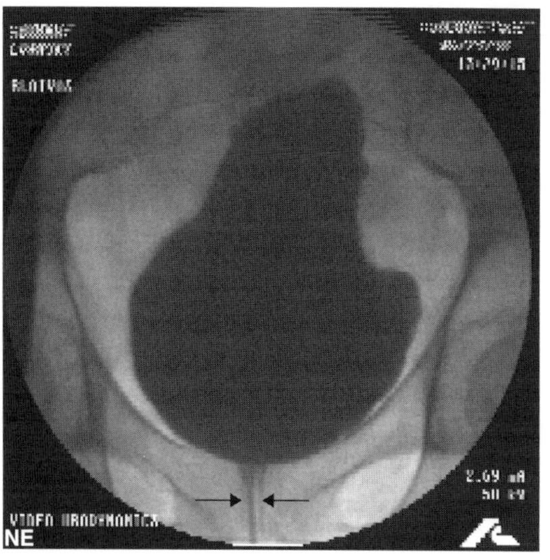

(B)

Fig. 14.5 Detrusor areflexia, low bladder compliance, and open bladder neck at rest associated with a T10–11 spinal fracture suffered 5 years prior to this study. The patient was a 41-year-old paraplegic male who had been treated with a Foley catheter. Renal ultrasound showed bilateral hydronephrosis and cortical atrophy. The hydronephrosis resolved and his kidneys have stabilized over the ensuing decade once he was started on intermittent catheterization. (A) Urodynamic tracing. During bladder filling, there is a steep rise in detrusor pressure and when filling is stopped, Pdet falls showing that this is due to low bladder compliance and not a detrusor contraction. The sporadic bursts of EMG activity are movement artifacts as each burst is accompanied by an increase in Pabd and Pves. (B) X-ray shows an open bladder neck (arrows).

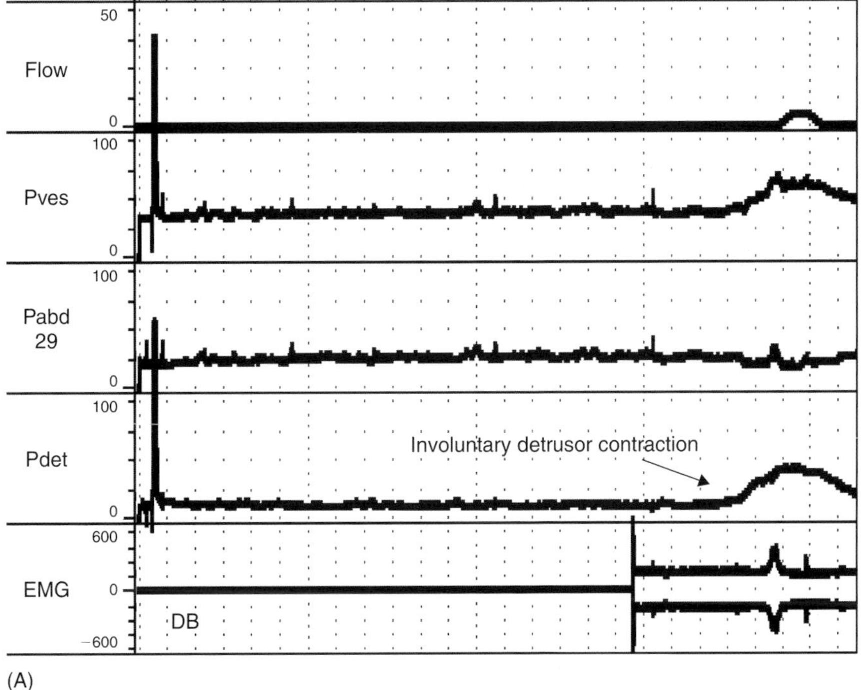

(A)

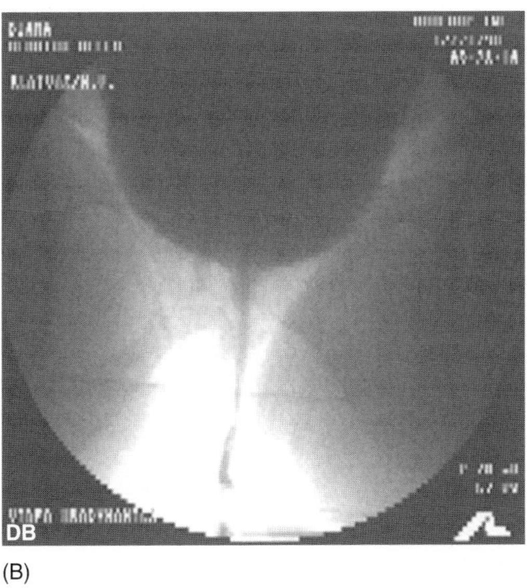

(B)

Fig. 14.6 Detrusor hyperreflexia (type 4 OAB) in 48-year-old woman diagnosed with MS 12 years previously. Her chief complaint is urge incontinence and she has been on intermittent self-catheterization for the last 10 years. (A) Urodynamic tracing. FSF = 229 ml, 1st urge = 305 ml, and severe urge = 363 ml synchronous with an involuntary detrusor contraction (arrow). She was unable to contract her sphincter and voided uncontrollably. The EMG tracing was not working properly; the tracing is all artifact. Q_{max} = 6 ml, Pdet@Q_{max} = 43 cmH_2O, Pdetmax = 44 cmH_2O, voided volume = 113 ml, and PVR = 271 ml. This documents grade 1 urethral obstructi on the Blaivas grouty Nomogram. (B) X-ray obtained at Q_{max} shows a reasonably normal configuration of the urethra. Since the distal segment is the narrowest portion of the urethra, and the pressure flow study documents urethral obstruction, this is consistent with either DESD or some other cause of distal urethral obstruction.

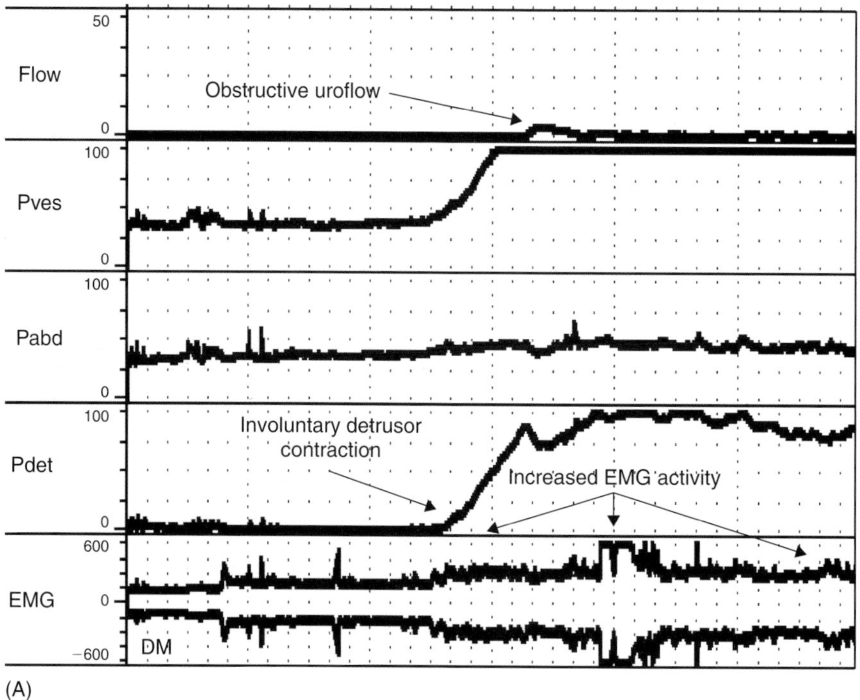

(A)

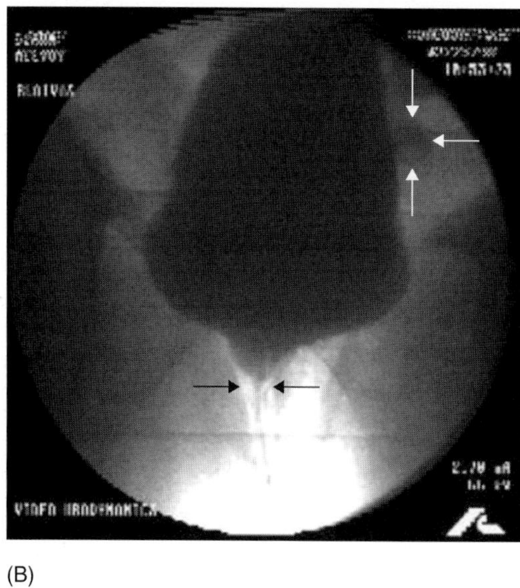
(B)

Fig. 14.7 DESD in a 53-year-old woman with chronic progressive MS. She complains of urinary frequency, urgency, and urge incontinence, saturating large pads on a daily basis. She was treated with intermittent catheterization and anticholinergics, and remained continent on that regimen.

(A) Urodynamic tracing. During bladder filling, there is a sustained involuntary detrusor contraction at a bladder volume of 353 ml. Increased EMG activity precedes and persists throughout the detrusor contraction (type 3 DESD), Q_{max}=5 ml/s, and Pdet@Q_{max}=75 cmH_2O. This corresponds to grade 2 urethral obstruction on the Blaivas grouty nomogram.

(B) X-ray obtained at Q_{max} shows the classic picture of DESD in a woman – a dilated proximal urethra that is obstructed in its distal third by the contracting sphincter (black arrows). The bladder has a "Christmas tree" shape and there is a bladder diverticulum on the left (white arrows).

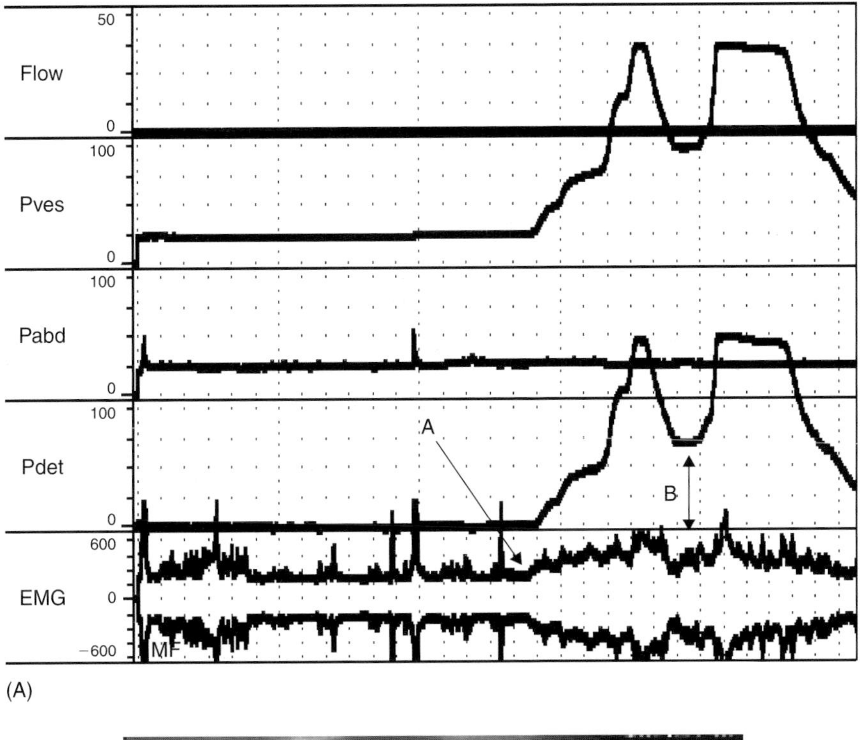

(A)

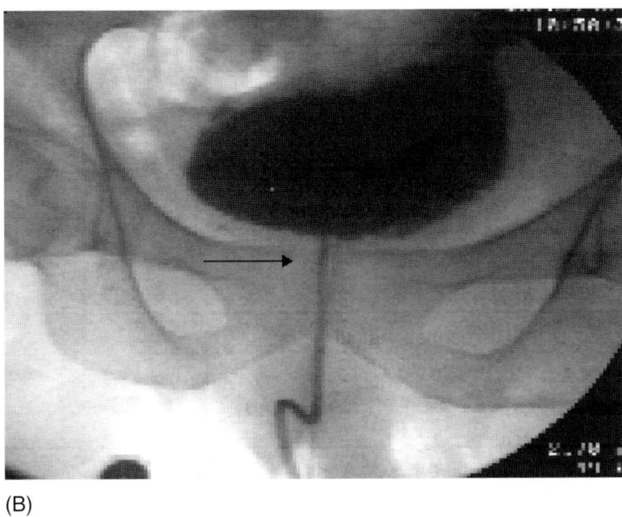

(B)

Fig. 14.8 DESD and prostatic/bladder neck obstruction in a 37-year-old quadriplegic man with chronic progressive MS of about 12 years duration. He wears diapers and has failed an empiric trial of oxybutynin, but, incredibly enough, has never been evaluated before. Renal ultrasound showed bilateral grade 3 hydronephrosis. (A) Urodynamic tracing. During bladder filling, at a volume of only about 75 ml, there is an increase in EMG activity (arrow A) followed in several seconds by an involuntary detrusor contraction to 150 cmH_2O. For the first half of the detrusor contraction there is no flow at all, then the sphincter relaxes and flow begins (arrow B) and then the sphincter contracts again and flow ceases. The examination was performed in the supine position, so uroflow was not obtained, but a dribbling stream was observed. (B) X-ray obtained at Pdetmax at the apex of the increased EMG activity shows no contrast in the urethra arrow and a heavily trabeculated bladder. The likeliest explanation is DESD and secondary bladder neck obstruction although from a strictly radiologic viewpoint there could be concomitant prostatic obstruction.

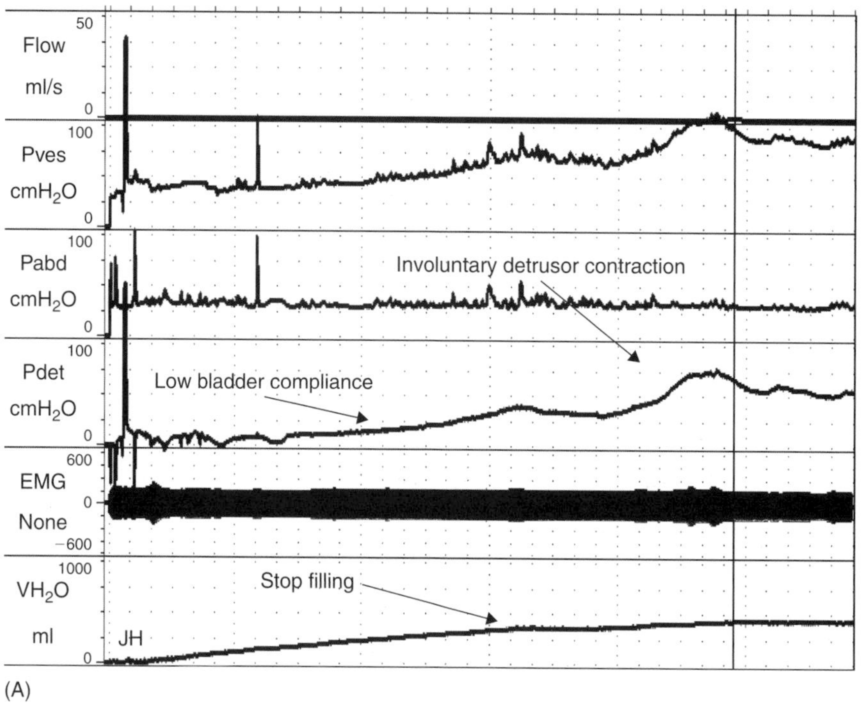

(A)

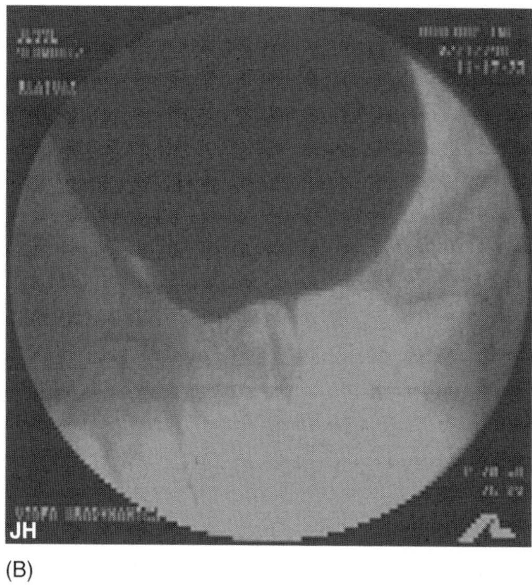

(B)

Fig. 14.9 Low bladder compliance and detrusor hyperreflexia in a 56-year-old man with chronic (slowly) progressive MS. His chief complaint is incontinence . . . "The biggest thing is at night. . . I fall asleep and I wake up wet."
(A) Urodynamic tracing. During bladder filling, there is a steep rise in Pdet that reaches 47 cmH_2O at a bladder volume of 325 ml. Bladder compliance = 325/47 = 6.9 ml/cmH_2O, Q_{max} = 2 ml/s, and Pdet@Q_{max} = 68 cmH_2O (vertical line). This corresponds to a Schafer grade 4 urethral obstruction. The EMG tracing shows little variation and is likely artifact.
(B) X-ray obtained at Q_{max} shows faint visualization of a narrowed proximal urethra. These findings are consistent with benign prostatic urethral obstruction, but it is not possible to determine whether or not there is associated DESD on the basis of this tracing.

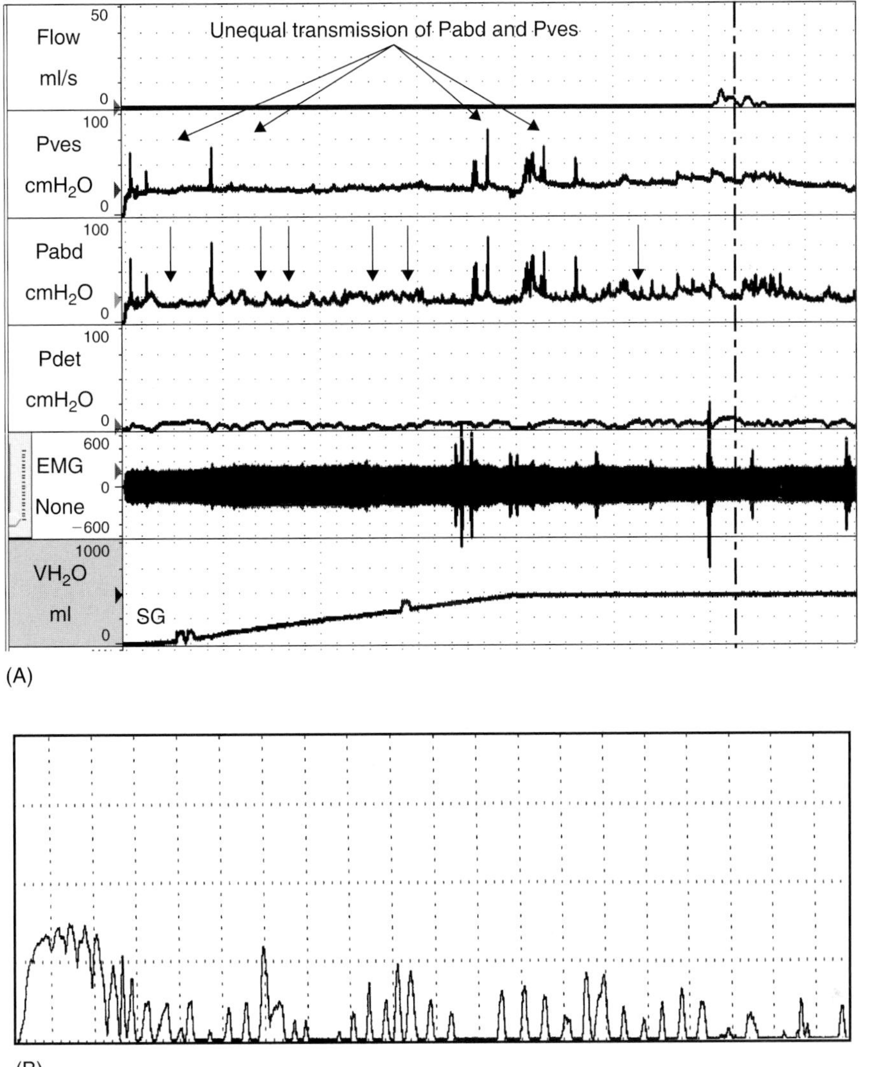

Fig. 14.10 Impaired detrusor contractility in a 55-year-old married woman with chronic progressive MS of 14 years duration. Her chief complaint is daily urinary urgency and urge incontinence. She ordinarily voids more than once an hour during the day and has nocturia about every 2–3 hours. After each void, she usually needs to urinate again within minutes. (A) Urodynamic tracing. FSF = 100 ml, 1st urge = 229 ml, severe urge = 365 ml, and bladder capacity was 506 ml. During bladder filling there were two problems that make the tracing difficult to interpret. Firstly, during coughing and straining there is unequal registration of abdominal and vesical pressure – abdominal pressure rises more than vesical pressure. Secondly, there are multiple rectal contractions (small arrows). The net effect is artifactual decreases in detrusor pressure and an irregular detrusor pressure tracing. At the vertical line there is a low magnitude voluntary detrusor contraction and low flow. Pdet/Q study: Q_{max} = 1 ml, Pdet@Q_{max} = 11 cmH_2O, Pdetmax = 13 cmH_2O, voided volume = 16 ml, and PVR = 490 ml. The low flow accompanied by low detrusor pressure indicates impaired detrusor contractility. (B) Unintubated flow: VOID: 14/347/201.

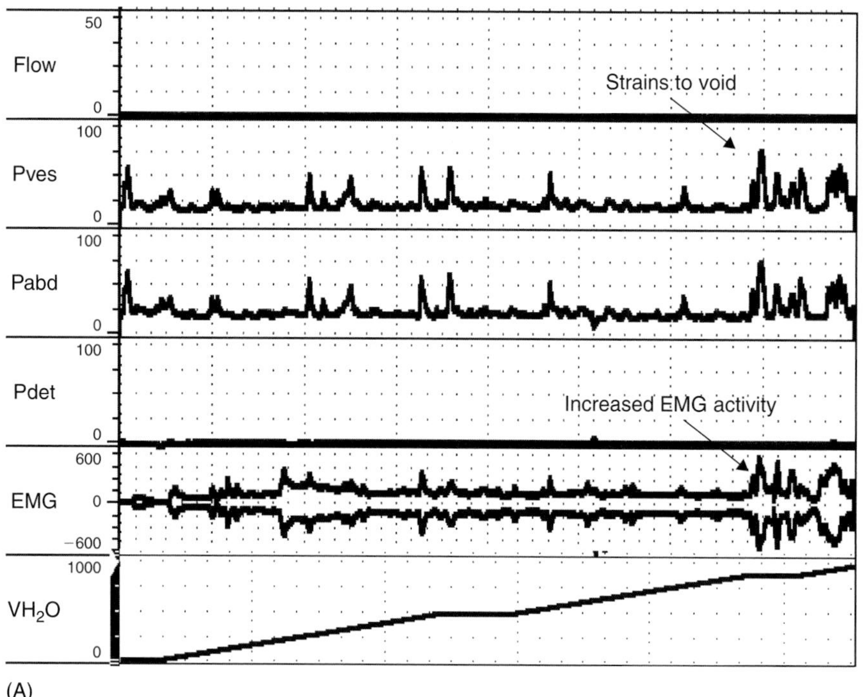

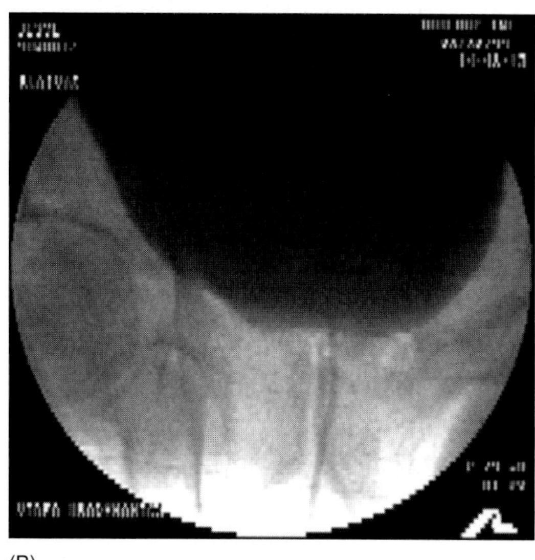

Fig. 14.11 End stage diabetic cystopathy in a 68-year-old type 1 diabetic man who denied LUTS until he presented with acute urinary retention and was catheterized for nearly 2l. This urodynamic study was done 1 month after he was started on intermittent self-catheterization. (A) Urodynamic tracing. FSF = 332 ml, 1st urge=640 ml, and severe urge=900 ml. Once he felt the severe urge he was asked to try to void, but could only push and strain. During straining, the sphincter EMG increased and he was unable to void. (B) While straining to void the bladder neck remains closed.

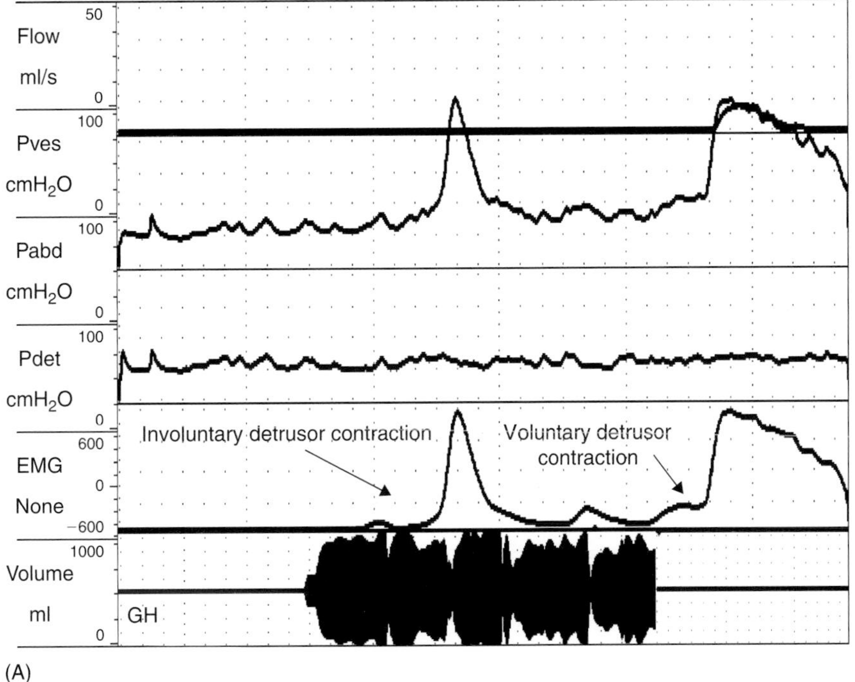

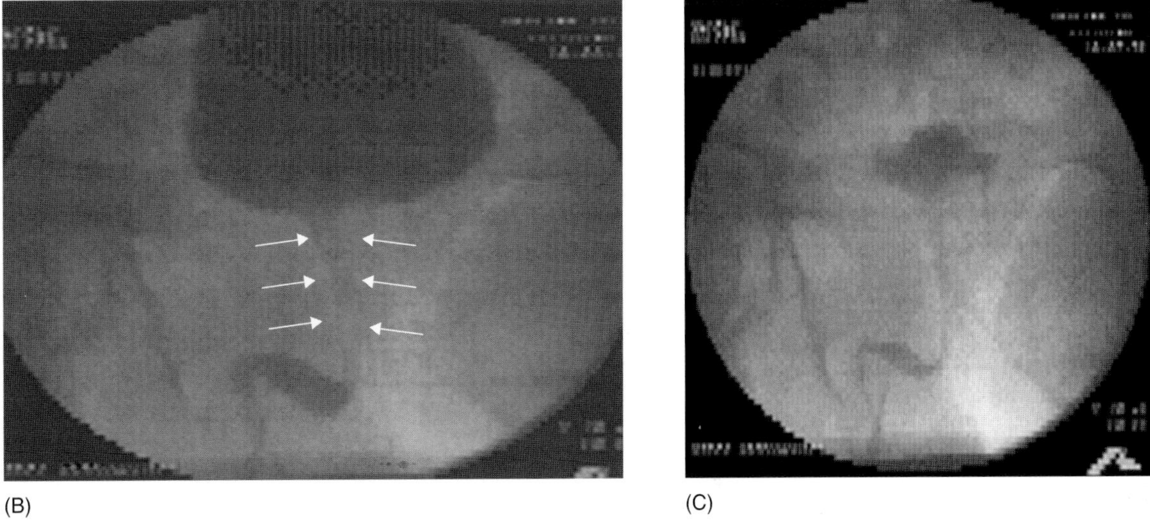

Fig. 14.12 Detrusor hyperreflexia (type 2 OAB) and grade 4 prostatic obstruction in 68-year-old juvenile onset, type 1 diabetic man. He also has severe peripheral neuropathy. It is not possible to determine the relative contributions of prostatic obstruction, BPH, and diabetic neuropathy from this urodynamic study. (A) Urodynamic study. FSF (first sensation of filling)=70 ml, 1st urge=105 ml, severe urge=240 ml, and bladder capacity=504 ml. There was an involuntary detrusor contraction at a volume of 105 ml. He perceived the contraction as an urge to void, was able to voluntarily interrupt the stream and was able to abort the contraction. At capacity, he had a voluntary detrusor contraction. Q_{max}=10 ml/s, Pdet@Q_{max}=90 cmH_2O, voided volume=534 ml, and PVR = 6 ml. (B) X-ray obtained a Q_{max} shows a poorly visualized prostatic urethra (arrows). (C) X-ray obtained at the end of micturition.

Stress Incontinence in Women

15

Stress incontinence refers to both a symptom and a condition [1]. The symptom is the complaint of involuntary leakage of urine on exertion or on sneezing or coughing. The condition is due to either sphincter weakness (sphincteric incontinence) or stress induced detrusor overactivity (stress hyperreflexia). The ICS defines urodynamic stress incontinence as the involuntary leakage of urine during increases in abdominal pressure, in the absence of a detrusor contraction. Mixed urinary incontinence is the complaint of an involuntary leakage of urine associated with urgency and also with exertion, effort, sneezing or coughing [2]. Overall, pure stress incontinence accounts for 49%, mixed stress and urge incontinence (29%) and pure urge incontinence (21%) [3].

There are a number of theories about the pathophysiology of sphincteric incontinence. Some believe that sphincteric incontinence is due to unequal transmission of abdominal pressure to the bladder and urethra. According to this theory, the bladder neck and proximal urethra normally occupy a high retropubic position and increased intra-abdominal pressure is transmitted equally to both bladder and urethra. In cases of sphincteric incontinence, due weakness of pelvic floor support, the bladder neck and urethra rotate posteriorly and descend caudally. The increased abdominal pressure is then transmitted greater to the bladder than the urethra and stress urinary incontinence ensues [4–9].

Others have suggested that sphincteric incontinence is due to widening and shortening of the urethra or unequal movement of the anterior and posterior walls of the bladder neck and proximal urethra during stress (Figs. 15.1–15.3) [10–12]. The hammock theory posits that continence is maintained because the urethra lies in a position where it can be compressed against a hammock-like musculofascial layer on which the bladder and urethra rest [13].

In 1998, Petros and Ulmsten published the "integral theory" of stress and urge incontinence [14]. According to the theory, female stress and urge incontinence have a common etiology. Laxity of the anterior vaginal wall causes activation of stretch receptors in the bladder neck and proximal urethra which can trigger an inappropriate micturition reflex. This can result in detrusor overactivity.

Support of the anterior vaginal wall is provided by three separate mechanisms which work in conjunction. The anterior pubococcygeus muscle lifts the anterior vaginal wall to compress the urethra; the bladder neck is closed by traction of the underlying vaginal wall in a backward and downward fashion; and the pelvic floor musculature, under voluntary control draws the hammock upward, closing the bladder neck. Overall laxity of the anterior vaginal wall causes a dissipation of all of these forces, and stress incontinence develops.

All classification systems for sphincteric incontinence are anatomic, based on the degree of urethral mobility during increases in abdominal pressure [4,15–17]. According to the most recent iteration of the Blaivas/Green/McGuire classification [17], there are four types as described in Figures 15.3–15.7.

Although we find the anatomic classifications intellectually appealing, we believe they are too simplistic and we no longer classify patients according to anatomy alone. Rather, we characterize sphincteric incontinence by two parameters – the degree of urethral mobility as measured by the Q-tip test and the vesical leak point pressure (VLPP).

In the vast majority of women with sphincteric incontinence, the diagnosis is apparent by history and physical examination. In these patients, urodynamic testing is designed to answer more specific and sophisticated questions than a simple yes/no with respect to sphincter function. The first is to measure sphincter strength (LPP) and urethral mobility (X-ray) during cough and strain. The second is to determine whether or not there is associated detrusor overactivity and, if so, whether this contributes to the patient's incontinence. The third is to assess voiding mechanics – urethral obstruction or impaired detrusor contractility Figures 15.8–15.14 depict examples of videourodynamic studies of sphincteric incontinence that, illustrate these points.

Suggested Reading

1 Blaivas JG, Appell RA, Fantl JA, et al. Definition and classification of urinary incontinence: recommendations of the Urodynamics Society, *Neurourol Urodyn*, 6: 149–151, 1997.

2 Abrams P, Cardozo L, Fall M, et al. The standardisation of terminology in lower urinary tract function: report from the standardisation sub-committee of the International Continence Society, *Urology*, 61: 37–49, 2003.

3 Hunskaar S, Burgio K, Diokno AC, Herzog AR, Hjalmas K, Lapitan MC. Epidemiology and natural history of urinary incontinence (UI). In Abrams P, Cardozo L, Khoury S, Wein A (eds) *Incontinence* (2nd Edition 2005) 2nd International Consultation on Incontinence. Health Publications Ltd, Plymouth, England 2002, pp 165–201.

4 McGuire EJ. Herlihy E. The influence of urethral position on urinary continence. (Journal Article) Investigative Urology. 15(3):205–7.

5 Constantinou CE. Principles and methods of clinical urodynamic investigations. [Journal Article] Critical Reviews in Biomedical Engineering. 7(3):229–64, 1982.

6 Westby M. Asmussen M. Ulmsten U. Location of maximum intraurethral pressure related to urogenital diaphragm in the female subject as studied by simultaneous urethrocystometry and voiding urethrocystography. [Journal Article] American Journal of Obstetrics & Gynecology. 144(4):408–12, 1982.

7 Constantinou CE. Resting and stress urethral pressures as a clinical guide to the mechanism of continence in the female patient. [Journal Article] Urologic Clinics of North America. 12(2):247–58, 1985.

8 Bump RC. Copeland WE Jr. Hurt WG. Fantl JA. Dynamic urethral pressure/profilometry pressure transmission ratio determinations in stress-incontinent and stress-continent subjects. [Journal Article] American Journal of Obstetrics & Gynecology. 159(3):749–55, 1988.

9 Theofrastous JP. Bump RC. Elser DM. Wyman JF. McClish DK. Correlation of urodynamic measures of urethral resistance with clinical measures of incontinence severity in women with pure genuine stress incontinence. The Continence Program for Women Research Group. [Journal Article] American Journal of Obstetrics & Gynecology. 173(2):407–12.

10 Yang A, Mostwin JL, Rosenshein N, Zerhouni EA. Pelvic floor descent in women: dynamic evaluation with fast MR imaging and cinematic display, *Radiology*, 179: 25–33, 1991.

11 Yang A, Mostwin JL, Genadry R, Sanders R. Patterns of prolapse demonstrated with dynamic fast scan MRI: reassessment of conventional concepts of pelvic floor weakness, *Neurourol Urodyn*, 12: 310–311, 1993.

12 Mostwin JL, Yang A, Sanders R, Genadry R. Radiography, sonography, and magnetic resonance imaging for stress incontinence, *Urol Clin North Am*, 22: 539–549, 1995.

13 DeLancey JO. Structural support of the urethra as it relates to stress urinary incontinence: the hammock hypothesis, *Am J Obstet Gynecol*, 170: 1713–1720, 1994.

14 Petros PP, Ulmsten U. An integral theory of female urinary incontinence: experimental and clinical

considerations, *Acta Obstet Gynecol Scand Suppl*, 153:7–31, 1990.
15 Green TH. The problem of urinary stress incontinence in the female: an appraisal of its current status, *Obstet Gynecol Surv*, 23: 603–634, 1968.
16 McGuire EJ, Lytton B, Pepe V, Kohorn EI. Stress urinary incontinence, *Obstet Gynecol*, 47: 255–264, 1976.
17 Blaivas JG, Olsson CA. Stress incontinence: classification and surgical approach, *J Urol*, 139: 727–731, 1988.
18 Bradley CS, Rovner ES. Urodynamically defined stress urinary incontinence and bladder outlet obstruction coexist in women, *J Urol*, 171: 757–761, 2004.
19 Constantinou CE, Govan DE. Contribution and timing of transmitted and generated pressure components in the female urethra. In *Female Incontinence*, New York: Alan R. Liss, 1981, pp. 113–120.
20 DeLancey JO. Anatomy and physiology of urinary continence, *Clin Obstet Gynecol*, 33: 298–307, 1990.
21 Fleischman N, Flisser AJ, Blaivas JG, Panagopoulos G. Sphincteric urinary incontinence: relationship of vesical leak point pressure, urethral mobility and severity of incontinence, *J Urol*, 169: 999–1002, 2003.
22 Flisser AJ, Wamsley K, and Blaivas JG. Urodynamic classification of patients with symptoms of overactive bladder, *J Urol*, 169: 529–533, 2003.
23 Govier FE, Pritchett TR, Kornman JD. Correlation of the cystoscopic appearance and functional integrity of the female urethral sphincteric mechanism, *Urology*, 44: 250–253, 1994.
24 Green, TH. Development of a plan for the diagnosis and treatment of urinary stress incontinence, *Am J Obstet Gynecol*, 83: 632, 1962.
25 Hodgkinson CP. Metallic bead-chain urethrocystography in preoperative and postoperative evaluation of gynecologic urologic problems, *Clin Obstet Gynecol*, 21: 725–735, 1978.
26 Hunskaar S, Lose G, Sykes D, Voss S. The prevalence of urinary incontinence in women in four European countries, *Br J Urol Int*, 93: 325–330, 2004.
27 McGuire EJ. Urodynamic findings in patients after failure of stress incontinence operations. In Zinner NR, Sterling AM (eds) *Female Incontinence* New York: Alan R. Liss, 1980, pp. 351–360.
28 McGuire EJ, Fitzpatrick CC, Wan J, et al. Clinical assessment of urethral sphincter function, *J Urol*, 150: 1452–1454, 1993.
29 Mostwin J, Bourcier A, Haab F, Koelbl H, Rao S, Resnick N, Salvatoire S, Sultan A, Yamaguchi O. Pathophysiology of urinary incontinence, fecal incontinence and pelvic organ prolapse. In Abrams P, Cardozo L, Khoury S, Wein A (eds) *Incontinence* (2nd Edition 2005) 2nd International Consultation on Incontinence. Health Publications Ltd, Plymouth, England 2002, pp 423–484.
30 Nitti VW, Combs AJ. Correlation of Valsalva leak point pressure with subjective degree of stress urinary incontinence in women, *J Urol*, 155: 281–285, 1996.
31 Petros PP, Ulmsten U. An anatomical classification – a new paradigm for management of female lower urinary tract dysfunction, *Eur J Obstet Gynecol Reprod Biol*, 80: 87–94, 1998.
32 Versi E, Cardozo L, Studd JW, et al. Internal urinary sphincter in maintenance of female continence. *Br Med J*, 292: 166–167, 1986.
33 Walters MD, Jackson GM. Urethral mobility and its relationship to stress incontinence in women, *J Reprod Med* 35: 777, 1990.

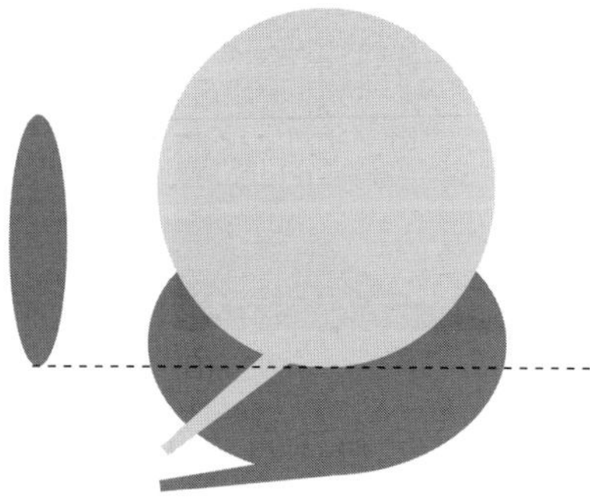

Fig. 15.1 Urethral hypermobility without incontinence. There is rotational descent of the bladder base and urethra during cough, but no incontinence. Light shading: bladder and urethra at rest; dark shading: bladder and urethra during cough or strain; dotted line: level of pubis.

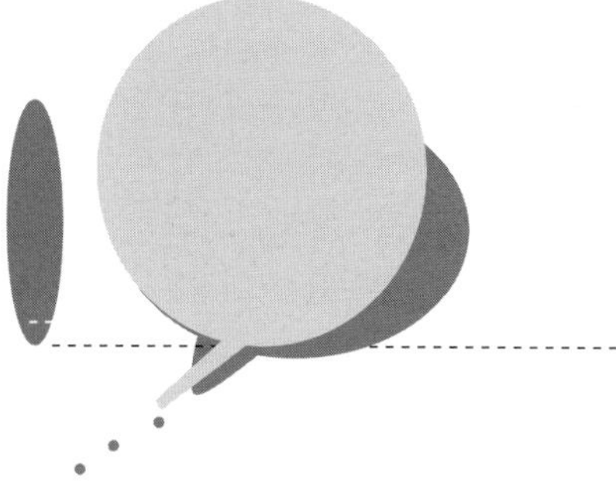

Fig. 15.2 Urethral hypermobility with incontinence. There is downward descent of the bladder base and urethra during cough, the urethra widens and shortens and incontinence ensues. Light shading: bladder and urethra at rest; dark shading: bladder and urethra during cough or strain; dotted line: level of pubis.

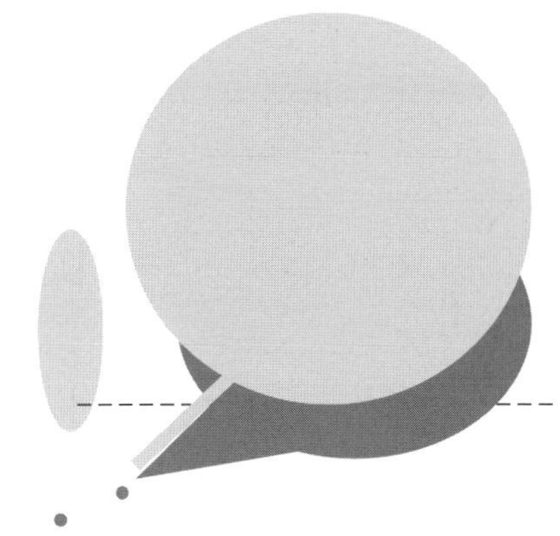

Fig. 15.3 Urethral hypermobility with incontinence. There is downward descent of the bladder base and urethra during cough, the posterior wall of the urethra moves more than the anterior wall pulling the urethra open and incontinence ensues. Light shading: bladder and urethra at rest; dark shading: bladder and urethra during cough or strain; dotted line: level of pubis.

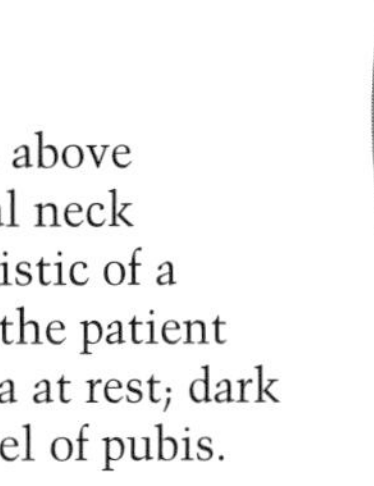

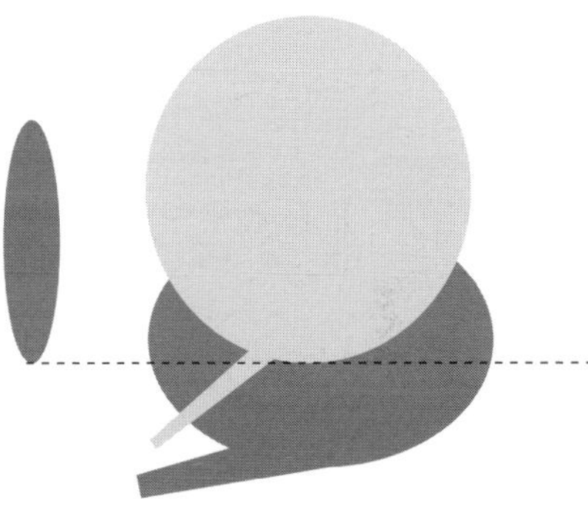

Fig. 15.4 Type 0 SUI: The vesical neck is closed at rest and situated above the inferior margin of the symphysis pubis. During stress the vesical neck and proximal urethra open and there is rotational descent characteristic of a cystourethrocele, but there is no incontinence despite the fact that the patient complains of stress incontinence. Light shading: bladder and urethra at rest; dark shading: bladder and urethra during cough or strain; dotted line: level of pubis.

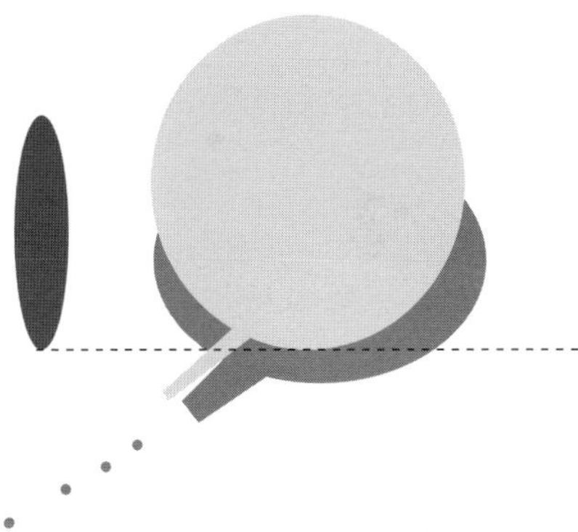

Fig. 15.5 Type 1 SUI: The vesical neck is closed at rest and situated above the inferior margin of the symphysis. During stress the vesical neck and proximal urethra open and descend <2cm and urinary incontinence is apparent during periods of increased abdominal pressure. There is little or no cystocele. Light shading: bladder and urethra at rest; dark shading: bladder and urethra during cough or strain; dotted line: level of pubis.

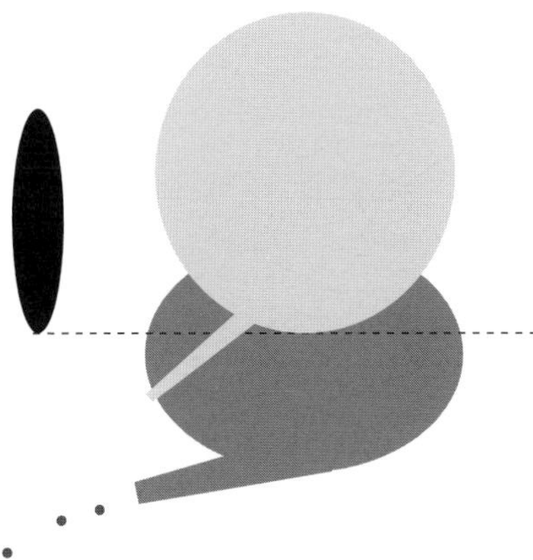

Fig. 15.6 Type 2 SUI: The vesical neck is closed at rest and situated above the inferior margin of the symphysis pubis. During stress the vesical neck and proximal urethra open and there is rotational descent characteristic of a cystourethrocele. Urinary incontinence is apparent during periods of increased intra-abdominal pressure. Light shading: bladder and urethra at rest; dark shading: bladder and urethra during cough or strain; dotted line: level of pubis.

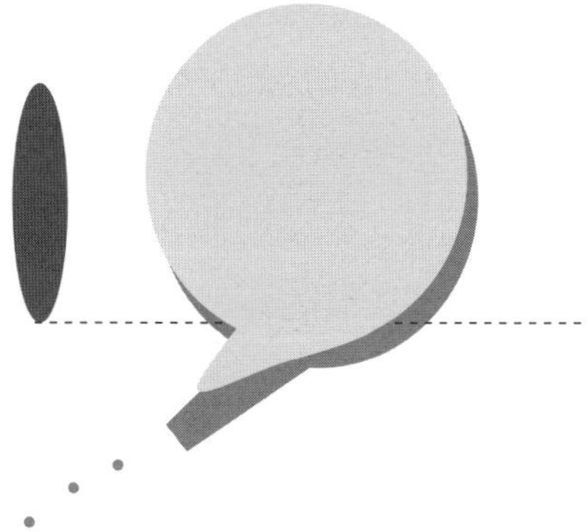

Fig. 15.7 Type 3 SUI: The vesical neck and proximal urethra are open at rest in the absence of a detrusor contraction. The proximal urethra no longer functions as a sphincter. There is obvious urinary leakage which may be gravitational in nature or associated with minimal increases in intravesical pressure. Light shading: bladder and urethra at rest; dark shading: bladder and urethra during cough or strain; dotted line: level of pubis.

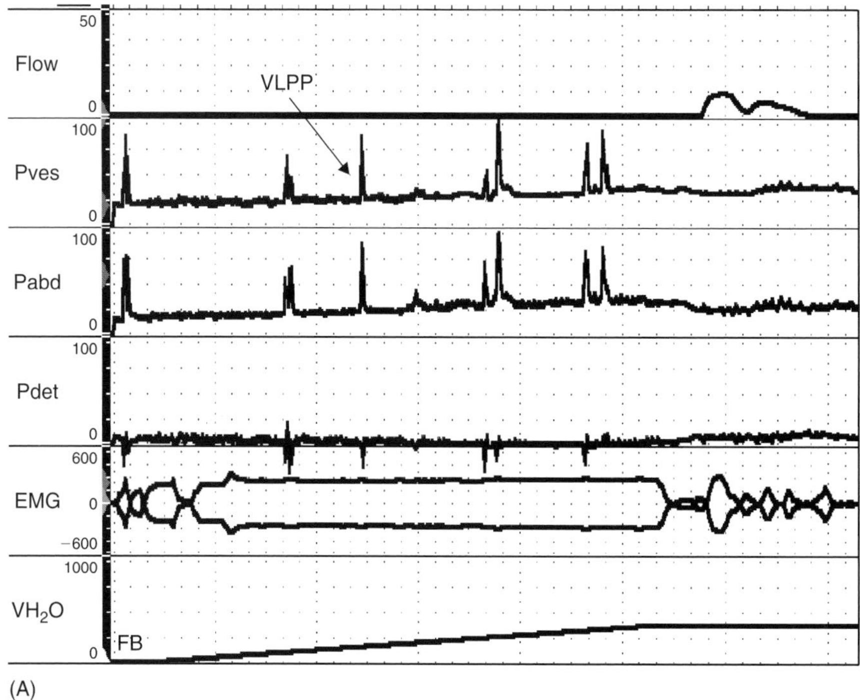

Fig. 15.8 Stress incontinence without urethral hypermobility. This corresponds to type 1 SUI according to the Blaivas/Green/McGuire classification system. FB is an 82-year-old woman who complains of mixed stress and urge incontinence. QtipwAs 0° > 0°. (A) Urodynamic tracing. FSF = 215, 1st urge = 371 ml, severe urge = 375 ml, bladder capacity = 381 ml, and bladder compliance = 96 ml/cmH_2O. When she voids, there is no appreciable rise in detrusor pressure because all of the force of detrusor contraction is converted to uroflow. There is an inexplicable fall in Pves and Pabd during voiding. Pabd falls more than vesical pressure resulting in an artifactual rise in detrusor pressure. VLPP = 42 cmH_2O, unintubated Q_{max} = 9 ml/s, voided volume = 267 ml, and post-void residual (PVR) = 32 ml.

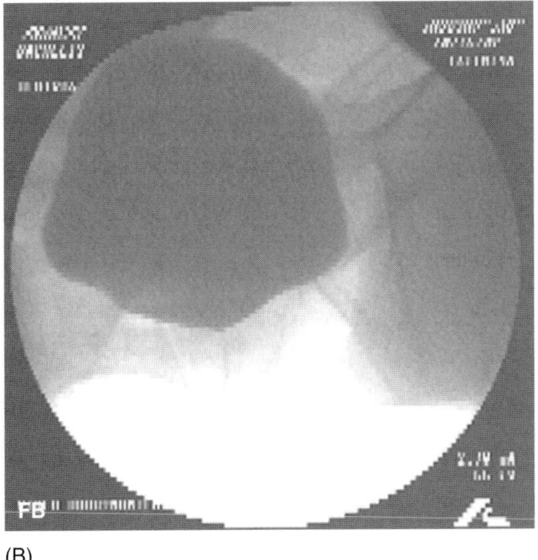

(B)

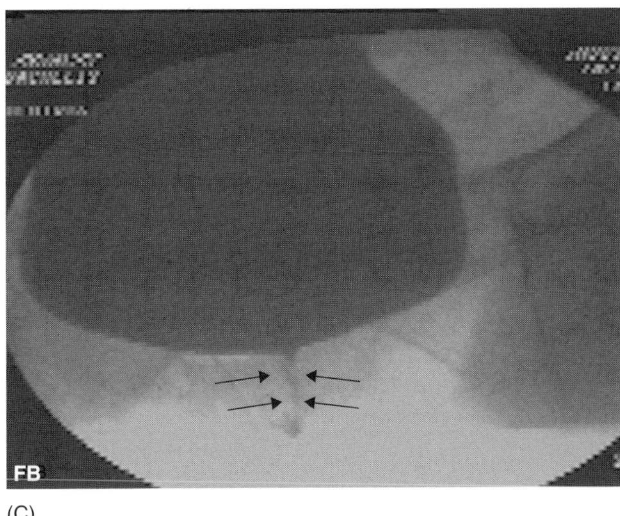

(C)

Fig. 15.8 (continued) (B) X-ray exposed just prior to VLPP at a bladder volume of 270 ml. Note that the bladder appears to have descended well below the pubis. This is an artifact because, with the patient in a sitting position, the C-arm needs to be tilted in order to obtain a good view of the urethra. (C) X-ray obtained at VLPP. There is contrast in the urethra without any urethral mobility (arrows). The bladder is still in the same position and has not descended at all during cough. Comment: Although her chief complaint was overactive bladder, urodynamics showed severe sphincteric incontinence and subsequently, her symptoms became "a nightmare" for her. In fact, a pad test showed over 100 grams of urinary loss but she considered this not to be a problem, probably because the large pads she wore, kept her dry. She elected treatment for the OAB symptoms only and was treated with a combination of anticholinergics and behavior modification and is pleased with the results, but diary and pad test showed only moderate improvement.

This case underscores the importance of clinical acumen of that combines history, urodynamics, cystoscopy, diary and pad test and highlights the shortcomings of relying on any one aspect of the evaluation. The patient was successfully treated to her own level of expectation with little impact on the underlying pathophysiology and little improvement in measurable signs. From her perspective something got better, but nothing we could measure other than her statement that "I feel like I have better bladder control."

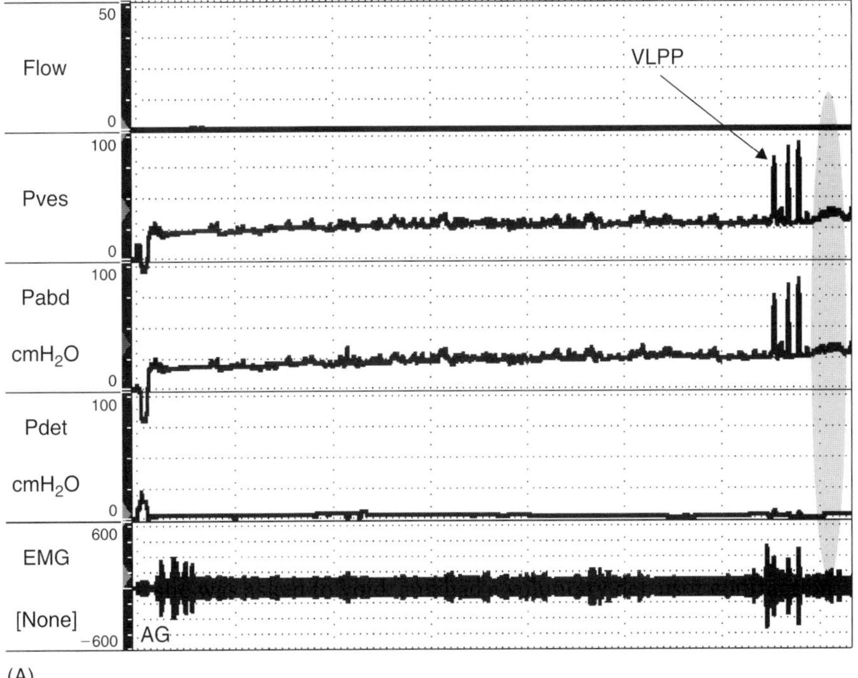

(A)

Fig. 15.9 Stress incontinence with urethral hypermobility and type 1 OAB. This corresponds to type 2 SUI according to the Blaivas/Green/McGuire classification. AG is a 51-year-old white woman with a chief complaint of gradually worsening stress incontinence of 10 years duration. About once or twice a month she soaks her clothes when she has been walking or does high impact aerobics. She wears one mini-pad all day which, at the end of the day is damp; "sometimes they're wetter than others". She also gets urgency and urge incontinence when she puts the key in her door lock, but has learned to control this by voiding beforehand. (A) Urodynamic tracing. FSF = 10 ml, 1st urge = 251 ml, severe urge = 492 ml, VLLP = 85 cmH_2O, bladder capacity = 585 cmH_2O. When asked to void, she strained a bit, but could not generate a detrusor contraction and was unable to void (shaded oval).

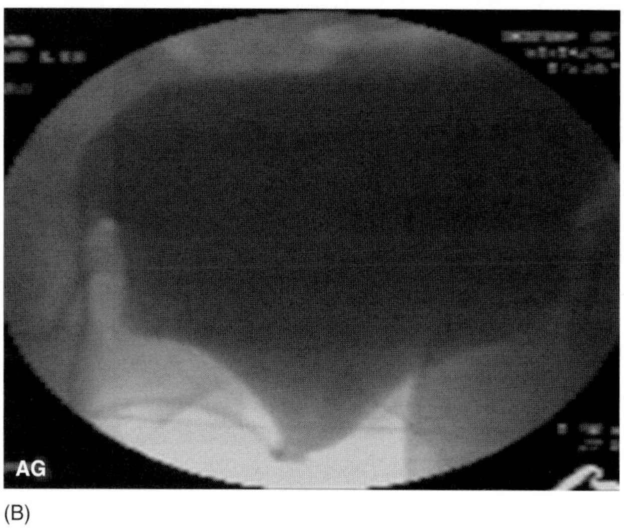

(B)

Fig. 15.9 (continued) (B) X-ray exposed at VLPP shows rotational descent of the urethra and incontinence. Q-tip angle was 65°. Comment: AG has classic type 2 stress incontinence and would likely do well after antiincontinence surgery, but when advised of the remote possibility of urinary retention, elected behavioral therapy.

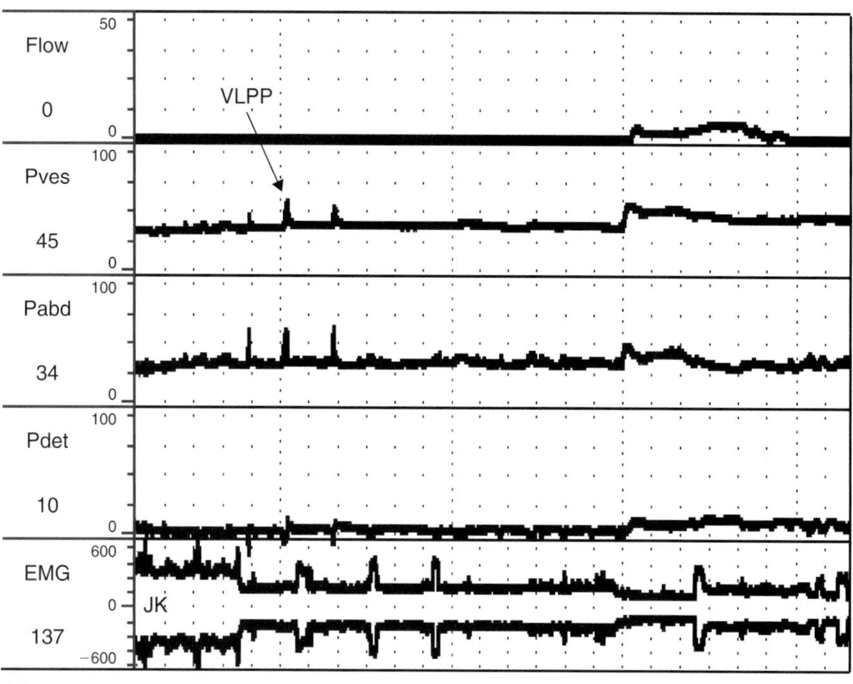

(A)

Fig. 15.10 Stress incontinence with urethral hypermobility. This corresponds to type 3 SUI according to the Blaivas/Green/McGuire classification. JK is a 31-year-old woman with persistent urinary incontinence after undergoing vaginal wall sling 18 months previously. After surgery, her incontinence was worse. She wears pads all the time, day and night and changes them 4–5 times a day and they are wet when she changes them. She complains of stress incontinence when she coughs and sneezes and sometimes when she just walks around, picking up her children, walking up stairs, playing sports, etc. Q-tip = 0 > 50°. At cystoscopy the urethra was abnormal. There was a distal circumferential scar and then a depression and then the vesical neck. The ureteral orifices were ectopic, just inside the vesical neck. There was no identifiable trigone. (A) Urodynamic study. FSF = 153 ml, 1st urge = 193 ml, severe urge = 306 ml. VLPP = 34 cmH_2O, VOID: 32/246/0 Pdet/Q: Q_{max} = 7 ml, Pdet@Q_{max} = 14 cmH_2O, Pdetmax = 15 cmH_2O, voided volume = 305 ml, and PVR = 0 ml.

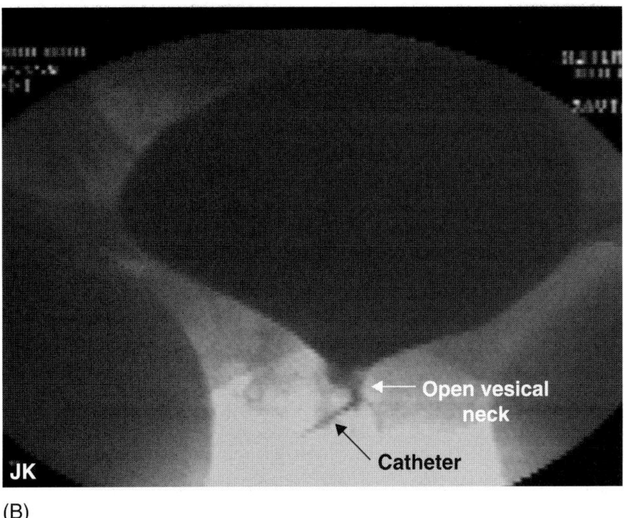

(B)

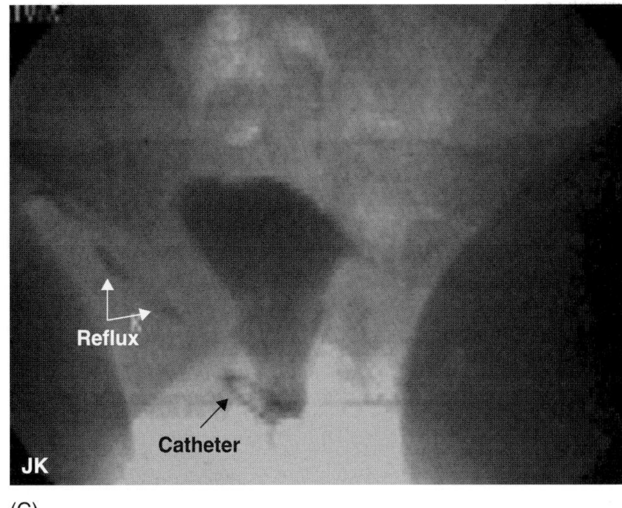

(C)

Fig. 15.10 (continued) (B) X-ray obtained at a bladder volume 200 ml shows an open vesical neck. (C) X-ray obtained just prior to the completion of voiding shows a wide-open urethra and grade 1 right vesicoureteral reflux (white arrows). The projection of the X-ray is nearly in anterior–posterior. This accounts for the looped appearance of the urethra catheter (black arrow).

Comment: It is impossible to determine whether her open vesical neck and reflux are the result of her prior surgery or the cause of failure. The fact that she has ectopic ureters and vesicoureteral reflux suggests the latter, but her persistent urethral hypermobility and abnormal urethral anatomy suggests the former. It would have been nice to know what she was like preoperatively, but videourodynamics were not done. She elected to undergo periurethral collagen injection because she was planning to become pregnant in the near future. After injection she was completely dry for about 6 months, then gradually the incontinence recurred and she moved to another city and was lost to follow-up.

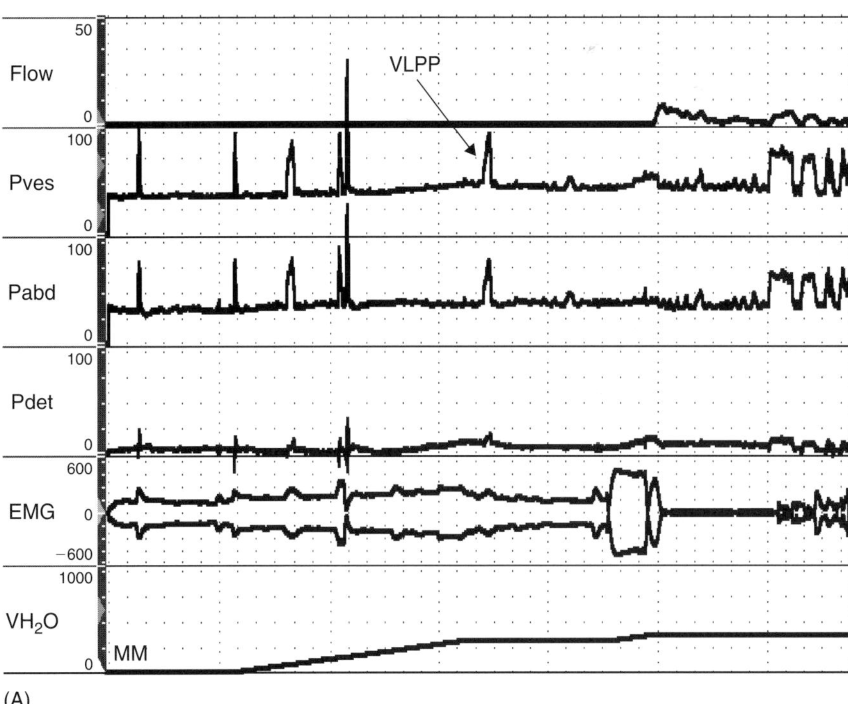

(A)

Fig. 15.11 "Pipe stem urethra" and impaired detrusor contractility in a 70-year-old woman who had previously undergone a vaginal hysterectomy, modified Pereyra, prolapse repair, TVT and SPARC in the course of 4 years. This corresponds to type 3 SUI according to the Blaivas/Green/McGuire classification. She complained "Incontinence . . . it happens all the time . . . its rare that I'm dry". (A) Urodynamic study. FSF = 103 ml, 1st urge = 138 ml, severe urge = 311 ml, bladder capacity = 381 ml, VLPP = 78 cmH_2O. VOID: 19/251/0 Pdet/Q study= impaired detrusor contractility, Q_{max} = 9 ml, Pdet@Q_{max} = 7 cmH_2O, Pdetmax = 16 cmH_2O, voided volume = 395 ml, PVR= 0 ml.

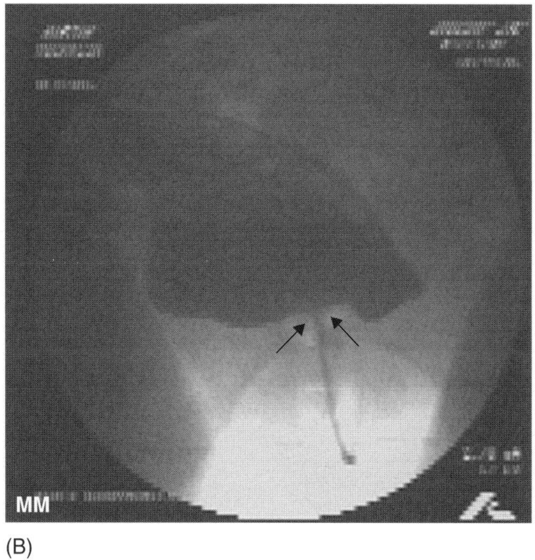

(B)

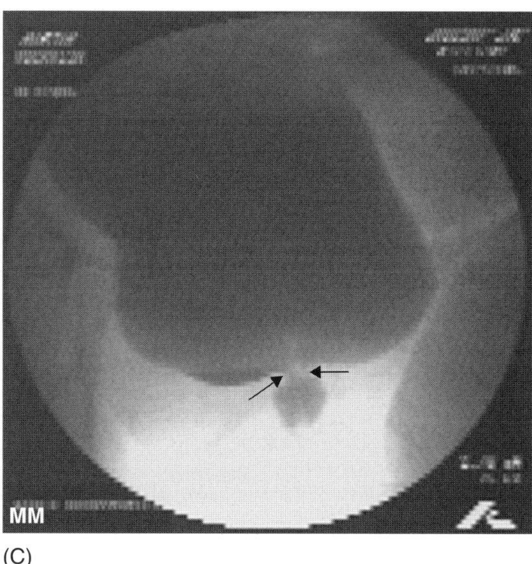

(C)

Fig. 15.11 (continued) (B) X-ray exposed during bladder filling shows a slightly open vesical neck (arrows) and an indentation on the bladder base likely a consequence of all of her prior surgeries. (C) X-ray exposed at the VLPP shows a narrowed vesical neck (arrows) and wide open proximal two-thirds of the urethra distal to the vesical neck. No contrast is seen in the distal urethra because air between her legs made it impossible to adjust the X-ray parameters properly.

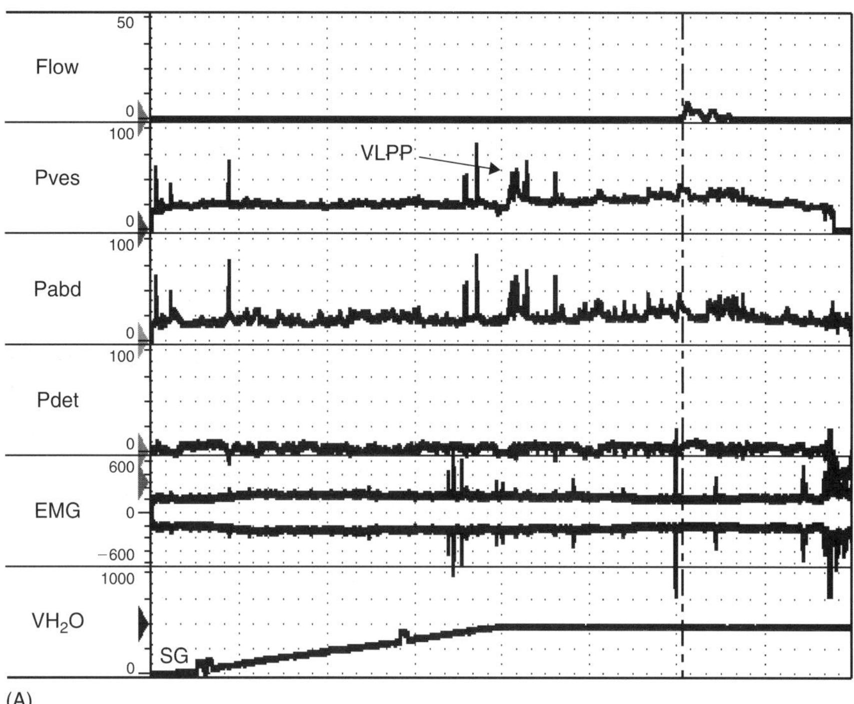

(A)

Fig. 15.12 Sphincteric incontinence, type 1 OAB and impaired detrusor contractility. SG is a 40-year-old woman (G2P1A1) who complains of stress incontinence and urinary frequency, urgency and urge incontinence during the latter part of each menstrual cycle. She underwent vaginal wall sling 2 years previously. (A) Urodynamic tracing. FSF = 224 ml, 1st urge = 400 ml, severe urge = 477 ml, VLPP = 62 cmH_2O, VOID: 18/375/0. Pdet/Q study: Q_{max} = 7 ml/s, Pdet@Q_{max} = 9 cmH_2O, Pdetmax = 12 cmH_2O, voided volume = 120 ml, and PVR= 374 ml.

Comment: The Pdet/Q study clearly demonstrates impaired detrusor contractility, but her unintubated uroflow was quite normal. Logic would dictate that this is because her urethral resistance is low (VLPP = 62 cmH_2O), but urethral compliance is also low and the urethral catheter is causing obstruction. She underwent autologous fascial pubovaginal sling and, with a 4 year follow-up, is cured of stress incontinence, but still has episodic, troublesome OAB symptoms. Urodynamics was not done, but uroflow and PVR remain normal.

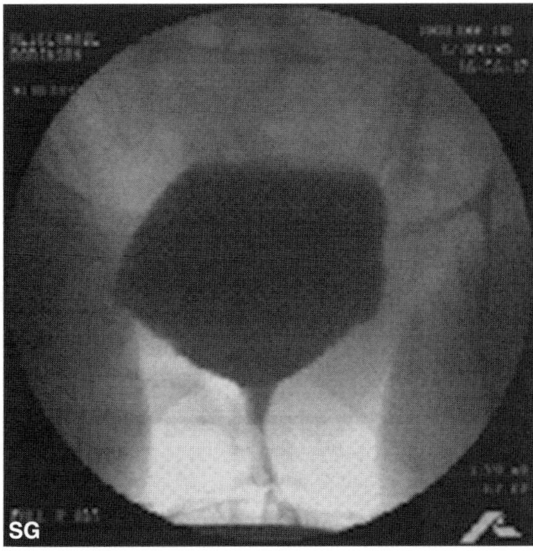

(B)

Fig. 15.12 (continued) (B) X-ray obtained at VLPP in a nearly AP projection, shows the entire urethra to be wide open during an episode of stress incontinence. The apparent (artifactual) descent of the bladder base and urethra is due to vertical rotation of the "C" arm necessary to visualize the urethra.

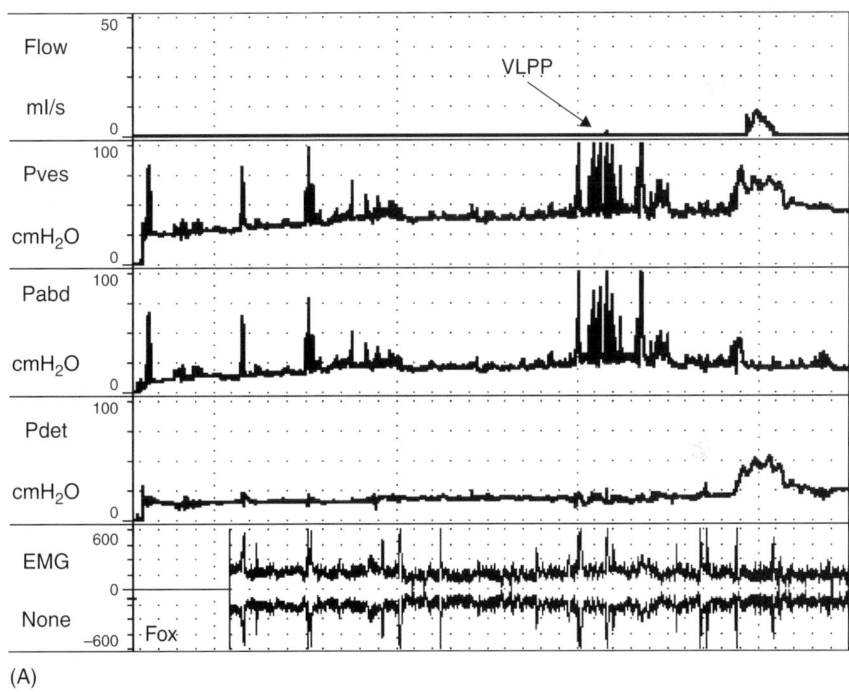

(A)

Fig. 15.13 Mixed stress and urge incontinence and grade 1 urethral obstruction. The patient is a 65-year-old woman who developed recurrent mixed incontinence after undergoing modified Peyrera operation 5 years ago and collagen injection 2 years ago. On examination, there was no clinical evidence of prolapse, but Q-tip angle was 0 > 70°. (A) Urodynamic tracing. VLPP = 88 cmH_2O. Pdet/Q study: Q_{max} = 11 ml/s, Pdet@Q_{max} = 50 cmH_2O, and Pdetmax = 50 cmH_2O.

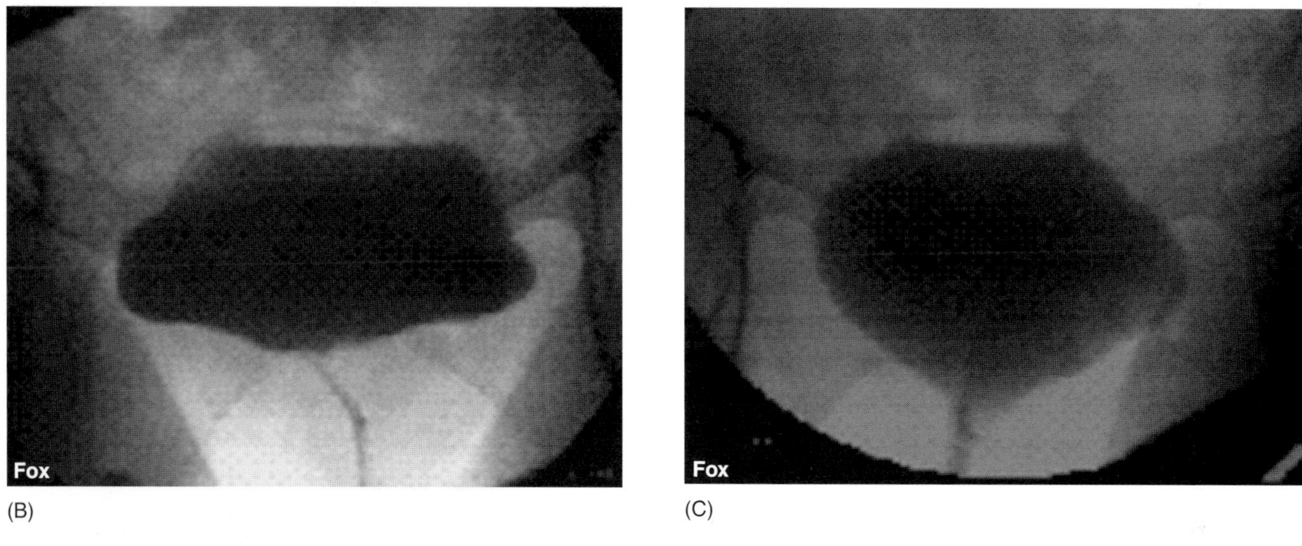

(B) (C)

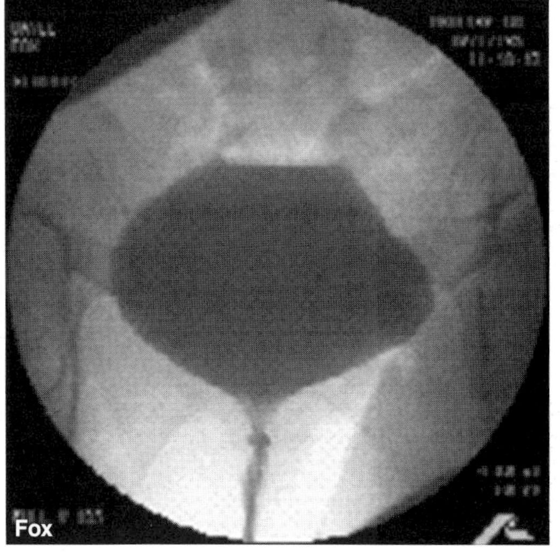

(D)

Fig. 15.13 (continued) (B) X-ray exposed just prior to the VLPP shows the vesical neck is closed. (C) X-ray exposed at VLPP shows an open vesical neck and urethra. (D) X-ray exposed during voiding in the AP position.

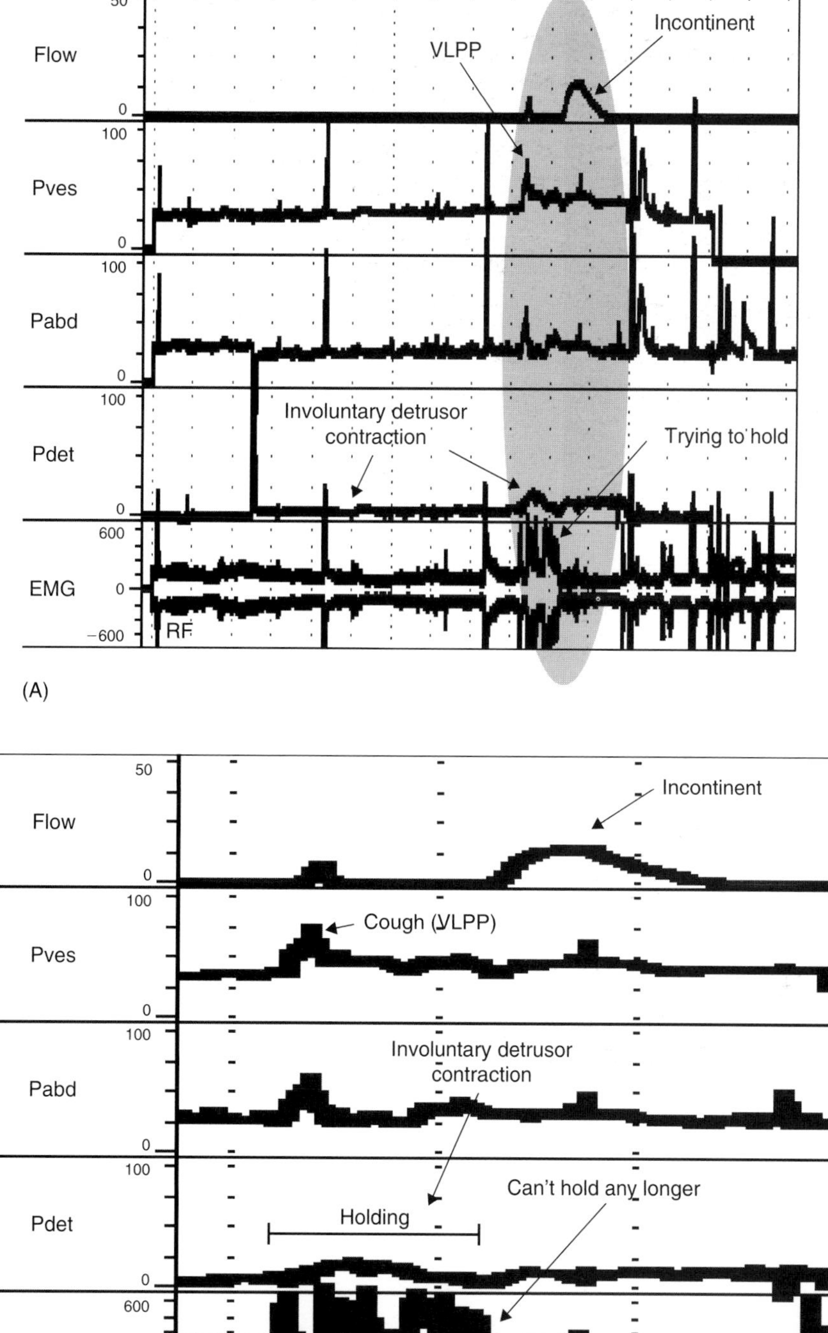

Fig.15.14 Sphincteric incontinence and stress hyperreflexia. RF is a 73-year-old woman who complains of both stress and urge incontinence that occur with about equal frequency and bother. (A) Urodynamic tracing. FSF = 182 m, 1st urge = 188 ml, severe urge = 200 ml. Bladder capacity was 312 ml. There was an involuntary detrusor contraction at a volume of 200 ml. She perceived the contraction as urge, was able to contract her sphincter and prevent incontinence.

VLPP = 88 cmH_2O. Just after the cough (shaded oval), she had another IDC and voided involuntarily. She contracted her sphincter and temporarily prevented further incontinence, but when she could no longer hold back, she voided (involuntarily) to completion. Pdet/Q: Q_{max} = 13 ml/s, Pdet@Q_{max} = 14 cmH_2O, Pdetmax = 15 cmH_2O, voided volume = 306 ml, and PVR = 0 ml.

(B) Expanded view of the tracing outlined by the shaded oval in the preceding figure.

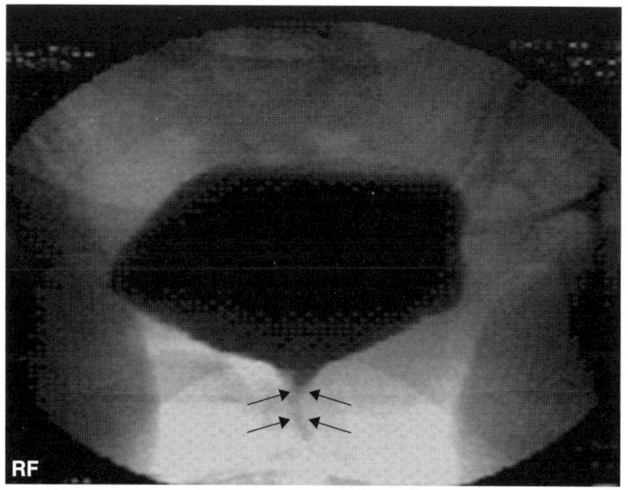

(C)

Fig. 15.14 (continued) (C) X-ray obtained at leak point pressure shows contrast in the urethra (arrows). Comment: Over the course of two years she underwent 4 periurethral collagen injections and was pleased with the outcome. The success of each injection lasted 3–6 months. Despite the subjective success, diaries and pad tests showed that she was never completely dry and still had urgency and urge incontinence. We believe that the most efficacious treatment for stress hyperreflexia is surgical, but there are no meaningful studies in the peer review literature to document our opinion.

16 Genital Prolapse

Introduction

Abnormal descent of the pelvic viscera into the vagina is termed pelvic organ prolapse (POP). Organs that can prolapse include bladder (cystocele), urethra (urethrocele), rectum (rectocele), intestine (enterocele), or uterus. However, it is not always apparent on examination which organs are involved in the prolapse, so it is preferred to describe the anatomic location of the prolapse (anterior, apical, posterior) [1]. Prolapse is graded by the maximum degree of pelvic organ descent. A simple classification describes the prolapse in relation to the hymenal ring. In grade 1, the inferior margin of the descent is above and in grade 2, at the hymenal ring. Grade 3 protrudes beyond the ring and grade 4 is well beyond it [2]. A more precise description of POP is offered by the POP-Q [3].

Women with genital prolapse may present with a plethora of lower urinary tract symptoms (LUTS) including urinary frequency, urgency, hesitancy, incomplete emptying, and incontinence. These symptoms may or may not be related to the prolapse, but with careful clinical and urodynamic investigation it is usually possible to determine the underlying pathophysiology with a high degree of accuracy.

Effect of genital prolapse on micturition

Genital prolapse can affect the lower urinary tract in a number of ways [3–9]. Firstly, it can cause, or at least be associated with, sphincteric incontinence (Fig. 16.1). Secondly, the prolapse itself can mechanically obstruct the urethra (Figs. 16.2 and 16.3). Thirdly, it may mask sphincteric incontinence because of compression of the urethra. Reduction of the cystocele with a pessary or sponge unmasks such "occult incontinence." (Fig. 16.4). Fourth, it can cause ureteral obstruction. The mechanism of ureteral obstruction has not been elucidated, but we hypothesize that in some patients, the trigone and ureters descend as part of the cystocele and can become compressed (Figs. 16.5 and 16.6). Figure 16.7 depicts a large cystocele in which the ureteral orifices do not descend with the cystocele. Finally, POP may be the cause of overactive bladder (OAB) with or without detrusor overactivity (Figs. 16.2, 16.4, and 16.8).

Of course not all LUTS in women with prolapse are due to the prolapse. Other common causes include urinary tract infection, detrusor instability, impaired detrusor contractility, bladder outlet obstruction, polyuria, and sensory urgency.

Urodynamic evaluation

The purpose of the urodynamic evaluation in women with genital prolapse is (1) to determine the precise etiology of the patient's LUTS, (2) to "unmask" occult incontinence in women with no incontinence symptoms, (3) to evaluate detrusor function (impaired detrusor contractility, detrusor overactivity), and (4) to determine the degree that cystocele and urethrocele are contributing to the prolapse (insofar as the bladder and urethra are directly visualized by X-ray).

To this end, we perform two urodynamic studies: the first without any reduction of prolapse and the second with the prolapse reduced with a ring pessary (see Fig. 16.4). Among urodynamicists, the concern has been raised that pessary reduction may cause artifactual urethral obstruction. In order to examine this possibility, we evaluated 60 women who had genital prolapse with LUTS and/or incontinence with videourodynamics to assess the effects of prolapse on micturition [9]. The women were divided into two groups based on the degree of descent – small cytocele (grade 1 or 2) and large cystocele (grade 3 or 4). Pressure-flow analysis, leak point pressure (LPP), and free flow were measured in all women. Those in the severe group also underwent repeat free flow analysis and LPP determination with mechanical reduction of their cystocele with a ring pessary.

Urodynamic data was sorted according to presence or absence of bladder outlet obstruction, impaired detrusor contractility, detrusor instability, and stress incontinence. Women with large cystoceles (grade 3–4) were much more likely to be obstructed on urodynamics (72%) as opposed to women with small ones (grades 1–2) (6%) ($P < 0.05$). Following pessary placement, 91% of those with large cystoceles and obstruction had normal free flowmetry, presumably because the prolapse itself was causing obstruction which was relieved after reduction. Of the 25 women with large cystoceles, 80% had occult stress incontinence. Following pessary placement all patients had a significant decrease in their LPP. Our study confirms the findings of other investigators and highlights the need to evaluate for the presence of urethral obstruction and occult stress incontinence in all women with prolapse, regardless of the symptom history. It is clear from this and other studies that reduction of genital prolapse during urodynamic evaluation is a valuable aid in unmasking occult stress incontinence.

Suggested Reading

1 Kenton K, Shott S, Brubaker L. Vaginal topography does not correlate well with visceral position in women with pelvic organ prolapse, *Int Urogynecol J Pelvic Floor Dysfunct*, 8(6): 336–339, 1997.

2 Baden WF, Walker TA. Physical diagnosis in the evaluation of vaginal relaxation, *Clin Obstet Gynecol*, 15: 1060–1065, 1972.

3 Bump RC, Mattiasson A, Bo K, Brubaker LP, DeLancey JO, Klarskov P, Shull BL, Smith AR. The standardization of terminology of female pelvic organ prolapse and pelvic floor dysfunction. I. *Am J Obstet Gynecol*, 175(1): 10–17, 1996.

4 Fianu S, Kjaeldgaard A, Larson B. Preoperative screening for latent stress incontinence in women with cystocele, *Neurourol Urodyn*, 4: 3–7, 1985.
5 Ghoneim GM, Walters F, Lewis V. The value of the vaginal pack test in large cystoceles. *J Urol*, 152: 931–934, 1993.
6 Mattox TF, Bhatia NN. Urodynamic effects of reducing devices in women with genital prolapse, *Int Urogynecol J*, 5: 283–286, 1994.
7 Bump RC, Fantl JA, Hurt WG. The mechanism of urinary continence in women with severe uterovaginal prolapse: results of barrier studies, *Obstet Gynecol*, 72: 291–295, 1988.
8 Coates KW, Harris RL, Cundiff GW, Bump RC. Uroflowmetry in women with urinary incontinence and pelvic organ prolapse, *Br J Urol*, 80: 217–221, 1997.
9 Romanzi LJ, Chaikin DC, Blaivas JG. Effect of genital prolapse on voiding, *J Urol*, 161: 581–586, 1999.
10 Rosenzweig BA, Pushkin S, Blumenfeld D, Bhatia NN. Prevalence of abnormal urodynamic test results in continent women with severe genitourinary prolapse, *Obstet Gynecol*, 79: 539–542, 1992.

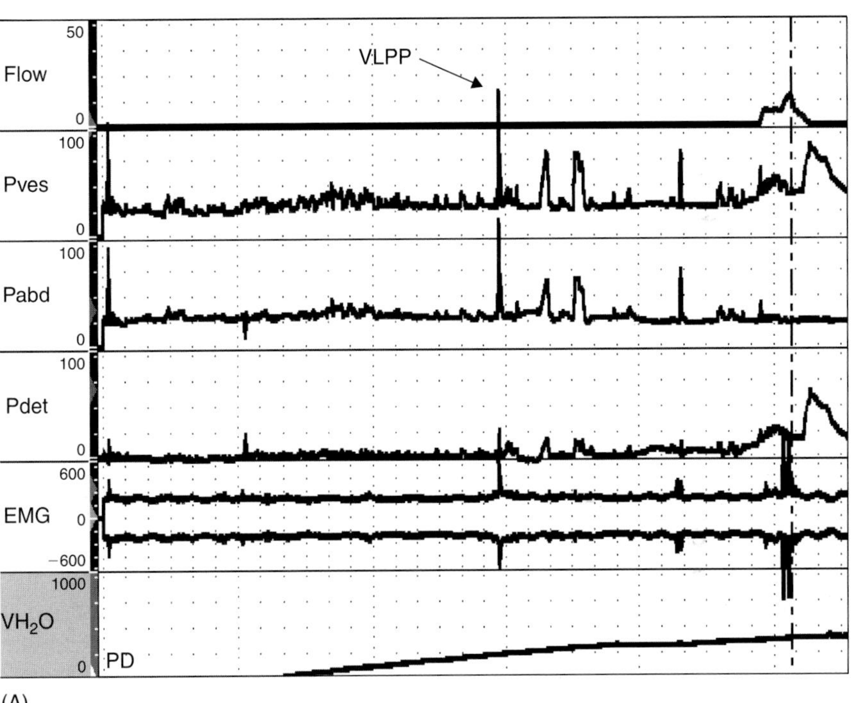

Fig. 16.1 Grade 1 anterior wall POP and sphincteric incontinence in a 53-year-old post-menopausal women. She has a large uterine leiomyoma. Q-tip test was −20° >+30°. (A) Urodynamic tracing. VLPP = 78 cmH_2O, Q_{max} = 15 ml/s, Pdet@ Q_{max} = 18 cmH_2O (vertical dotted line), Pdetmax=64 cmH_2O, voided volume=262 ml, and PVR = 148 ml. Note that there is a detrusor after contraction. These are considered to be of no clinical consequence, but one wonders why she left a 148 ml PVR. Prior to the urodynamic study PVR was nil.

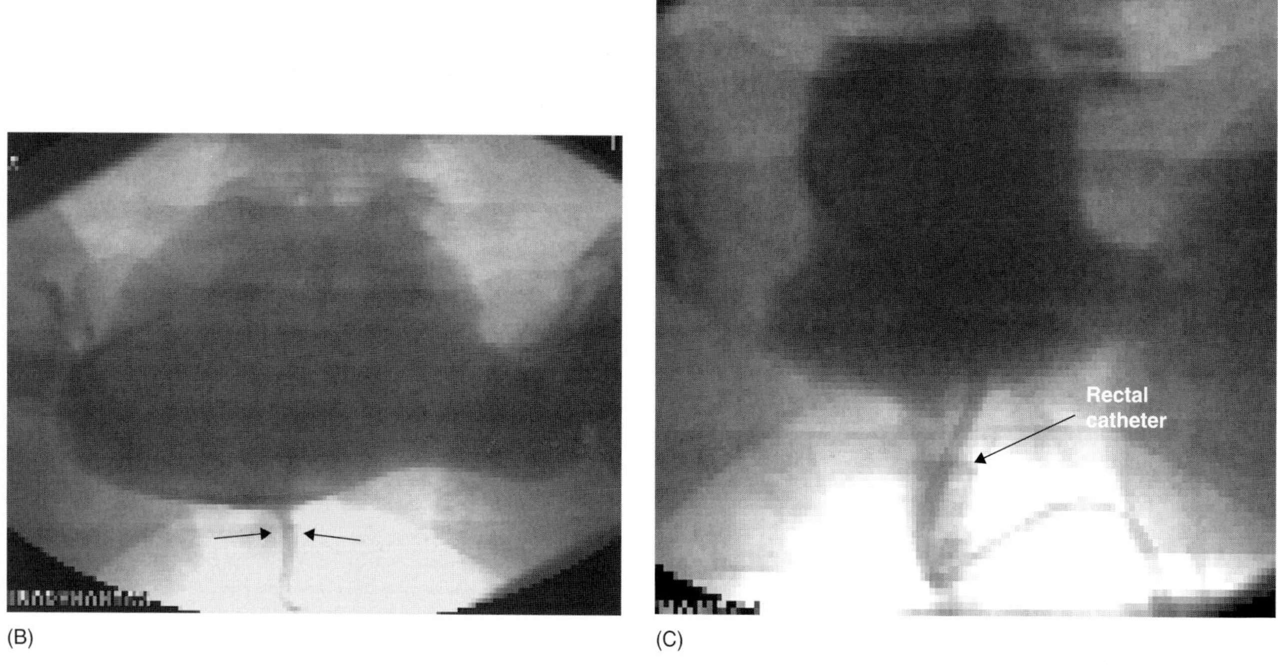

Fig. 16.1 (continued) (B) X-ray exposed at the VLPP (arrow) shows sphincteric incontinence (arrows). (C) X-ray exposed at maximum uroflow (vertical line) shows a wide open, unobstructed urethra. The rectal catheter is superimposed over the urethra.

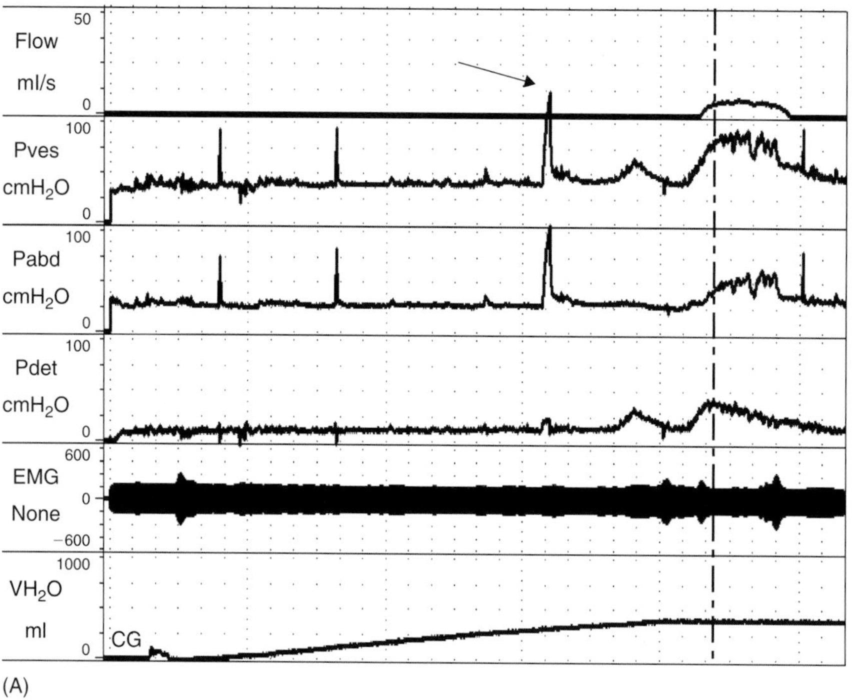

Fig. 16.2 Grade 2 POP, type 2 OAB, and grade 1 urethral obstruction in a 68-year-old woman with urgency, urge incontinence, and recurring urinary tract infections. (A) Urodynamic tracing with prolapse in its most dependent position. During cough and straining, there is no incontinence with vesical pressures as high as 132 cmH_2O (arrow). During voiding there is grade 1 obstruction according to the Blaivas–Groutz nomogram. Q_{max} = 8.3 ml/s, Pdet@Q_{max} = 36 cmH_2O (vertical dotted line), Pdetmax = 42 cmH_2O, voided volume = 376 ml, and PVR (post-void residual) = 13 ml.

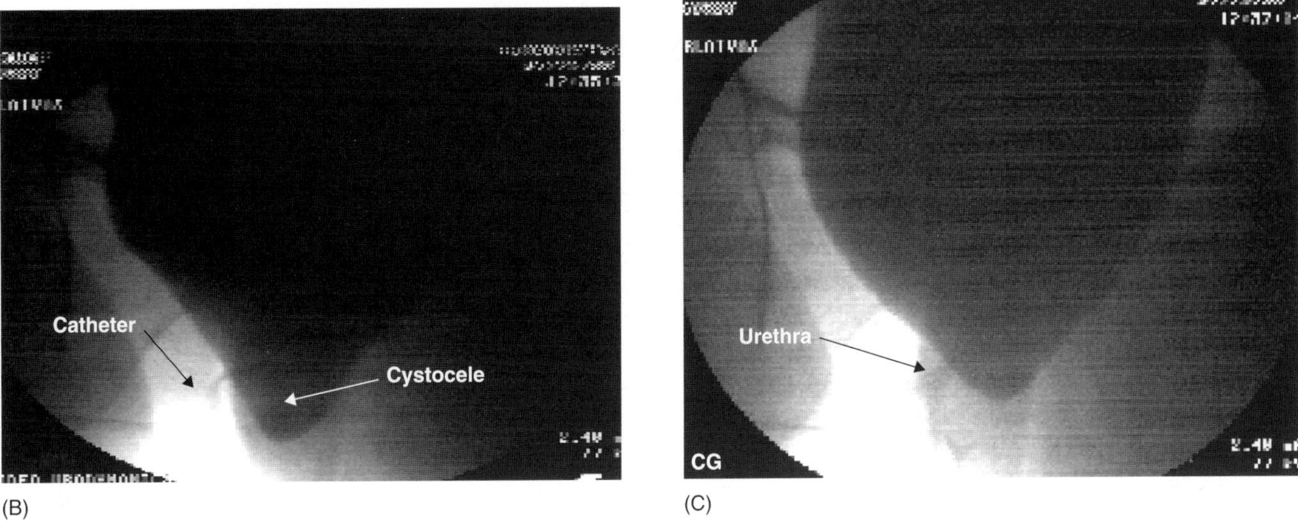

Fig. 16.2 (continued) (B) X-ray exposed during cough. (C) X-ray exposed during voiding. There is only faint visualization of the urethra.

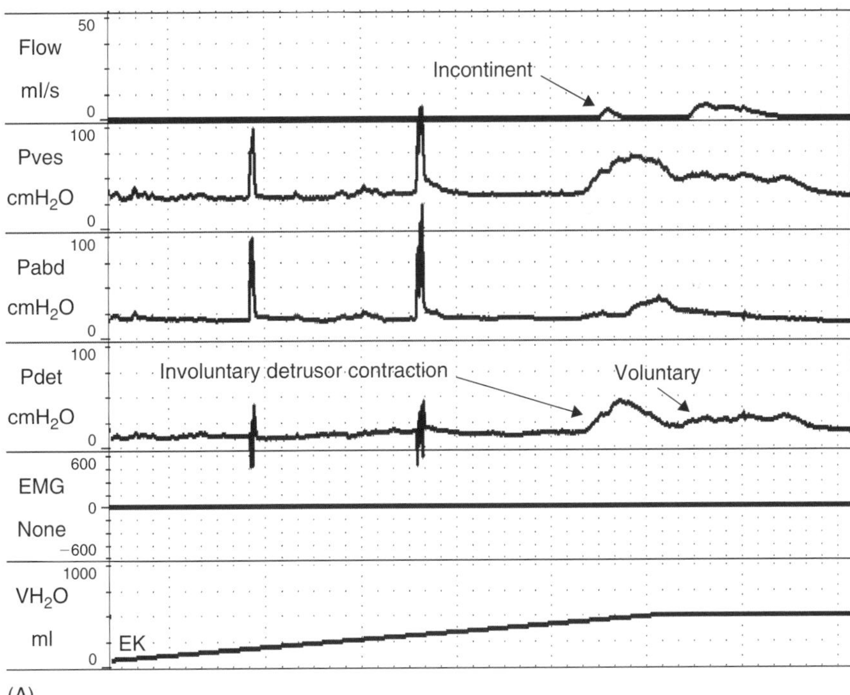

Fig. 16.3 Grade 3 prolapse grade 2 urethral obstruction and type 3 OAB in a 76-year-old woman. Her chief complaint is OAB and "a dropped bladder." Cystoscopy showed that the bladder prolapsed posterior to the trigone. The ureteral orifices did not descend with the cystocele. (A) Urodynamic study. FSF = 269 ml, 1st urge = 302 ml, and severe urge = 426 ml. IDC@448 ml, Bladder capacity = 510 ml, Q_{max} = 6 ml/s, Pdet@Q_{max} = 28 cmH_2O, Pdetmax = 45 cmH_2O, voided volume = 160 ml, and PVR = 344 ml. The EMG channel was not working.

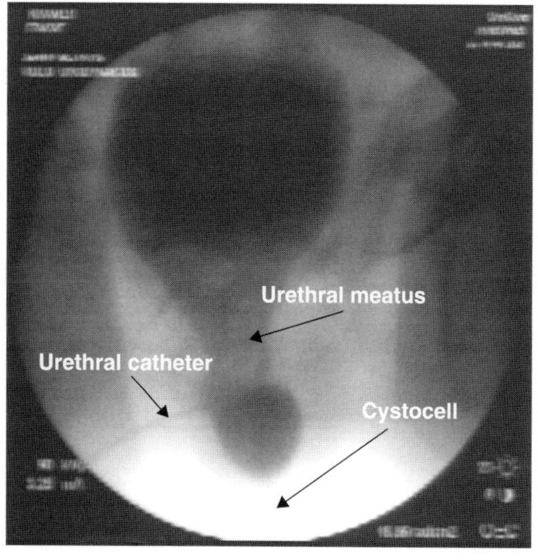

(B)

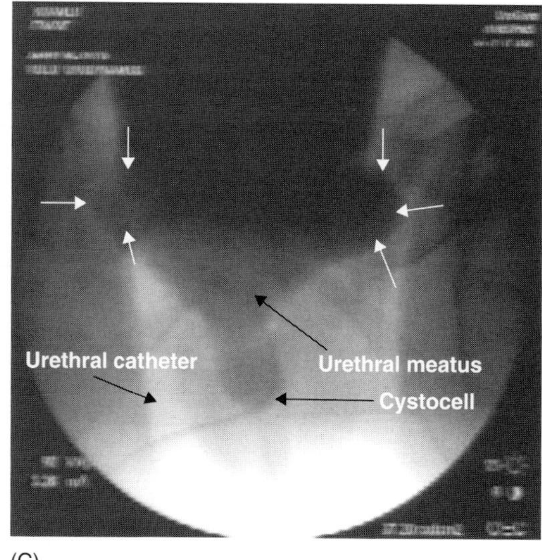

(C)

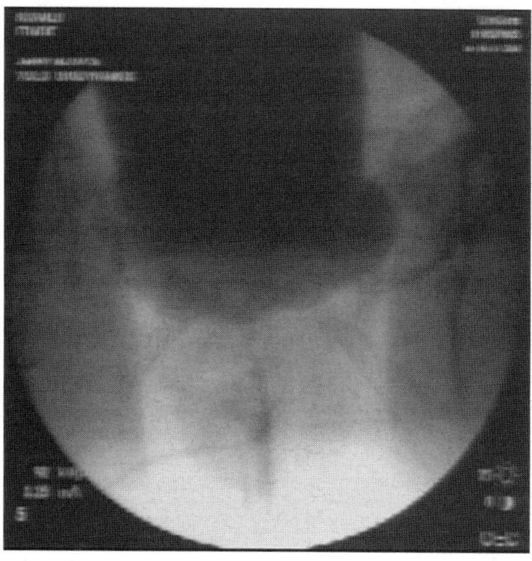

(D)

Fig. 16.3 (continued) (B) X-ray exposed just prior to the onset of micturition. (C) X-ray exposed at Q just after the onset of micturition. The white arrows point to bilateral bladder diverticula. (D) X-ray exposed at Q_{max} shows only faint visualization of the urethra. Note that the cystocele has completely reduced.

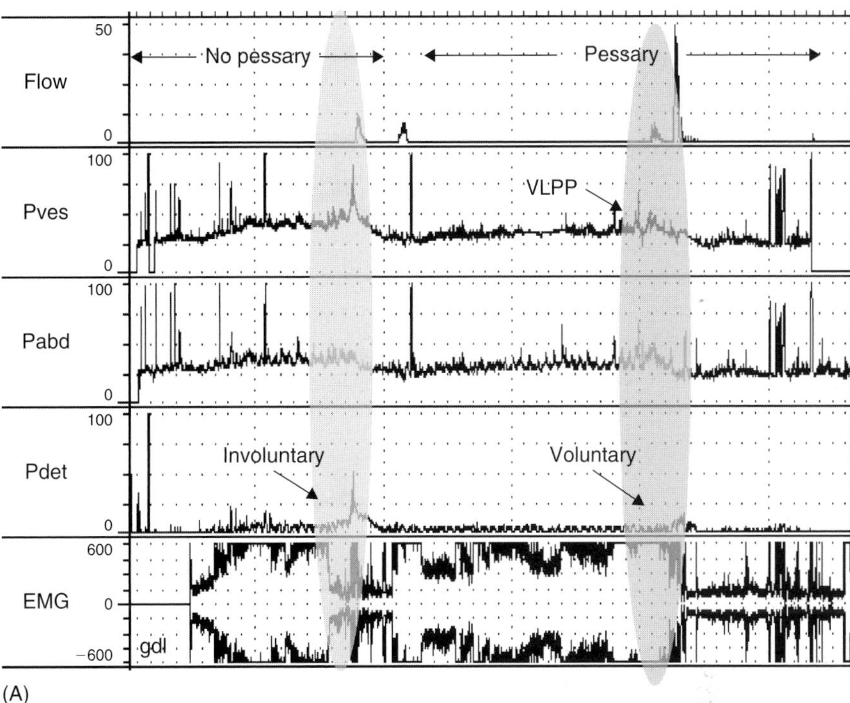

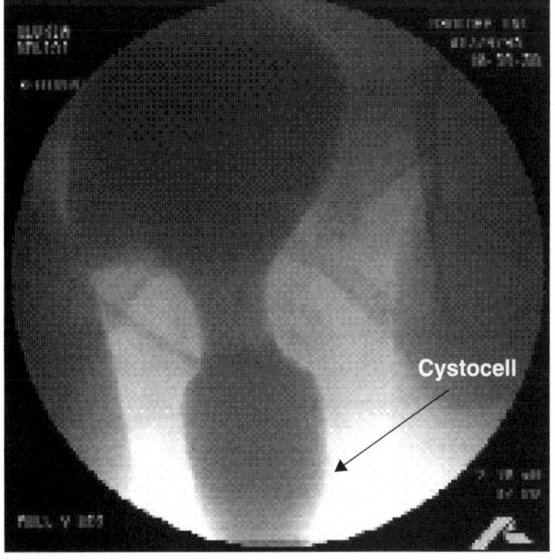

Fig. 16.4 Grade 4 prolapse, detrusor overactivity, and occult sphincteric incontinence. (A) Urodynamic tracing. The examination was begun with the cystocele in a grade 4 position. FSF = 17 ml, 1st urge = 58 ml, and a severe urge occurred at 140 ml accompanied by an involuntary detrusor contraction (see Fig. 16.4(C)).

During bladder filling without the pessarys, she was asked to cough and strain and there was no incontinence. After the involuntary detrusor contraction, a #4 ring pessary was inserted. At bladder capacity (271 ml), bladder filling was stopped, she strained and was incontinent (valsalva leak point pressure, VLPP). Then she was asked to void and had a voluntary detrusor contraction and voided normally. (B) X-ray exposed during cough to 100 cmH_2O shows the cystocel.

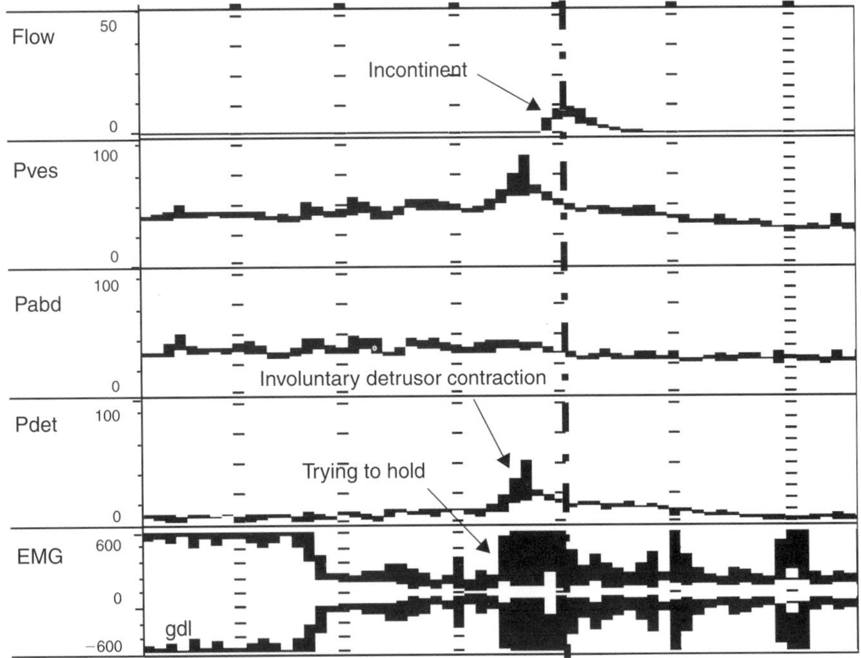

(C)

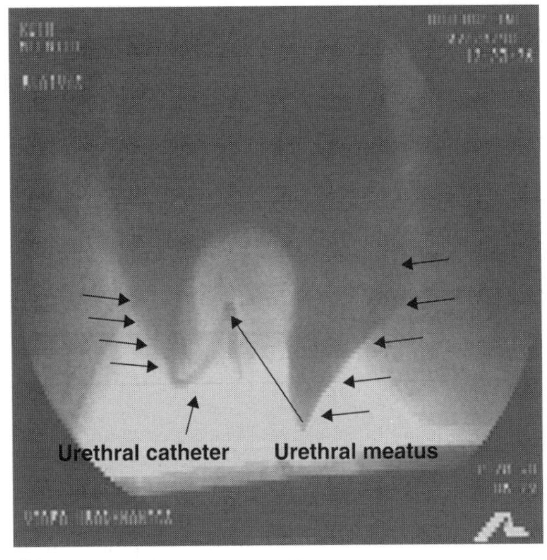

(D)

Fig. 16.4 (**continued**) (C) Expanded view of the involuntary detrusor contraction marked by the shaded oval in Figure 16.4(A) without the pessary. She perceived the contraction as an urge to void and was able to temporarily prevent incontinence by contracting the sphincter, but once she fatigued, she was incontinent. Pressure flow without pessary at vertical line, Pdet@Q_{max} = 15 cmH_2O, Q_{max} = 10 ml/s, and PVR = 0. (D) X-ray exposed at the LPP with the pessary in place shows some prolapse of the bladder around the pessary (arrows).

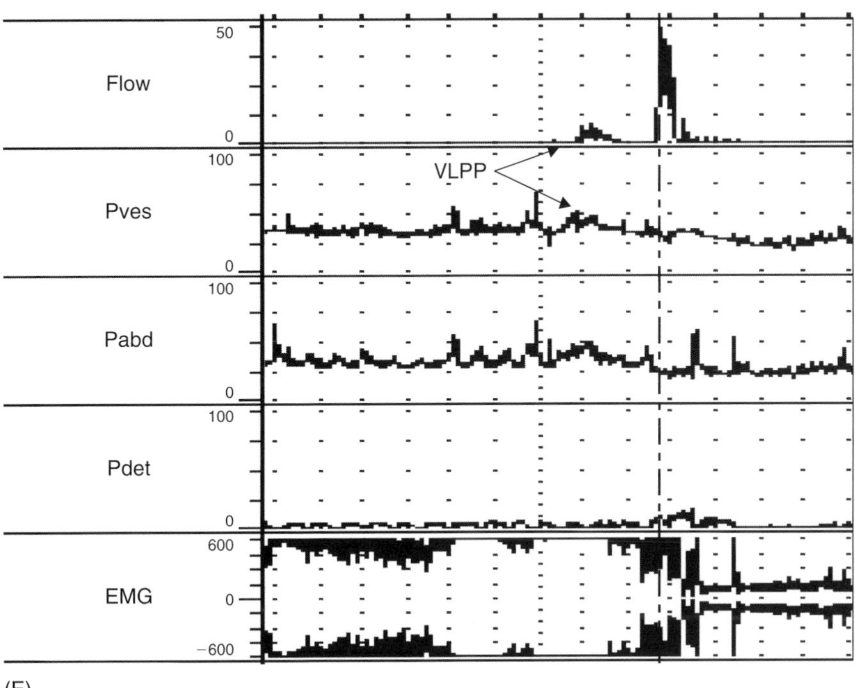

Fig. 16.4 (continued) (E) Expanded view of the 2nd shaded oval. Incontinence occurred at a VLPP=50 cmH_2O. Voluntary voiding occurred with a Pdet@ Q_{max}=6 cmH_2O and Q_{max}=48 ml/s (vertical line). Comment: at first glance, there appears to be urethral obstrctuion with the prolgesse at maximal descent. Closer inspection of the expanded molynomic tracing shows that the high Pdet is due to a voluntary sphincter contraction in an attempt to prevent incontinence during an involuntary detrusor contraction.

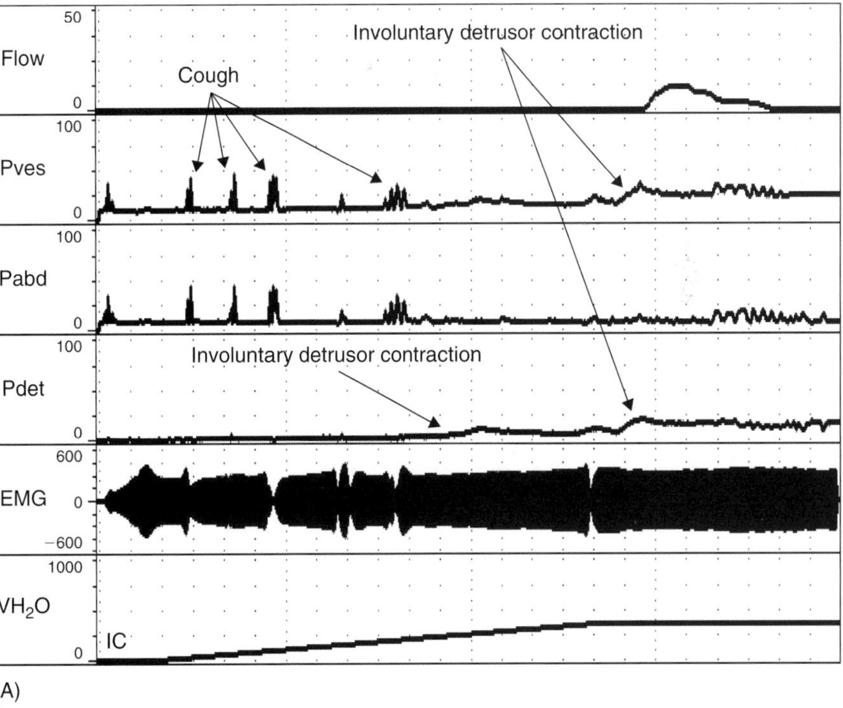

Fig. 16.5 Grade 3 cystocele in a 77-year-old woman who complains of pelvic discomfort and mixed stress and urge incontinence. She also notes that she has to push and strain to void. At cystoscopy, it was observed that the trigone and ureteral orifices descended with the bladder as part of the cystocele. (A) Urodynamic study. FSF = 236 ml, 1st urge = 277 ml, and severe urge = 283 ml. The severe urge was accompanied by an involuntary detrusor contraction, (type 2 OAB). She perceived the contraction as urge, was able to contract her shincter, abort the detrusor contraction, and prevent incontinence. At bladder capacity (377 ml), she was asked to void. and had a voluntary detrusor contraction. During multiple coughs and valsalvas, there was no incontinence. VOID: 24/312/0 Pdet/Q_{max}: Q_{max} = 12 ml/s, Pdet@Q_{max} = 16 cmH_2O, Pdetmax = 22 cmH_2O, voided volume = 371 ml, and PVR = 0 ml (no obstruction).

205

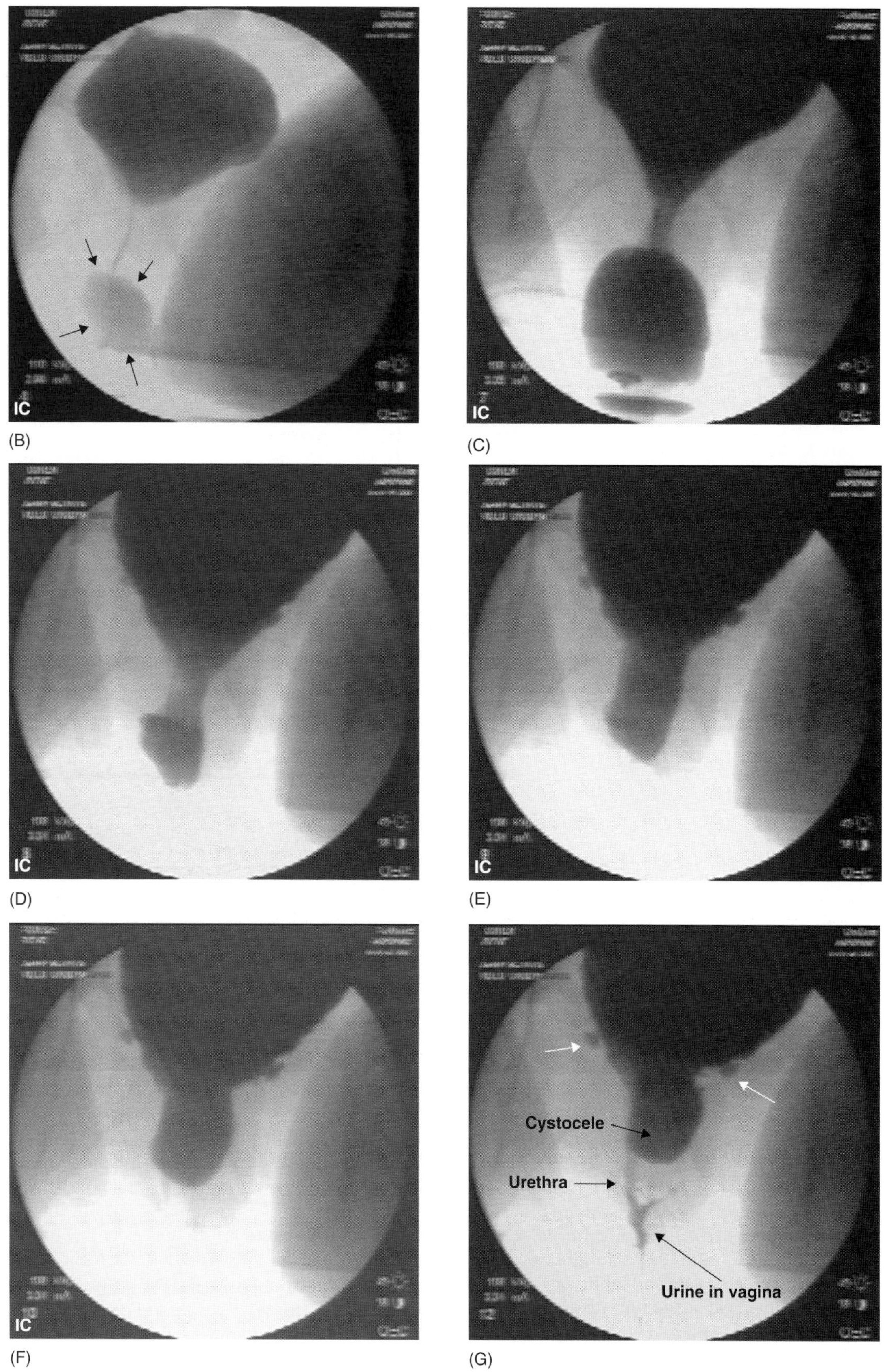

Fig. 16.5 (continued) (B) During early bladder filling the cystocele defect is already apparent (arrows). (C) During further filling the cystocele is more apparent. (D) As the bladder starts to contract, the cystocele is reducing. (E) As the bladder continues to contract and she voids, the cystocele is partially reduced. (F) Just prior to voiding. (G) Note that, in contradistinction to the patient depicted in Figure 16.7, the urethra opens and voiding begins even with the cystocele deformity still present. White arrows point to small bladder diverticula.

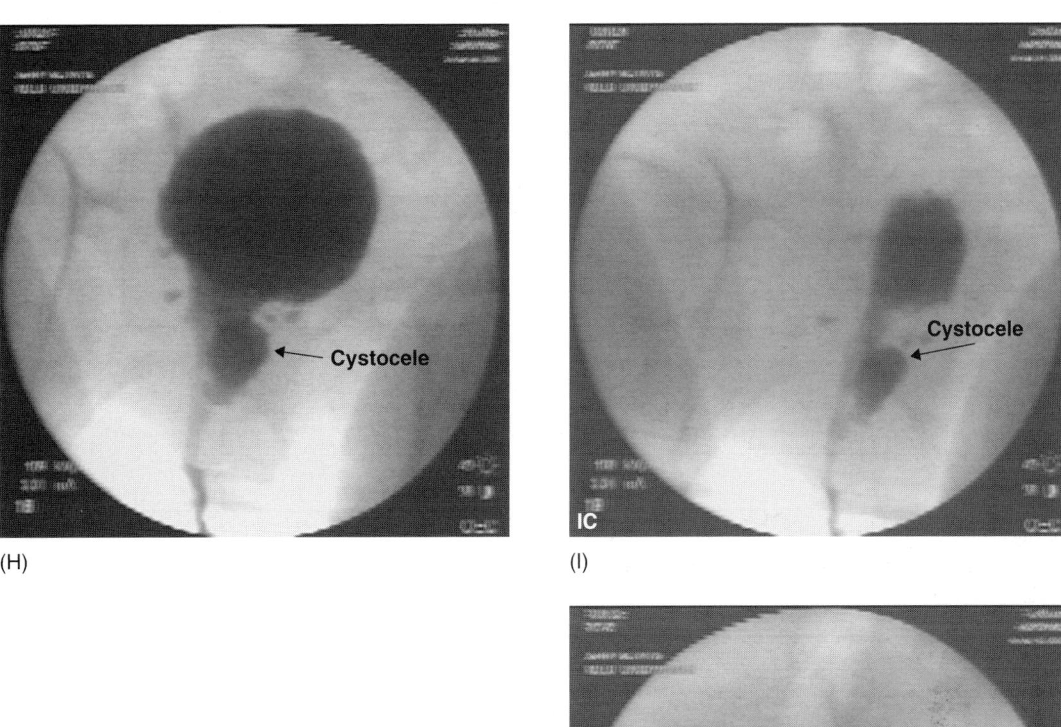

(H) (I)

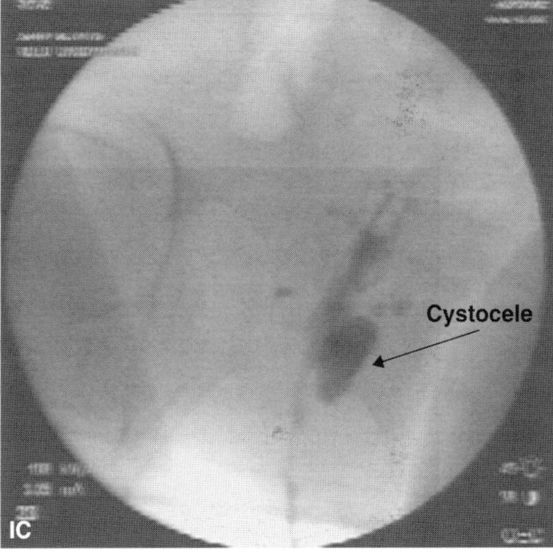

(J)

Fig. 16.5 (continued) (H) Voiding continues to occur despite persistence of the cystocele. (I) Even towards the end of micturition, the cystocele is still present. If the entire sequence of micturition was not observed, one could easily misinterpret this as a urethral diverticulum. (J) Even after micturition is completed almost all of the residual urine (10 ml) is in the remaining cystocele.

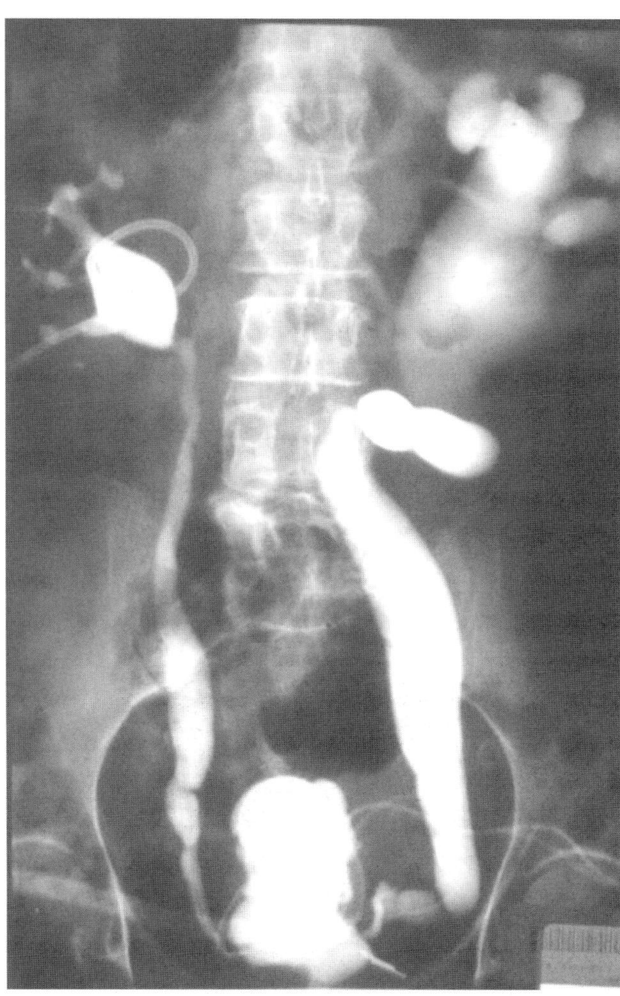

Fig. 16.6 Bilateral nephrostograms showing bilateral ureteral obstruction in a 72-year-old woman with longstanding grade 4 POP.

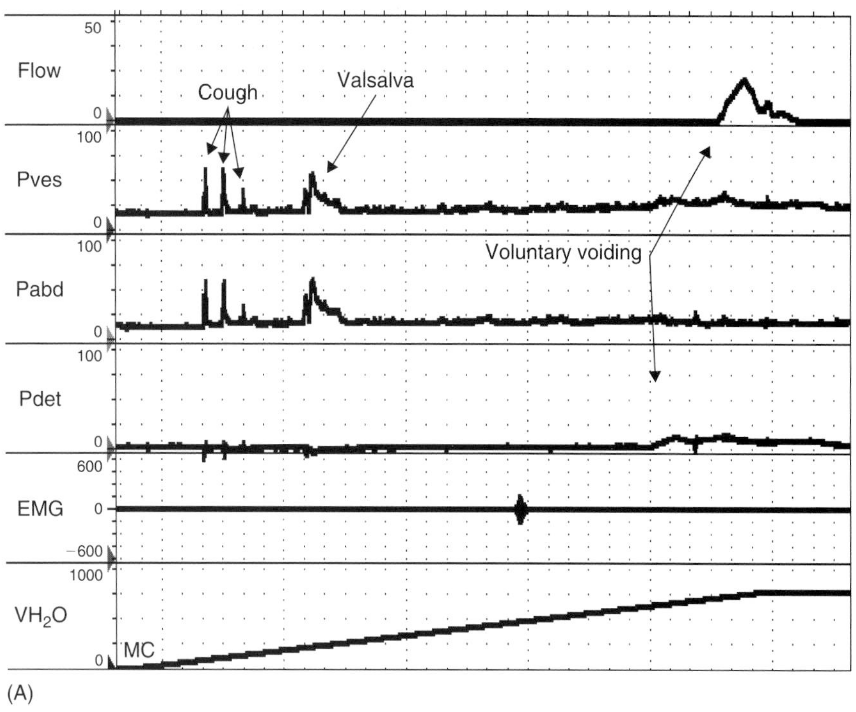

Fig. 16.7 A 64-year-old woman with grade 3 anterior wall and vault prolapse 28 days status post abdominal hysterectomy. Her chief complaint was urinary urgency, urge incontinence, and frequent urinary tract infections. Cystoscopy showed that the ureteral orifices and trigone did not descend with the cystocele. (A) Urodynamic Study. FSF = 439 ml, 1st urge = 633 ml, and severe urge = 725 ml. There was no incontinence during cough and valsalva. During bladder filling there were no spontaneous involuntary detrusor contractions. Bladder capacity was 771 ml. Pdet/Q study: Q_{max} = 24 ml/s, Pdet@Q_{max} = 10 cmH_2O, Pdetmax = 13 cmH_2O, voided volume = 388 ml, and PVR = 379 ml (no obstruction). It is not clear why she did not empty her bladder.

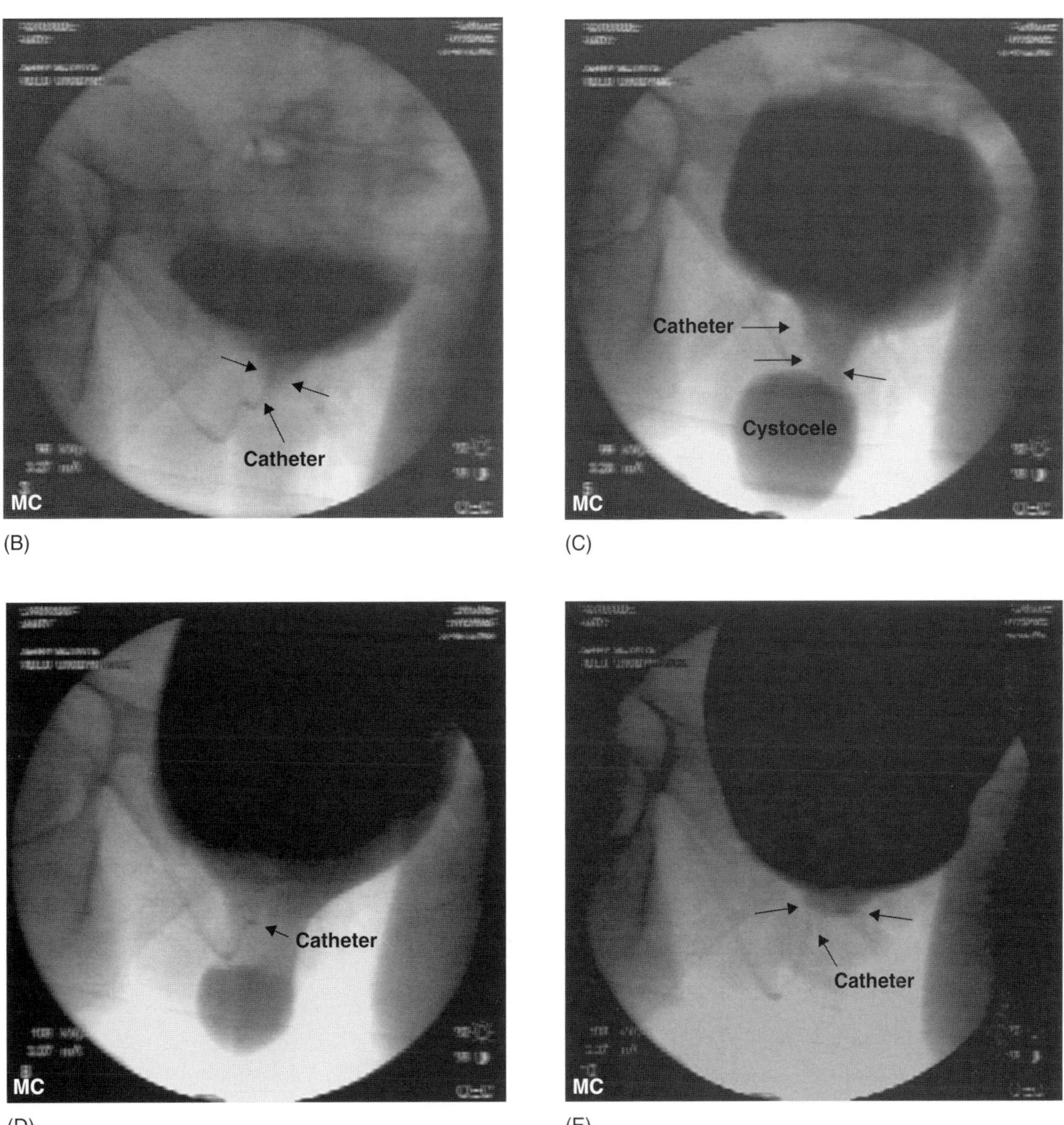

Fig. 16.7 (continued) (B) X-ray exposed during bladder filling with about 50 ml. At first glance it appears that the bladder neck is open (arrows), but this is actually the beginning of the cystocele defect. (C) X-ray exposed during bladder filling with about 200 ml. Note that the bladder base has descended into the vagina (cystocele) through a fairly narrow defect (arrows). (D) The bladder has just started to contract, but flow has not begun and the cystocele is beginning to recede; contraction of the detrusor draws the bladder base back into its normal anatomic position. (E) Just prior to the start of flow the bladder base has almost completely receded back into its normal anatomic position (arrows).

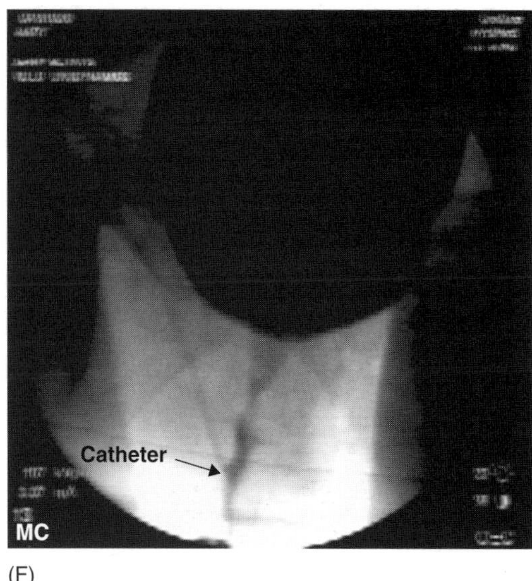

(F)

Fig. 16.7 (continued) (F) As she begins to void, the bladder base has receded to its normal anatomic position and the urethra opens normally.

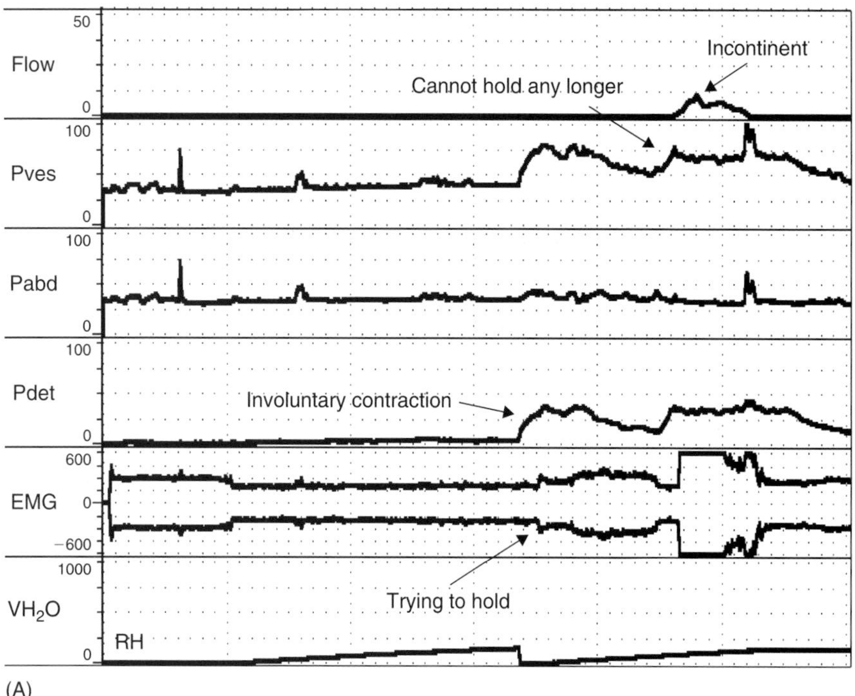

(A)

Fig. 16.8 Procidentia (grade 4 POP), type 3 OAB and grade 1 urethral obstruction in a 74-year-old woman. She complained of OAB with urge incontinence of 3 years duration and a vaginal bulge, pressure, and heaviness.

(A) Urodynamic study. Q_{max} = 11 ml/s, Pdet@Q_{max} = 31 cmH_2O, Pdetmax = 45 cmH_2O, voided volume = 176 ml, PVR = 55 ml.

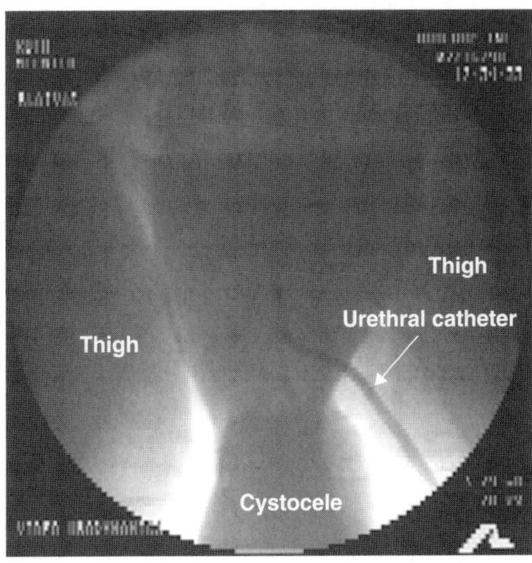

(B)

Fig. 16.8 (continued) (B) X-ray obtained with a full bladder just prior to the onset of the involuntary detrusor contraction.

17 Sphincteric Incontinence in Men and Other Complications of Prostate Cancer Treatment

Sphincteric incontinence in men is uncommon. By far the most common cause is radical prostatectomy for prostate cancer. Transurethral prostatectomy, particularly after radiotherapy for prostate cancer is probably the next most common cause [1]. Less common causes are neurologic conditions including thoraco-lumbar neurologic lesions such as spina bifda, multi-system atrophy (Shy–Drager syndrome) and after abdomino-perineal resection of the rectum.

In the vast majority of patients after radical prostatectomy, incontinence is transitory, usually spontaneously subsiding in a matter of months, although it may take as long as 1 year for full recovery. Sphincteric incontinence that occurs in men who have undergone radiation (external beam or brachytherapy), on the other hand, often does not spontaneously remit. Rather, if incontinence improves it is usually because of the development of a urethral stricture that begins a vicious cycle. Treatment of the stricture usually results in recurrent incontinence and treatment of the incontinence (sphincter prosthesis or male sling) is often complicated by the development of recurrent stricture [2,3].

From a diagnostic standpoint, most patients who complain of a constant, dribbling, gravitational, or stress induced incontinence have sphincteric malfunction, and most who complain of urinary frequency, urgency and urge incontinence have involuntary detrusor contractions. However, there may be considerable overlap between these two conditions and both may coexist in the same patient. Sphincter malfunction is the commonest cause of post-prostatectomy incontinence (PPI), accounting for about 95% of cases, but it may be accompanied by detrusor overactivity and/or low bladder compliance. As an isolated cause, detrusor overactivity causes about 5% of PPI [4–6].

On fluoroscopy, the classic appearance of post-radical prostatectomy stress incontinence is the funnel of bladder–urethral anastomosis at rest with contrast seen in the bulbar or distal urethra during increases in abdominal pressure (Fig. 17.1B). The presence of and size of the urodynamic catheter used to measure leak point pressure (LPP) may itself impact the recording and may mask sphincteric incontinence or suggest urethral obstruction when it is not clinically relevant (Fig. 17.2). Figure 17.3 shows a videourodynamic study in a man after successful implantation of a sphincter prosthesis for post-prostatectomy sphincteric incontinence.

In the majority of patients, the etiology of incontinence will be apparent after a careful history, physical examination, voiding diary, and pad test. However, detrusor overactivity and low bladder compliance can only be diagnosed with urodynamic studies (Figs. 17.4 and 17.5).

Recurrent incontinence and complications after implantation of sphincter prosthesis and male slings are not uncommon. The differential diagnosis includes sphincteric incontinence (due to atrophy of the urethra, from compression by the cuff), prosthetic malfunction, detrusor overactivity, low bladder compliance, and urethral erosion of the cuff [7]. These are depicted in Figures 17.6–17.9.

Complications after radiation treatment, both external beam and brachytherapy, even in the present era of careful urethral dosimetry, continue to be an occasional cause of devastating complications including recurring strictures, stones, urethral erosion, intractable overactive bladder (OAB), and pain [8–10] as depicted in Figures 17.8–17.11.

Suggested Reading

1 Schaeffer AJ. Prostatectomy incontinence, *J Urol*, 167 (2 Pt 1): 602, 2002.

2 Castle EP, Andrews PE, Itano N, Novicki DE, Swanson SK, Ferrigni RG. The male sling for post-prostatectomy incontinence: mean followup of 18 months, *J Urol*, 173 (5): 1657–1660, 2005.

3 Lagerveld BW, Laguna MP, Debruyne FM, De La Rosette JJ. Holmium:YAG laser for treatment of strictures of vesicourethral anastomosis after radical prostatectomy, *J Endourol*, 19 (4): 497–501, 2005.

4 Hellstrom P, Likkarinen O, Kontturi M. Urodynamics in radical retropubic prostatectomy, *Scand J Urol Nephrol*, 23: 21, 1989.

5 Foote J, Yun S, Leach GE. Postprostatectomy incontinence pathophysiology, evaluation, and management, *Urol Clin N Am*, 18: 229–241, 1991.

6 Groutz A, Blaivas JG, Chaikin DC, Verhaaren M. The pathophysiology of post radical prostatectomy incontinence: a clinical and videourodynamic study, *J Urol*, 163: 1767, 2000.

7 Webster GD, Sherman ND. Management of male incontinence following artificial urinary sphincter failure, *Curr Opin Urol*, 15 (6): 386–390, 2005.

8 Han BH, Demwl KC, Wallner K, Ellis W, Young L, Russell K. Patient reported complications after prostate brachytherapy, *J Urol*, 166: 962–963, 2001.

9 Moreira SG, Seigne JD, Orderica RC, et al. Devastating complications after brachytherapy in the treatment of prostate adenocarcinoma, *Br J Urol Int*, 93: 31–35, 2004.

10 Sarosdy MF. Urinary and rectal complications of contemporary permanent transperineal brachytherapy for prostate carcinoma with or without external beam radiation, *Cancer*, 101 (4): 754–760, 2004.

11 O'Donnell PD, Brookover T, Hewett M, al-Juburi AZ. Continence level following radical prostatectomy, *Urol*, 36: 511–512, 1990.

12 Pesti Jr JC, Schmidt RA, Narayan PA, Carroll PR, Tanagho EA. Pathophysiology of urinary incontinence after radical prostatectomy, *J Urol*, 143: 975–978, 1990.

13 Steiner MS, Morton RA, Walsh PC. Impact of anatomical radical prostatectomy on urinary continence, *J Urol*, 145: 512–514, 1991.

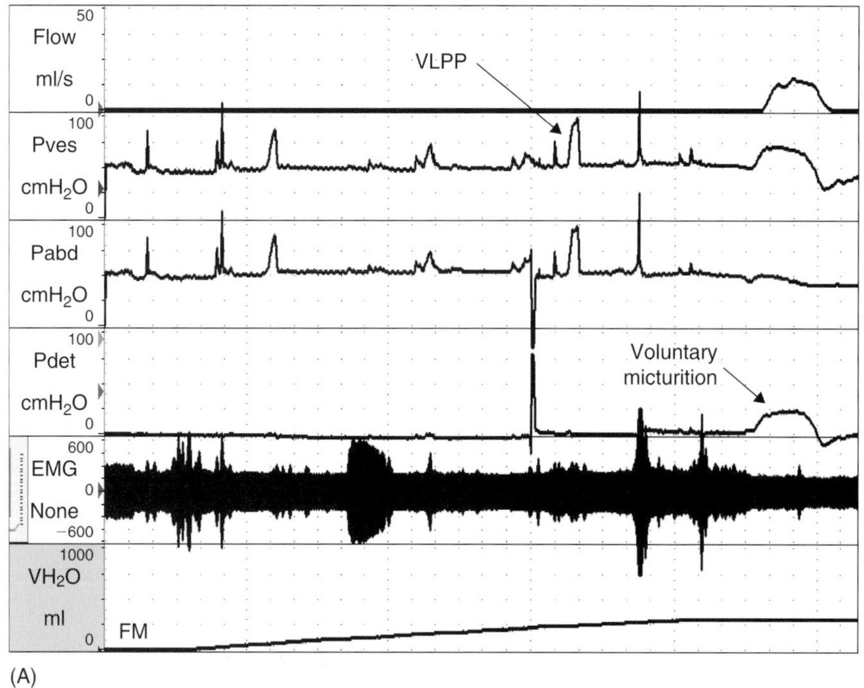

(A)

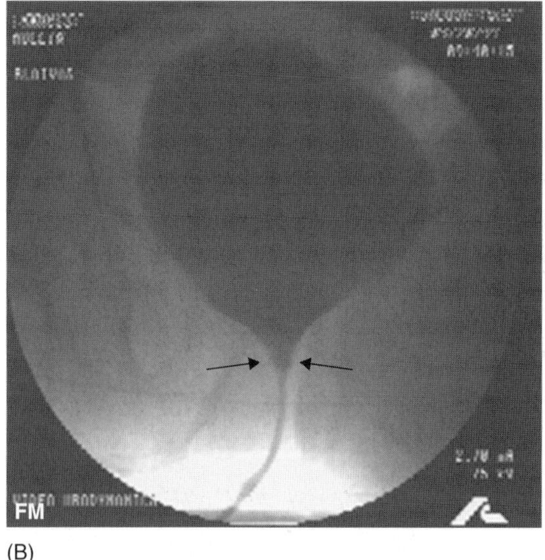

(B)

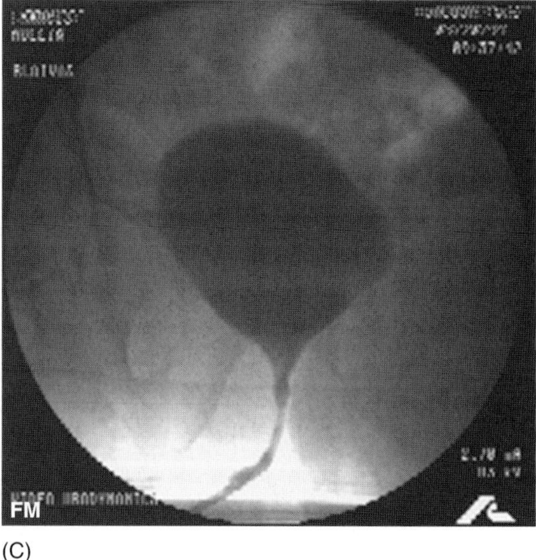

(C)

Fig. 17.1 Sphincteric incontinence after radical retropubic prostatectomy. FM is a 72-year-old man who is 7 years status post-radical prostatectomy. His only prior treatment was a collagen injection. He complains of pure stress incontinence which was reproduced on examination. He ordinarily voids every 3 hours during the day and has nocturia about every 2–3 hours at night. He wears absorbent pads daily, and he changes them 3 times per day. The pads are usually soaked through. His AUA symptom score is 10. (A) Urodynamic tracing. FSF = 211 ml, 1st urge = 299 ml, severe urge = 305 ml, bladder capacity = 311 ml, VLPP = 84 cmH_2O, Q_{max} = 16 ml/s, Pdet@Q_{max} = 23 cmH_2O, Pdetmax = 23 cmH_2O, voided volume = 317 ml, and PVR = 0 ml. (B) X-ray obtained with a full bladder, just prior to VLPP shows contrast in the proximal urethra (arrows). (C) X-ray obtained at VLPP shows contrast throughout the entire urethra.

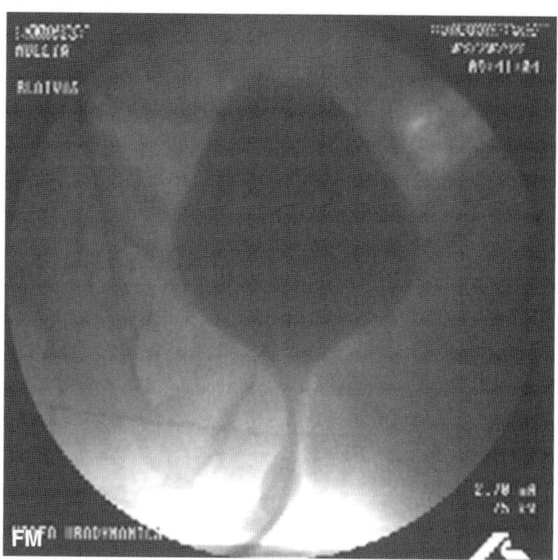

Fig. 17.1 (continued) (D) X-ray obtained during voiding.

(D)

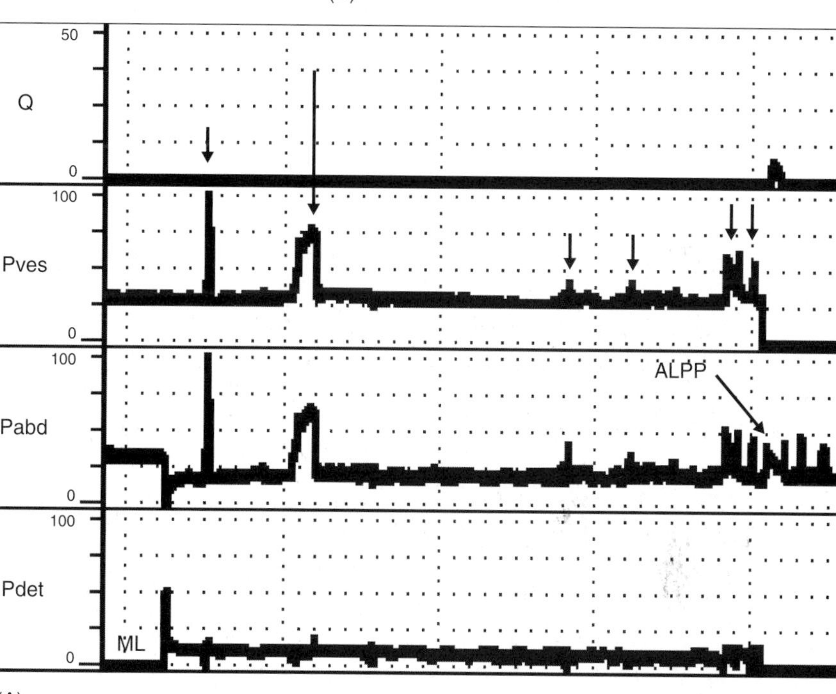

(A)

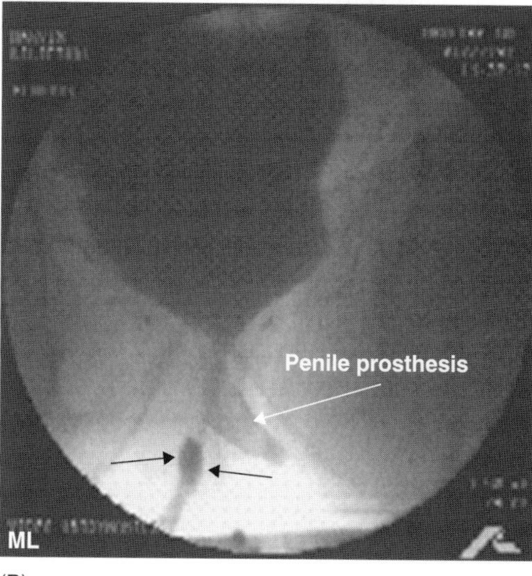

(B)

Fig. 17.2 Post-prostatectomy sphincteric incontinence masked by the presence of the urodynamic catheter. (A) Urodynamic tracing. During bladder filling he was asked to valsal va (large arrow) and cough (small arrows), but there was no leakage. At bladder capacity the urethral catheter was removed and he was incontinent with an ALPP = 48 cmH_2O. (B) X-ray exposed at the ALPP shows contrast throughout the entire urethra. The density just distal to the membranous urethra (arrows) is due to overlapping (*en face* appearance) of the bulb because the patient was not obliqued enough. He had previously undergone insertion of a penile prosthesis, but one of the cylinders had eroded through the urethra and was removed.

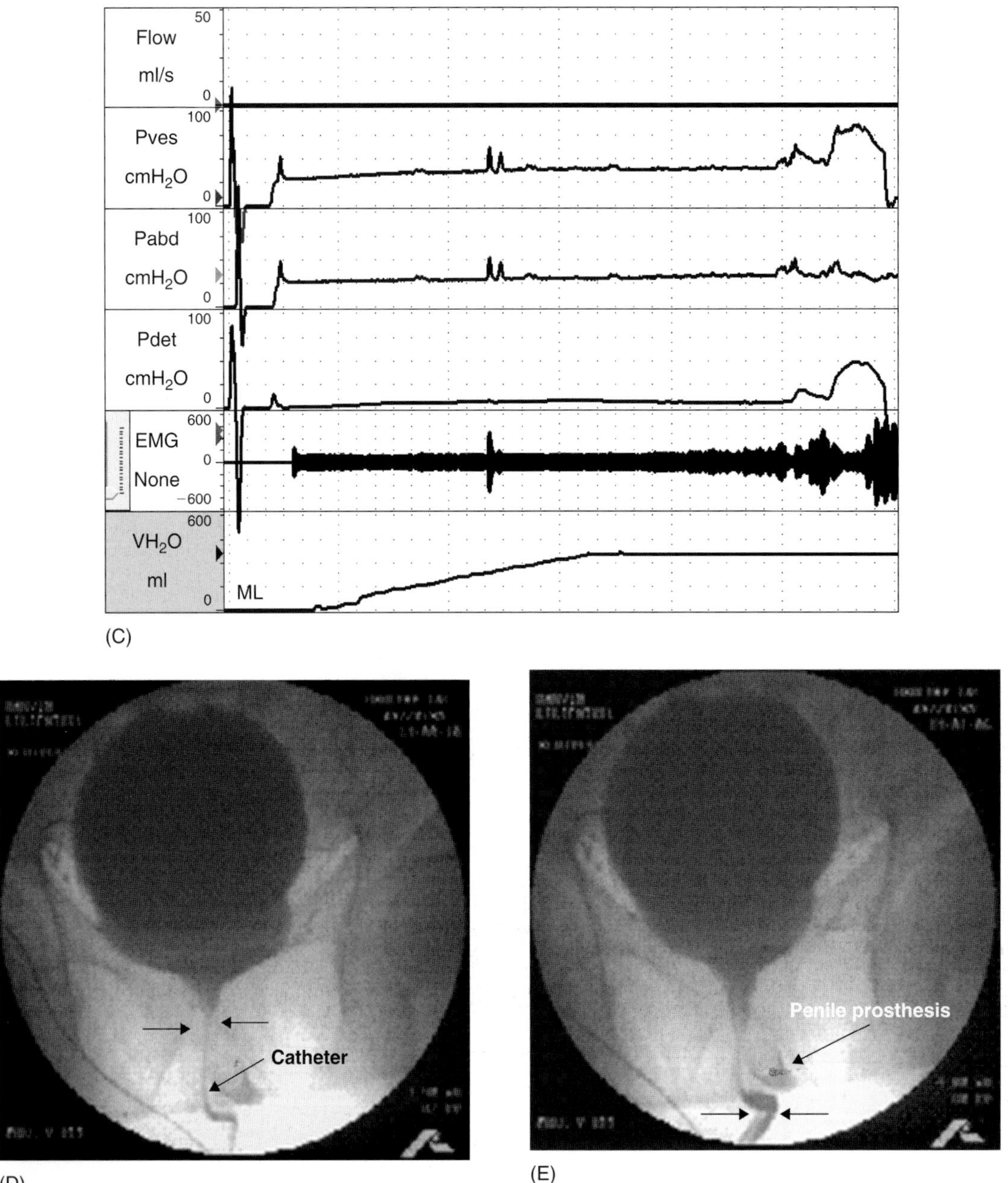

Fig. 17.2 (continued) (C) The bladder is refilled and he has a voluntary detrusor contraction to 50 cmH_2O, but there is no flow, suggesting urethral obstruction. (D) X-ray obtained with the urethra catheter in place shows obstruction at about the level of the membranous urethra (arrows). The double density seen in the bladder is due to unequal mixing of contrast with residual urine in the bladder. (E) X-ray obtained after removal of the urethral catheter shows contrast in the anterior urethra (arrows). Uroflow was normal.

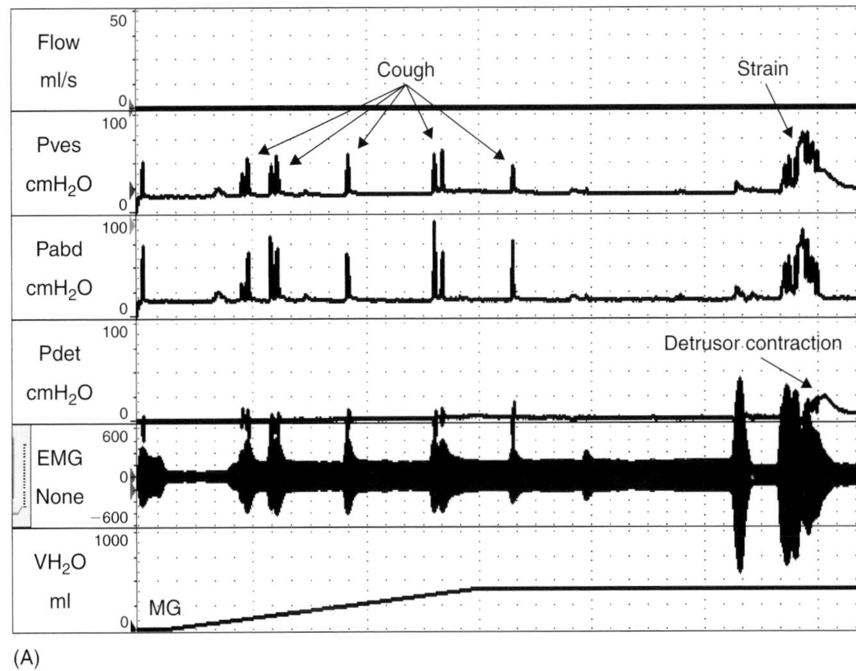

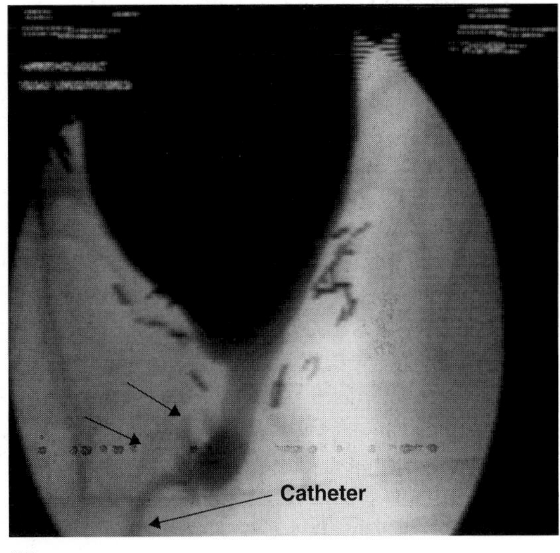

Fig. 17.3 Normal study 6 months after implantation of sphincter prosthesis in a 69-year-old man S/P radical retropubic prostatectomy and (unsuccessful) male sling. The study was repeated because of low bladder compliance on his preoperative urodynamic study. (A) Urodynamic tracing. There is no leakage despite multiple coughs. At the end of the procedure he strains and achieves a Pves = 80 cmH_2O. There is a detrusor contraction initiated by straining to 25 cmH_2O and he is still not incontinent. Note the appropriate increase in EMG activity during coughing and straining. (B) X-ray obtained during maximum straining shows that continence is maintained at the level of the sphincter prosthesis. The arrows point to contrast in the sphincter cuff. There are multiple surgical clips from his prior surgery.

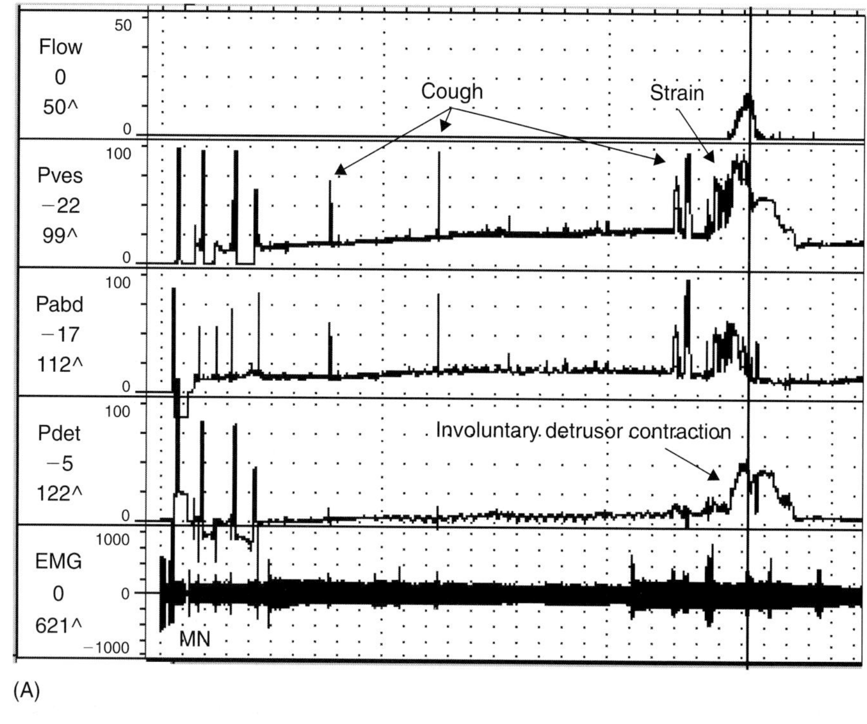

(A)

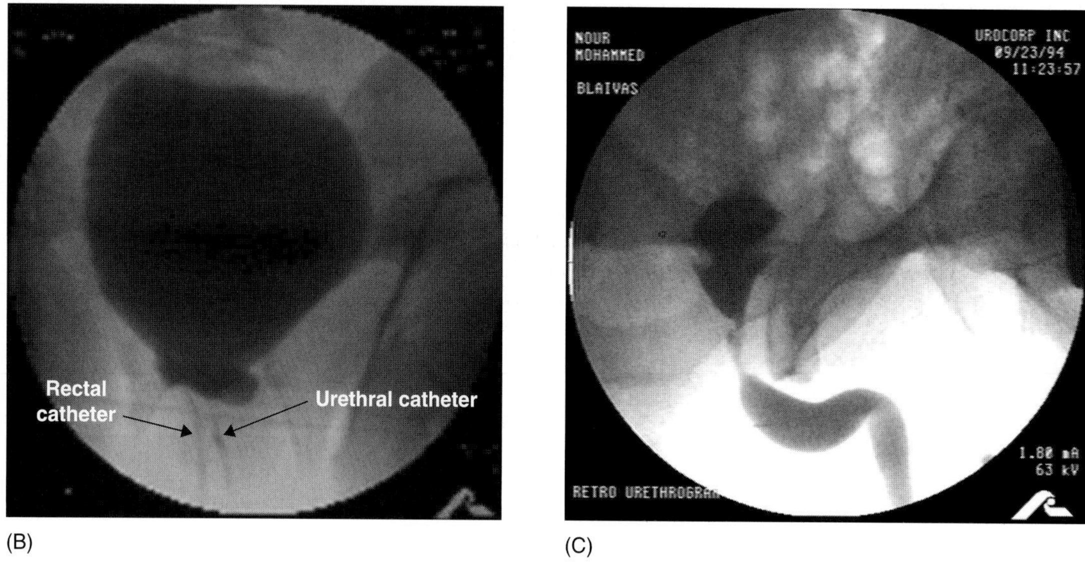

(B) (C)

Fig. 17.4 Post-prostatectomy incontinence due to detrusor overactivity. (A) Urodynamic study. There is no leakage when he coughs and strains, but immediately after straining, he has an involuntary detrusor contraction that he could not abort. (B) X-ray obtained during straining, just prior to the involuntary detrusor contraction. There is no leakage, but the posterior urethra has an unusual shape. (C) X-ray obtained towards the end of micturition.

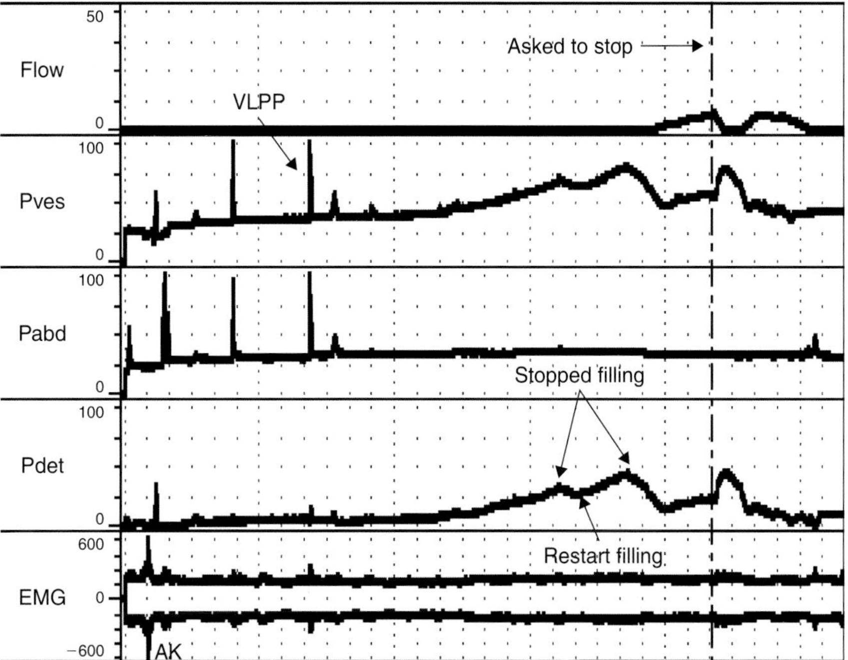

Fig. 17.5 Post-prostatectomy sphincteric incontinence and low bladder compliance. This is a 75-year-old man who underwent radical retropubic prostatectomy 3 years earlier. He developed postoperative stress incontinence immediately after removal of the catheter, but never underwent treatment for this. (A) Urodynamic study. FSF = 182 ml and 1st urge = 246 ml, during bladder filling there was a steep rise in Pdet. When filling was stopped, Pdet fell and when restarted it rose. Bladder compliance = 375 ml/48 cmH_2O = 7.8 ml/cmH_2O and bladder capacity was 390 ml. Vesical leak point pressure VLPP = 59 cmH_2O at bladder volume = 188 ml, Pdet/Q study: Q_{max} = 7 ml/s, Pdet@Q_{max} = 24 cmH_2O, Pdetmax = 46 cmH_2O, voided volume = 387 ml, and post-void residual (PVR) = 0 ml. On the Schafer nomogram, this represents grade 1 obstruction and impaired detrusor contractility. Preurodynamic uroflow, though was normal. Note that when he was asked to stop voiding, he interrupted his stream, flow fell to 0 and detrusor pressure rose. The only way this could happen is if he contracted his sphincter, yet the EMG was substantially unchanged. This once again demonstrates the fallibility of surface EMG recordings.

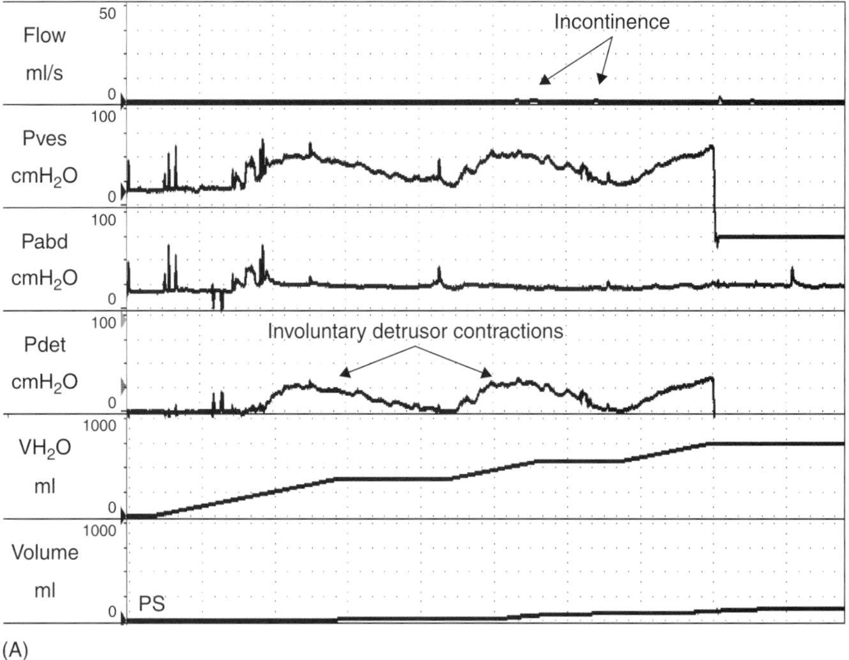

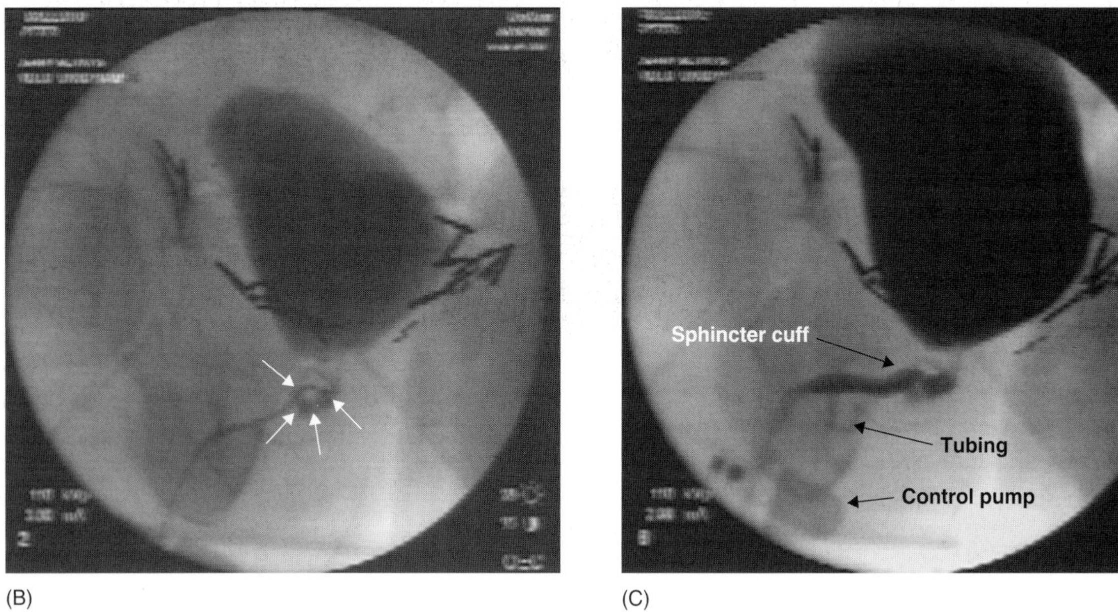

Fig. 17.6 Type 4 OAB and impaired detrusor contractility in a 70-year-old man 2 years S/P implantation of a sphincter prosthesis. He originally complained of mixed stress and urge incontinence and was also noted to have wide caliber anastomotic stricture. His symptoms were dramatically improved for several years postoperatively, then the urge incontinence worsened despite treatment with anticholinergics. (A) Urodynamic study. PVR = 0 ml, FSF = 124 ml, 1st urge = 238 ml, severe urge = 247 ml, bladder capacity = 750 ml. At a bladder volume of 247 ml there was an involuntary detrusor contraction. He perceived the contraction as urge, but was not able to contract his sphincter (EMG not used in this study). At bladder capacity, he was asked to void and voided the catheter out, but still could only generate a flow that barely activated the flowmeter. Unintubated uroflow: Q_{max} = 12 ml/s, voided volume = 159 ml, pattern = interrupted, PVR = 0 ml, Pdet/Q study, Q_{max} = 2.7 ml/s, Pdet@Q_{max} = 28 cmH_2O, Pdetmax = 28 cmH_2O, voided volume = 103 ml, and PVR = 647 ml. (B) X-ray obtained during bladder filling shows that the sphincter cuff (arrows) is closed (filled with contrast). (C) X-ray obtained at Q_{max} shows contrast getting past the sphincter during the involuntary detrusor contraction, causing incontinence, but the proximal urethra is barely visible. There are multiple surgical clips.

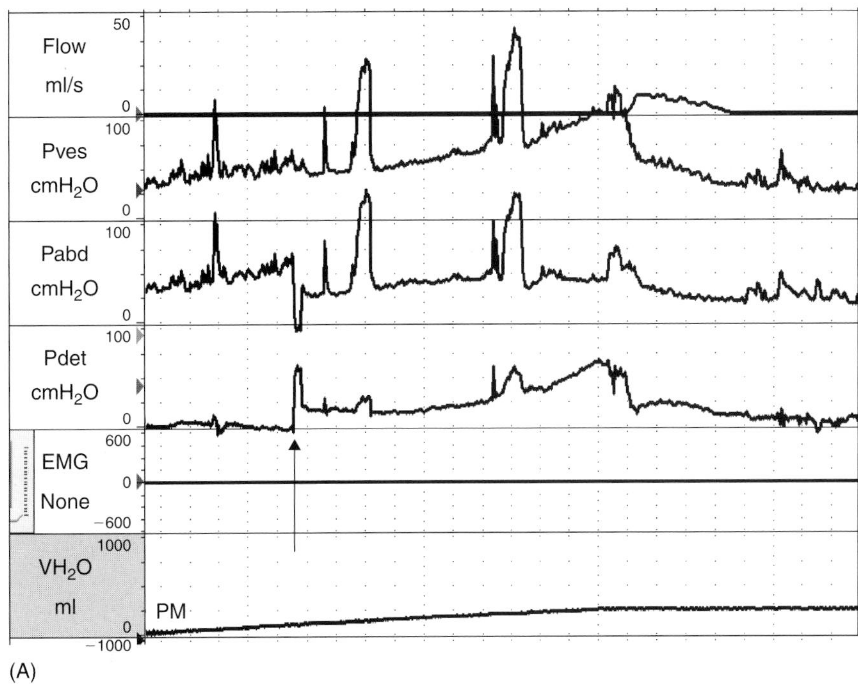

(A)

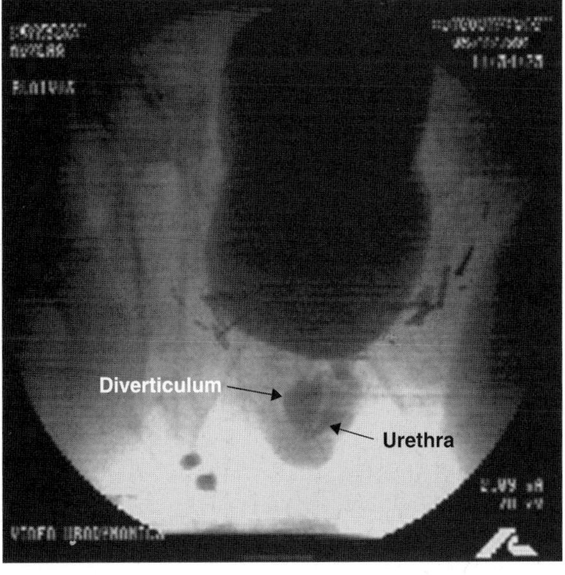

(B)

Fig. 17.7 Low bladder compliance and urethral diverticulum. This 72-year-old man underwent sphincter prosthesis about 5 years after radical retropubic prostatectomy. (A) Urodynamic tracing. FSF = 200 ml, 1st urge = 218 ml, severe urge = 265 ml. Bladder compliance was low (4 ml/cmH_2O). Note that at the arrow, the rectal pressure catheter fell out and the detrusor pressure artifactually rose. After rectal tube replacement, Pabd was lower than before the catheter fell out. This artifactually raised Pdet throughout the remainder of the tracing. There was no leakage during cough or strain to a Pvesmax = 194 cmH_2O, Pdet/Q study: Q_{max} = 10 ml/s, Pdet@Q_{max} = 22 cmH_2O, Pdetmax = 25 cmH_2O, voided volume = 271 ml, and PVR = 0 ml. (B) X-ray exposed during straining to 194 cmH_2O shows that there is no incontinence. There is urethral diverticulum proximal to the sphincter cuff.

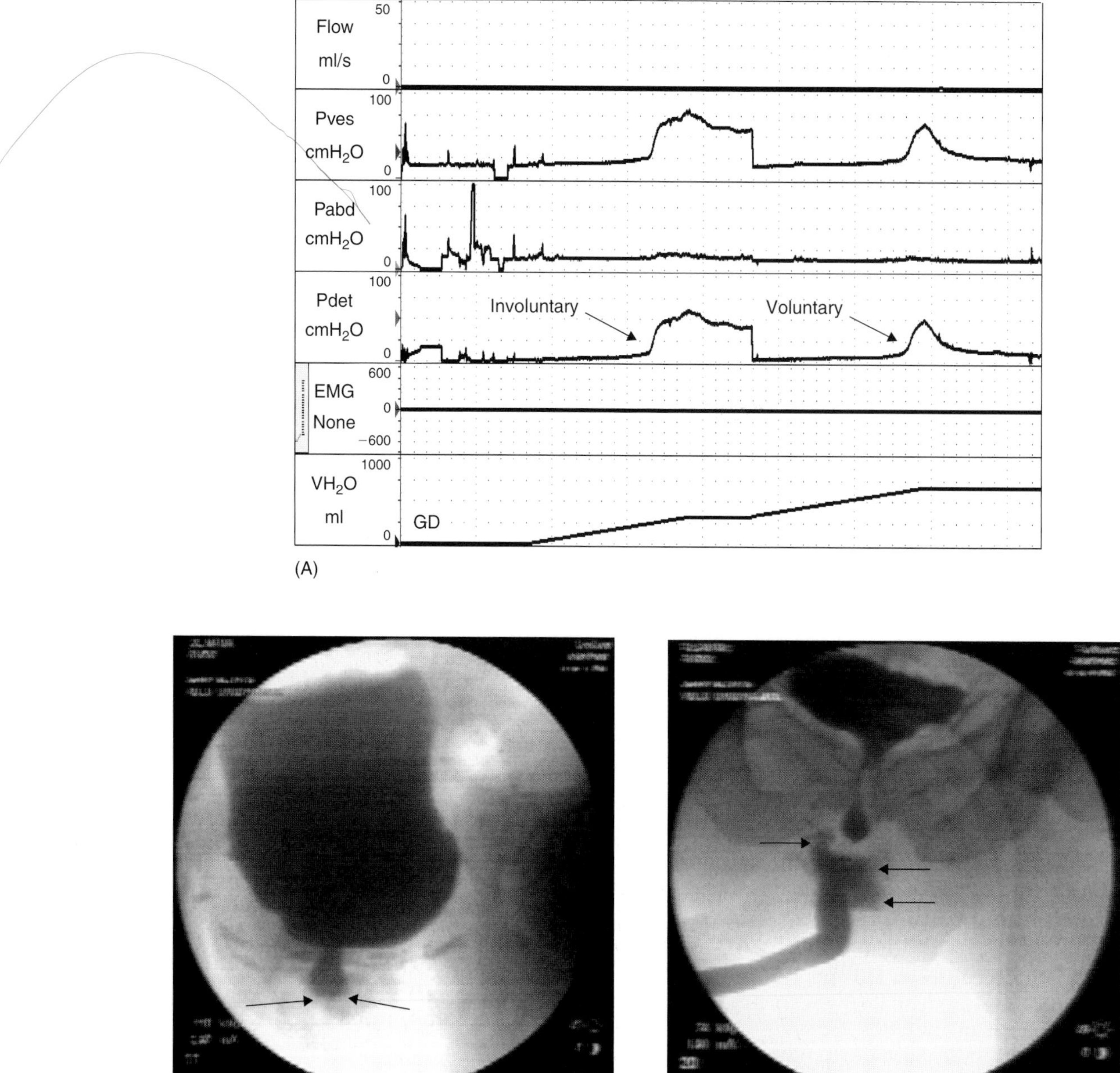

Fig. 17.8 Urethral erosion of male sling, detrusor overactivity and urethral obstruction. GD is a 63-year-old man S/P radical retropubic prostatectomy (1993) followed by external beam XRT. In status post he had mild incontinence until about 2004 which gradually worsened and he underwent three collagen injections followed by an InVance male sling. He developed urinary retention, was treated with a 14F Foley catheter and failed multiple voiding trials. (A) Urodynamic study. FSF = 178 ml, 1st urge = 201 ml, and severe urge = 326 ml coincident with an involuntary detrusor contraction. At bladder capacity (700 ml) he had a voluntary detrusor contraction to 50 cmH_2O, but only voided a small amount that barely activated the flowmeter. (B) X-ray obtained in the midst of the detrusor contraction shows obstruction at the membranous urethra (arrows). (C) X-ray obtained towards the end of the detrusor contraction shows extravasation of contrast along the sling (arrows).

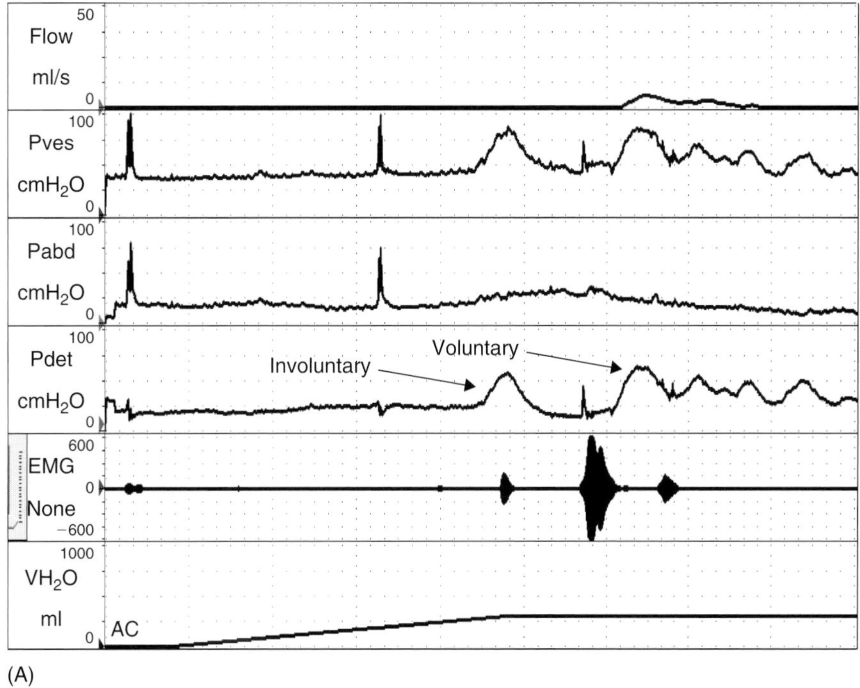

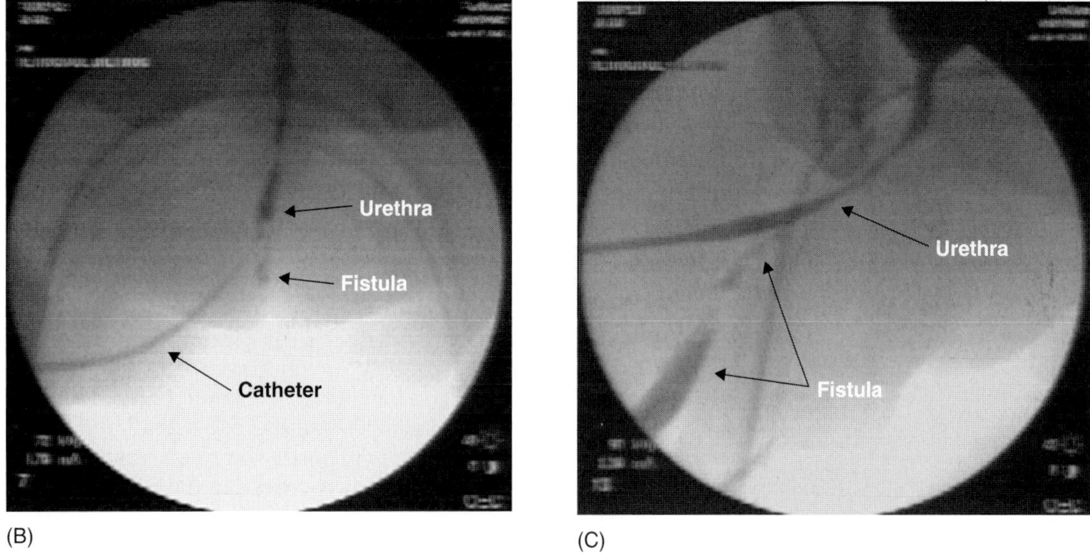

Fig. 17.9 Urethroscrotal fistula after erosion of sphincter prosthesis. AC is a 75-year-old man who underwent XRT for prostatic carcinoma followed by salvage prostatectomy 6 years later. He developed sphincteric incontinence and underwent sphincter prosthesis complicated by urethral erosion. After removal of the prosthesis, he developed this urethroscrotal fistula. (A) Urodynamic study. FSF = 101 ml, 1st urge = 201 ml, and severe urge = 296 ml. An involuntary detrusor contraction occurred at a bladder volume of 298 ml. He was able to contract his sphincter, prevent incontinence and abort the detrusor contraction. Note that the EMG channel was not recording very well. There was no leakage despite a cough to a Pves = 103 cmH_2O. Unintubated uroflow: Q_{max} 2 ml/s, voided volume: 336 ml, and PVR = 0 ml, Pdet/Q study: Grade 3 urethral obstruction, Q_{max} = 6 ml, Pdet@Q_{max} = 61 cmH_2O, Pdetmax = 64 cmH_2O, voided volume = 148 ml, and PVR = 144 ml. (B) X-ray obtained just as voiding begins shows a narrowed proximal urethra and a fistula. (C) X-ray obtained towards the end of micturition shows better visualization of the fistula.

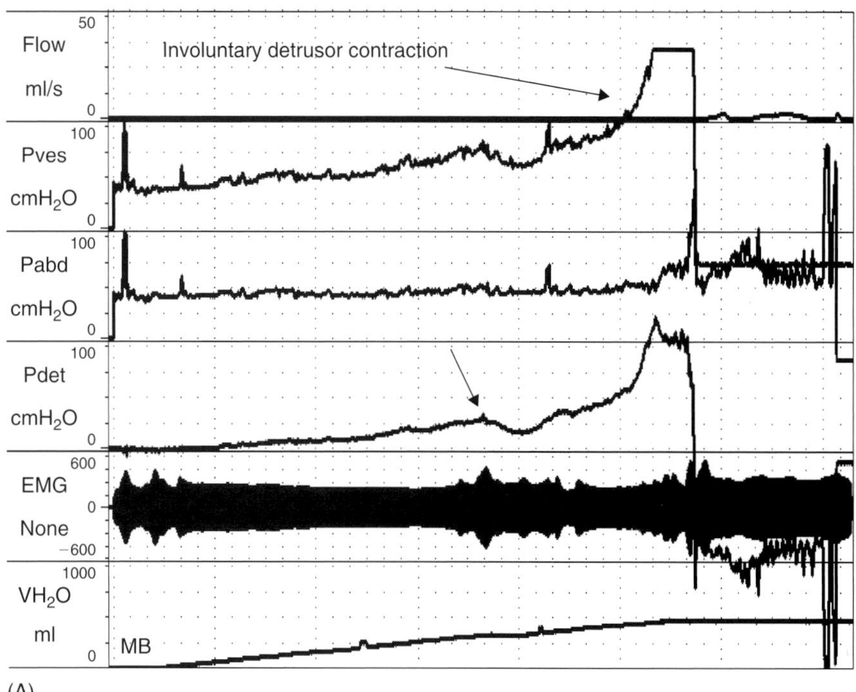

(A)

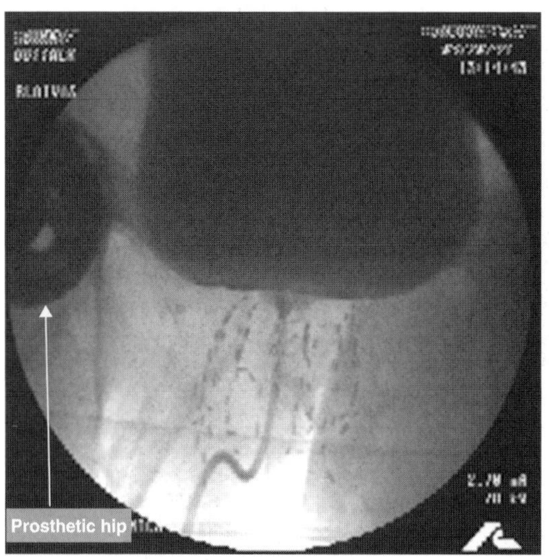

(B)

Fig. 17.10 Urethral obstruction, type 4 OAB and low bladder compliance after brachytherapy for prostate cancer. MB is a 66-year-old man who underwent brachytherapy 6 months previously. He complains of marked urinary frequency, urgency, urge incontinence, and difficulty voiding accompanied by weak stream. (A) Urodynamic study. During bladder filling there is a steep rise in Pdet. At a volume of 490 ml, he experienced an involuntary detrusor contraction that he could not abort and he voided the catheter out. At the short arrow bladder infusion was stopped and there was a fall in detrusor pressure confirming that the rise in pressure was due to compliance. (B) This X-ray was obtained just prior to expelling the catheter at the height of the rise in Pdet. There is complete obstruction just distal to the bladder neck. Note the multiple radiation seeds.

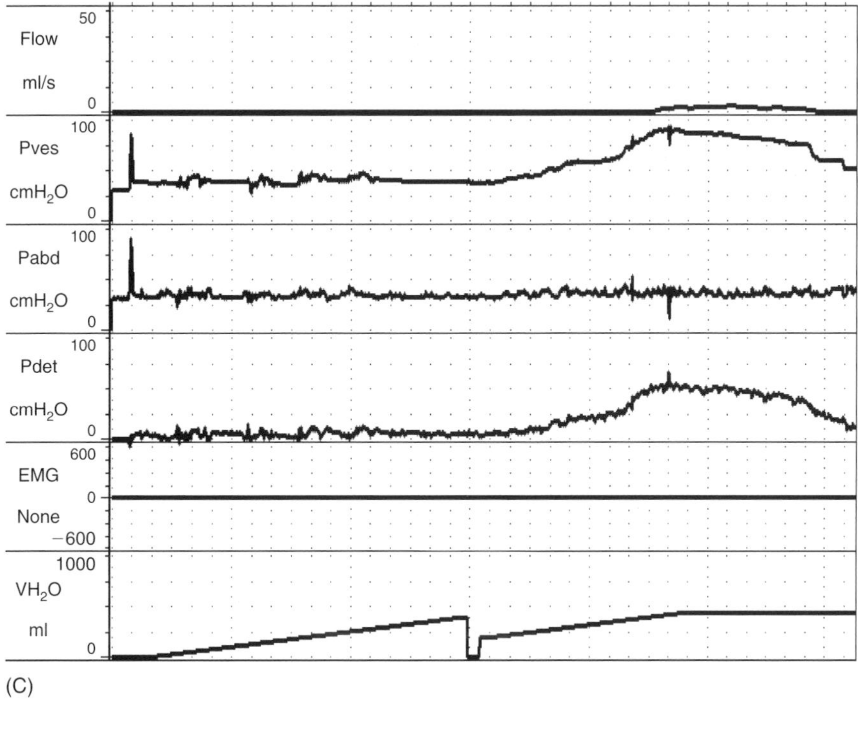

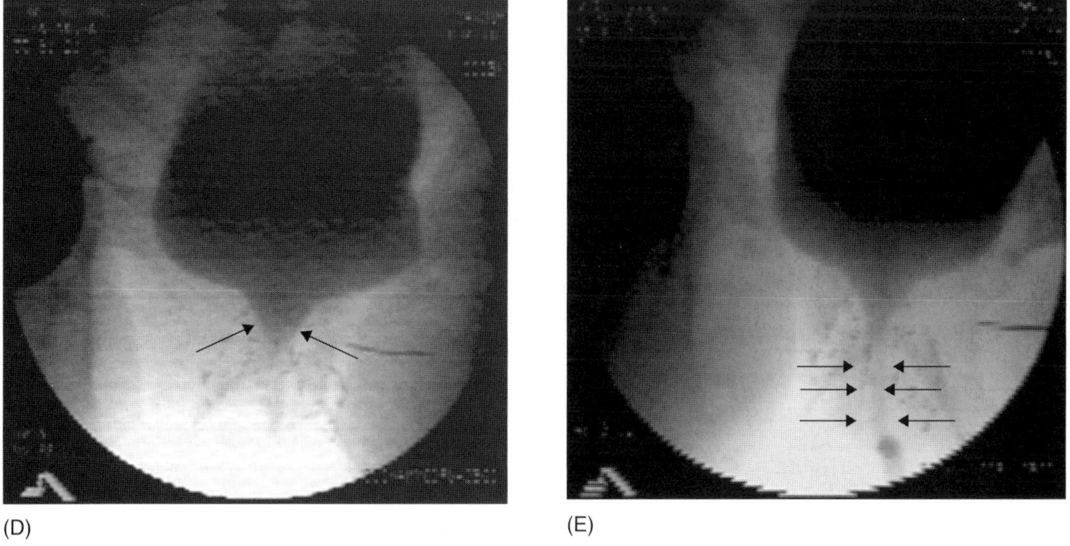

Fig. 17.10 (continued) (C) He underwent TURP and did well for about a year and then gradually developed worsening urinary frequency, urgency, urge incontinence, and difficulty voiding that culminated in urinary retention. Urodynamic study shows grade 3 urethral obstruction (Pdet@Q_{max} = 50 cmH_2O, Q_{max} = 4 ml/s). (D) X-ray obtained during bladder filling shows a TURP defect (arrows). (E) X-ray obtained during voiding shows that the obstruction is at the junction of the distal prostatic and membranous urethra (arrows). Cystoscopy showed that this was a stricture and after transurethral incision he developed sphincteric incontinence.

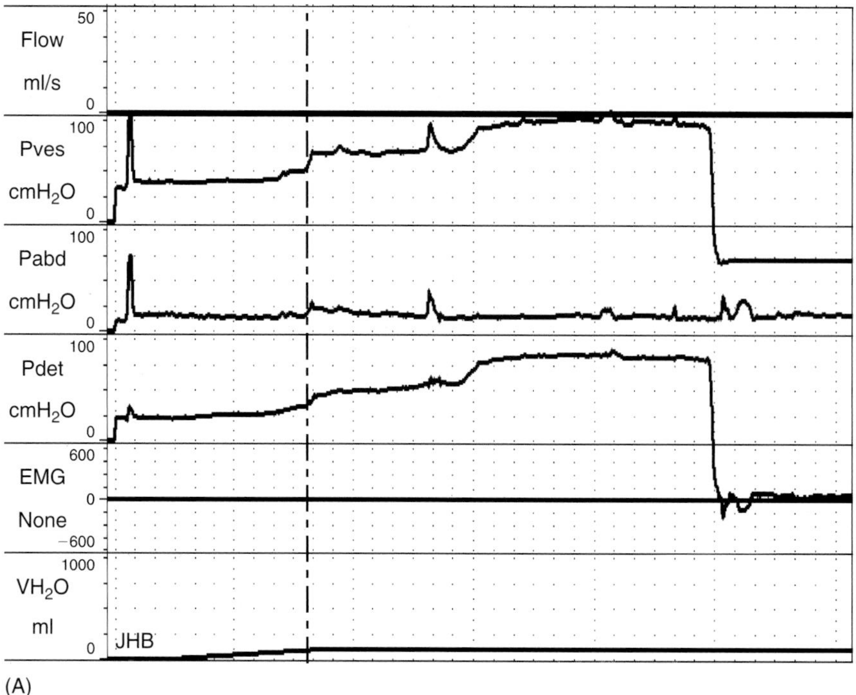

(A)

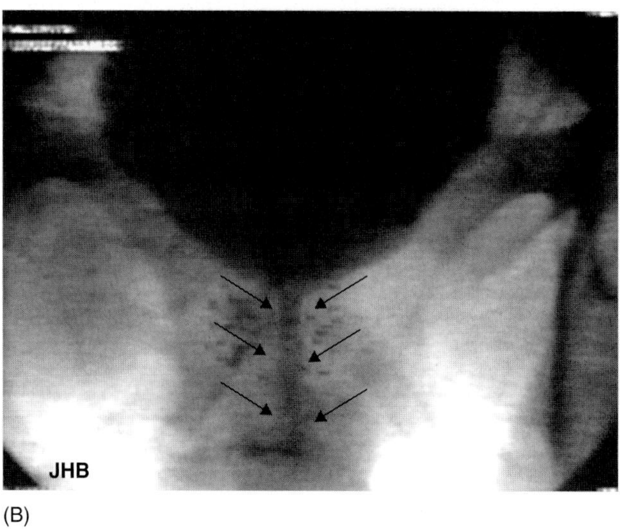

(B)

Fig. 17.11 Prostatic stricture and stone after brachytherapy for prostate cancer. JHB is a 77-year-old man who underwent brachytherapy 10 years ago because of T1c prostate cancer. He developed incontinence and 1½ years ago underwent TUR bladder neck contracture. Since then, the incontinence worsened. He's never able to void easily "I can squirt about a tablespoon full and then I do that over and over again." He ordinarily voids every hour during the day. He wears pads day and night and they are usually soaked. He was empirically treated with Ditropan and found that made it even more difficult to void. Cystoscopy showed a tight bladder neck contracture with an adherent stone. Subsequent to this study, he underwent KTP laser ablation of the stricture and removal of stone. Thereafter, he had severe sphincteric incontinence. (A) Urodynamic tracing. At a bladder volume of 108 ml there is an involuntary detrusor contraction that he could not abort. The sustained contraction reached a magnitude of 94 cmH_2O and flow was too low to activate the flowmeter. This corresponds to a grade 5 obstruction on the Schafer nomogram. Once the detrusor contraction began, bladder filling was stopped (vertical line). Detrusor pressure continued to rise proving that this was a detrusor contraction and not low bladder compliance. (B) X-ray obtained at Pdetmax shows multiple radiation seeds in the prostate and a narrowed, elongated prostatic urethra (arrows). When put in perspective with cystoscopic findings and the high detrusor pressure without measurable flow, the diagnosis is a long prostatic urethral stricture. The stone at the bladder neck is not visible on this X-ray.

18 Enterocystoplasty and Neobladder

Until the mid-1980's, there were few indications for enterocystoplasty and even the idea of creating a neobladder had not been formulated [1–4]. Low bladder compliance was not yet recognized as an important clinical entity and the "gold standard" for the treatment of end stage bladder was the ileal conduit, which has subsequently been shown to have a high complication rate [5,6]. Furthermore, from a psycho-social standpoint, it results in a less than satisfactory quality of life compared to treatments that do not require an external appliance [7].

In the 1980's neurogenic bladder was considered a relative contraindication to enterocystoplasty [1–4]; today it is one of the commonest indications, due primarily to the widespread acceptance of intermittent self catheterization as a means of bladder emptying [8–11]. It has been shown to be safe and effective for patients with refractory detrusor overactivity and low bladder compliance [9–12], but ineffective for patient with refractory interstitial cystitis [11]. Further, continent urinary diversion and neobladder have become the standard of care for patients undergoing cystectomy for bladder cancer; conduit diversion is mainly indicated for high risk patients [13–15].

The goal of enterocystoplasty and neobladder is to create a low pressure, high capacity urinary reservoir that can be emptied either by intermittent catheterization (Fig. 18.1), activation of the micturition reflex (Fig. 18.2) or by straining (Fig. 18.3). There are a number of different methods to construct a neobladder. We prefer the Studer technique (Fig. 18.4). Occasionally, augmentation cystoplasty can be utilized when patients require extensive partial cystectomy for bladder cancer (Fig. 18.5). When intermittent catheterization through the urethra is impractical or impossible, a continent catheterizable stoma has proven to be effective, but is still plagued by stomal complications [11,13,16]. If the patient is unable to catheterize at all, augmentation cystoplasty with and incontinent stoma (ileal chimney) can be considered [17,18].

Suggested Reading

1 Goodwin WE, Winter CC. Technique of sigmoidocystoplasty, *Surg Gynecol Obstet*, 108: 370–373, 1959.
2 Goodwin WE, Winter CC, Barker WF. "Cup-patch" technique of ileocystoplasty for bladder enlargement or partial substitution, *Surg Gynecol Obst*, 108: 200–248, 1959.
3 Hanley HG. Ileocystoplasty: a clinical review, *J Urol*, 62: 317–321, 1959.
4 Whitmore WF, Gittes RF. Reconstruction of the urinary tract by cecal and ileocecal cystoplasty – review of a 15 year experience, *J. Urol*, 129: 494–498, 1983.
5 Radomski SB, Herschorn S, Stone AR. Urodynamic comparison of ileum vs. sigmoid in augmentation cystoplasty for neurogenic bladder dysfunction, *Neurourol Urodynam*, 14(3): 231–237, 1995.

6 Madersbacher S, Schmidt J, Eberle JM, Thoeny HC, Burkhard F, Hochreiter W, Studer UE. Long-term outcome of ileal conduit diversion, *J Urol*, 169(3): 985–990, 2003.
7 Herschorn S, Hewitt RJ. Patient perspective of long-term outcome of augmentation cystoplasty for neurogenic bladder. *Urology*. 52(4):672–8, 1988.
8 Linder A, Leach GE, Raz S. Augmentation cystoplasty in the treatment of neurogenic bladder dysfunction, *J Urol*, 129: 491, 1983.
9 Goldwasser B, Webster GD. Augmentation and substitution enterocystoplasty, *J Urol*, 135: 215, 1986.
10 Luangkhot R, Peng B, Blaivas JG. Ileocecocystoplasty for the management of refractory neurogenic bladder: surgical technique and urodynamic findings, *J Urol*, 6: 1340–1344, 1991.
11 Blaivas JG, Weiss JP, Desai P, Flisser AJ, Stember D, Stahl P. Long term followup of augmentation enterocystoplasty and continent diversion in patients with benign disease, *J, Urol,* 173:1631–1634, 2005.
12 Sidi AA, Becher EF, Reddy PK, Dykstra DD. Augmentation enterocystoplasty for the management of voiding dysfunction in spinal cord injury patients, *J Urol*, 143: 83, 1990.
13 Benson MC, Olsson CA. Continent urinary diversion, *Urol Clin N A*, 26(1): 125–147, 1999.
14 Hautmann RE, de Petriconi R, Gottfried HW, Kleinschmidt K, Mattes R, Paiss T. The ileal neobladder: complications and functional results in 363 patients after 11 years of followup, *J Urol*, 161(2): 422–427, 1999.
15 Jonsson O, Olofsson G, Lindholm E, Tornqvist H. Long-time experience with the kock ileal reservoir for continent urinary diversion, *Eur Urol*, 40(6): 632–640, 2001.
16 De Ganck J, Everaert K, Van Laecke E, Oosterlinck W, Hoebeke P. A high easy-to-treat complication rate is the price for a continent stoma, *Br J Urol Int*, 90 (3): 240–243, 2002.
17 Schwartz SL, Kennelly MJ, McGuire EJ, Faerber GJ. Incontinent ileo-vesicostomy urinary diversion in the treatment of lower urinary tract dysfunction, *J Urol*,152: 99–102, 1994.
18 Atan A, Konety BR, Nangia A, Chancellor MB. Advantages and risks of ileovesicostomy for the management of neuropathic bladder. *Urology*, 54(4):636–40, 1999.
19 Flood HD, Malhotra SJ, O'Connell HE, Ritchey MJ, Bloom DA, McGuire EJ. Long-term results and complications using augmentation cystoplasty in reconstructive urology, *Neurourol Urodynam*, 14(4): 297–309, 1995.
20 Hautmann RE. Urinary diversion: ileal conduit to neobladder, *J Urol*, 169(3): 834–342, 2003.
21 Konety ABR, Nangia A, Chancellor MB. Advantages and risks of ileovesicostomy for the management of neuropathic bladder, *Urology*,54(4): 636–640, 1999.

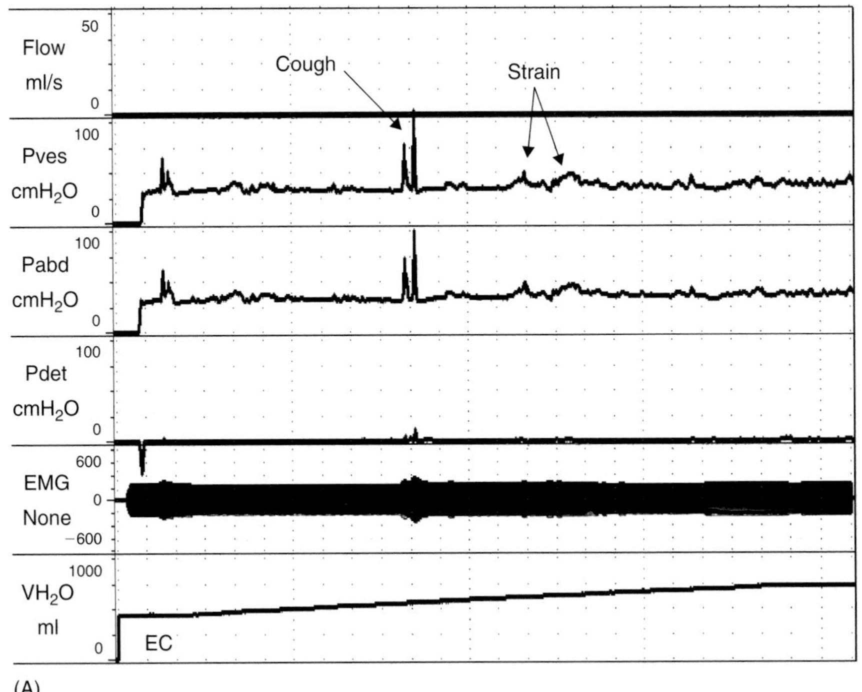

Fig. 18.1 Augmentation enterocystoplasty in a 35-year-old woman with exacerbating, remitting multiple sclerosis who underwent the operation 7 years earlier because of refractory detrusor-external sphincter dyssynergia (DESD). She is on intermittent catheterization 4 times a day and remains continent. (A) Urodynamic tracing shows and acontractile bladder with a capacity of over 750 ml, FSF = 435 ml, 1st urge = 650 ml, and severe urge = 750 ml. There is no incontinence despite coughing to over 100 cmH_2O.

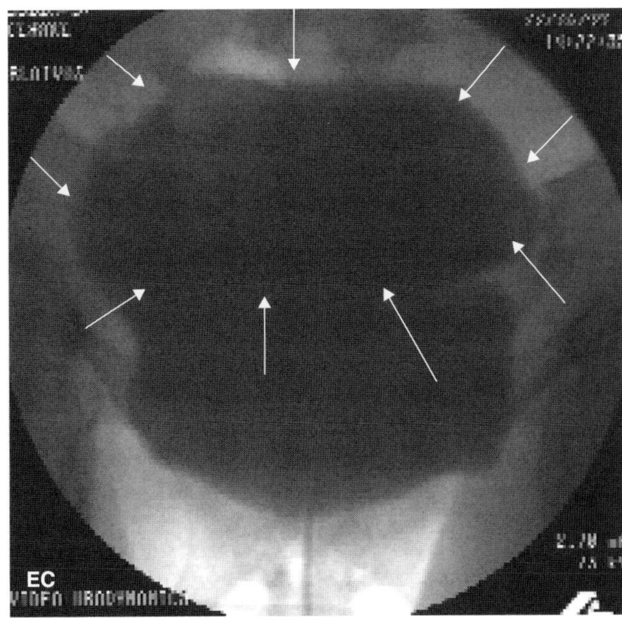

Fig. 18.1 (continued) (B) X-ray obtained at 550 ml shows that the augmented bladder has a somewhat irregular border, but the overall configuration is near normal. The arrows point to the ileal portion of the augmented bladder. (B)

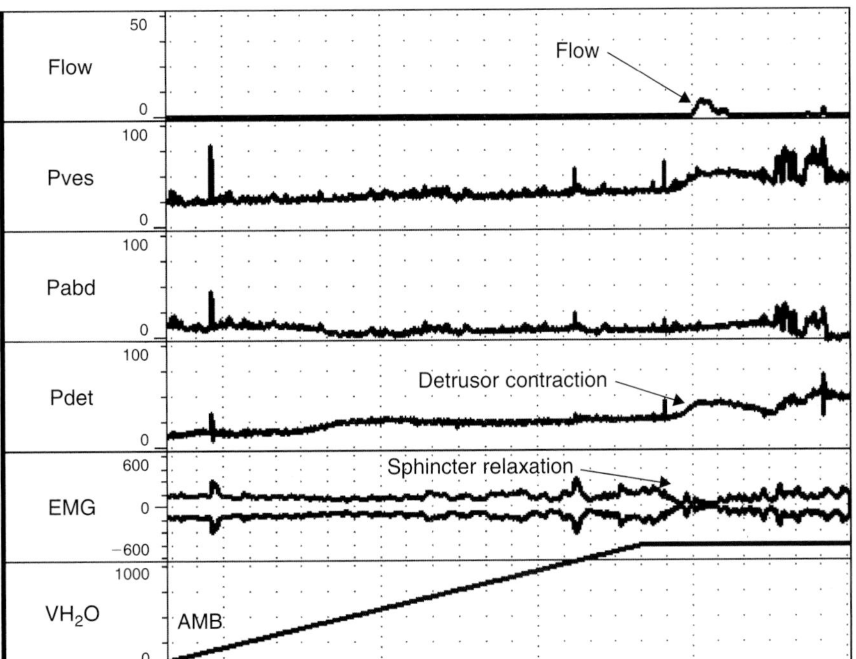

Fig. 18.2 Urodynamic study in a 43-year-old woman who underwent ileal augmentation cystoplasty 18 months earlier because of refractory idiopathic overactive bladder (OAB). Urodynamic study. FSF = 415 ml, 1st urge = 574 ml, and severe urge = 600 ml. Pressure flow study: Q_{max} = 8 ml/s, Pdet@Q_{max} = 43 cmH_2O, Pdetmax = 54 cmH_2O, voided volume = 216 ml, PVR = 975 ml. Note that she is able to void by voluntarily relaxing her sphincter and generating a voluntary detrusor contraction. She was only able to void, though, at a high bladder volume (1300 ml). After the catheter was removed, in the privacy of the bathroom, she voided to completion with a bell shaped curve and Q_{max} = 25 ml/s. VOID: 26/462/200. This corresponds to a mild grade 1 urethral obstruction on the Blaivas–Groutz nomogram.

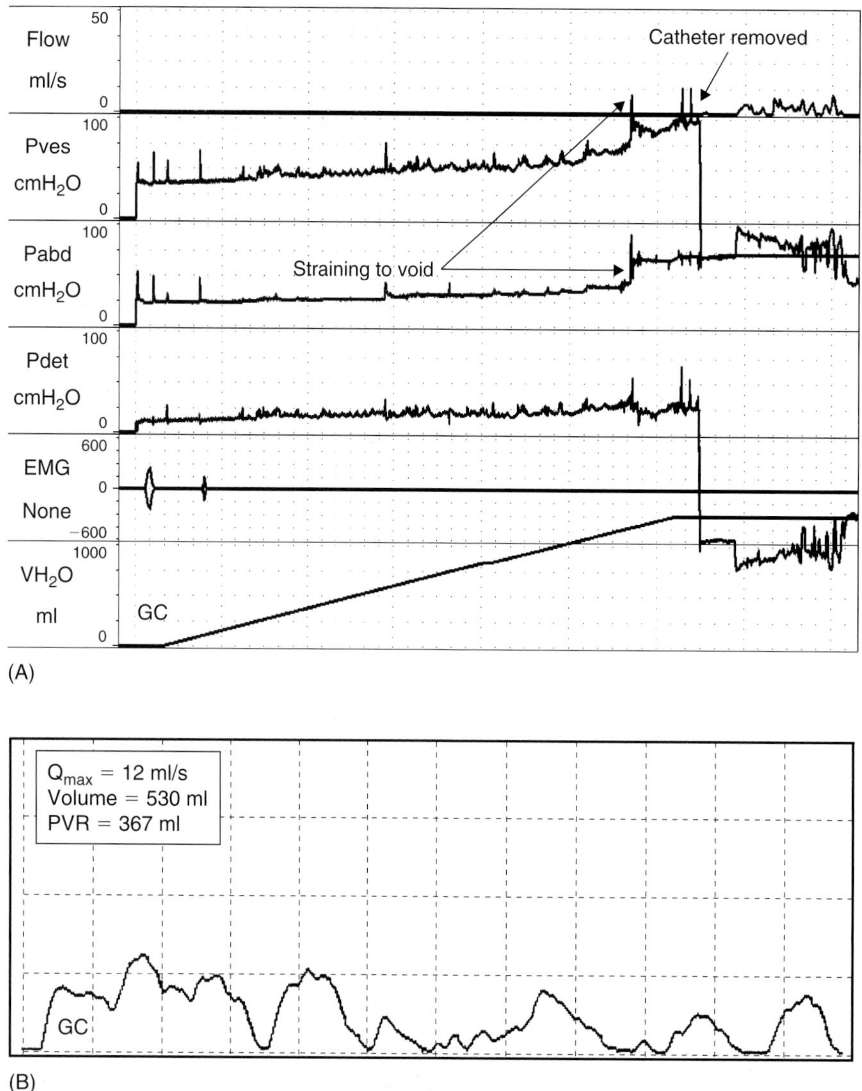

Fig. 18.3 Ileal neobladder. This is a 54-year-old man 2 years status post ileal (studer) neobladder for invasive bladder cancer. He voids by, straining, about every 4–6 hours during the day and does not have nocturia. He has occasional enuresis, but denies any other lower urinary tract symptoms (LUTS). (A) Urodynamic tracing. FSF = 559 ml, 1st urge = 1028 ml, severe urge = 1297 ml, and bladder capacity = 1311 ml. Note that when strains with the catheter in place, he was unable to void, but once the catheter was removed, he voided with an interrupted stream. The electromyography (EMG) channel was not working properly during this study. (B) Uroflow without the catheter shows a straining pattern.

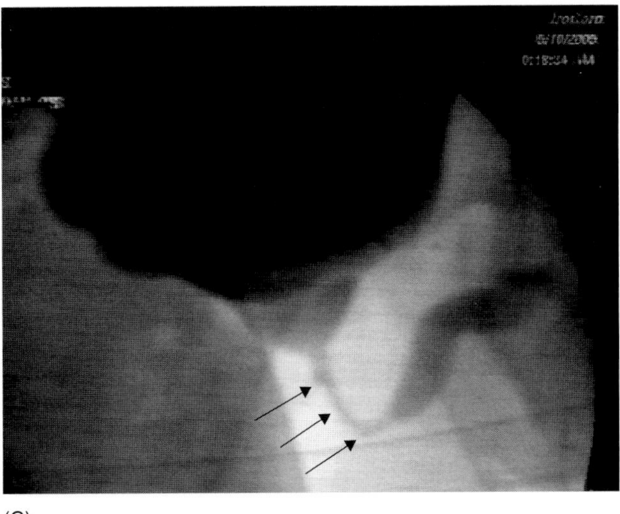

(C)

Fig. 18.3 (continued) (C) Straining to void. Note the narrowed bulbo-membranous urethra (arrows).

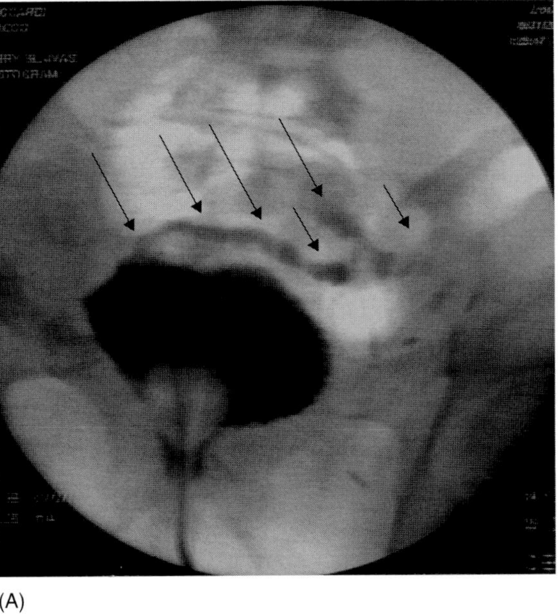

(A)

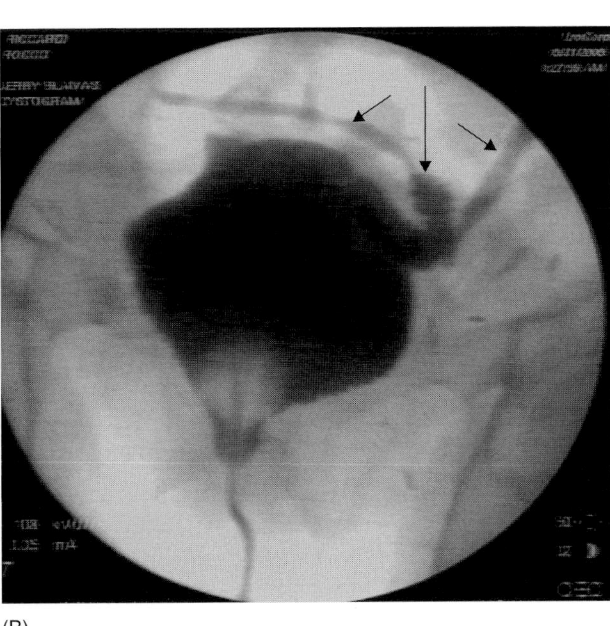

(B)

Fig. 18.4 Studer neobladder: 62-year-old man status post nerve sparing cystoprostatectomy and construction of ileal neobladder with Studer limb. He voids about 6 times a day, by design, but never senses an urge to void. He is never incontinent, day or night. (A) Cystogram obtained 3 weeks postoperatively with 100 ml in the bladder. The balloon of a Foley catheter is seen as a filling defect at the bladder base. The Studer limb is outlined by the arrows. (B) When he strains to void, there is bilateral vesicoureteral reflux (VUR) (small arrows). The Studer limb (large arrow) is comprised of a segment of ileum into which the ureters have been implanted.

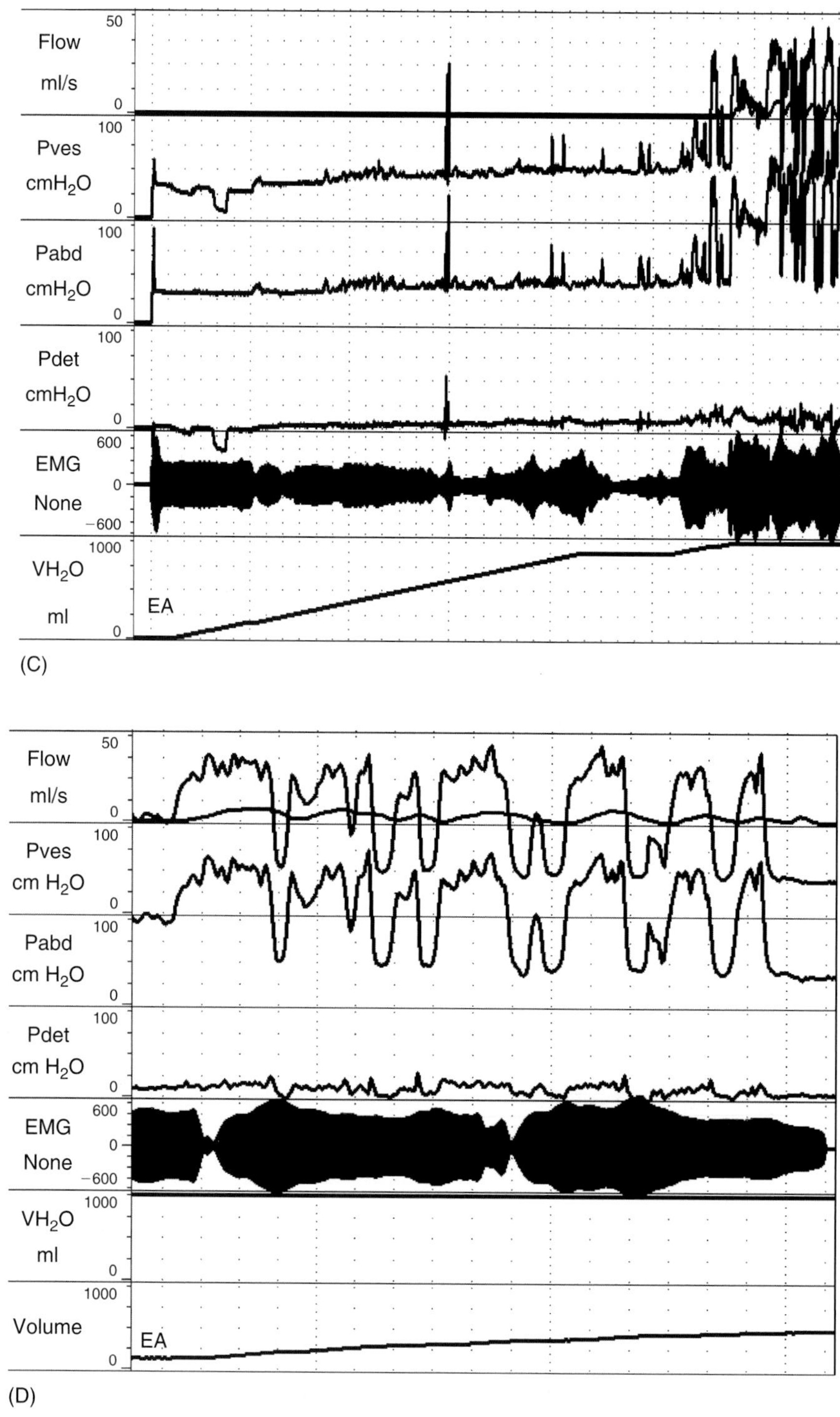

Fig. 18.4 (continued) (C) Urodynamic study obtained 3 years postoperatively in another patient who underwent ideal neobladder. In the filling phase of the study, he did not perceive the urge to void, but felt a vague fullness beginning at about 900 ml. He voided voluntarily by marked abdominal straining at a bladder volume of about 1 l. Q_{max} = 11 ml/s, voided volume = 492 ml, and post-void residual (PVR) = 510 ml. (D) A magnified view during voiding shows that flow occurs by abdominal straining, without a meaningful detrusor contraction. During each rise in vesical pressure, flow increases and when he stops straining, flow falls.

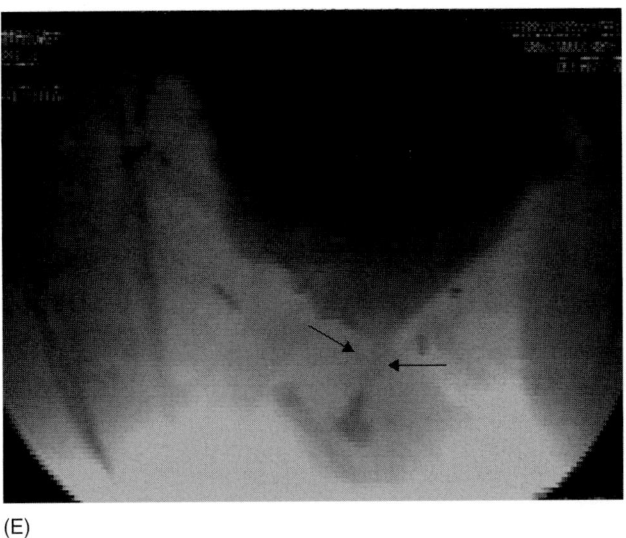

(E)

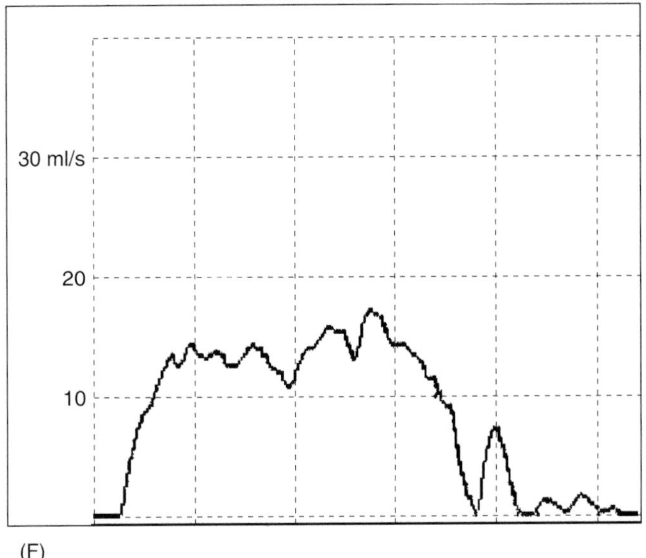

(F)

Fig. 18.4 (continued) (E) X-ray obtained during uroflow shows a somewhat irregular shape to the neobladder, although, overall, it looks pretty much like a bladder. The urethra just distal to the anastomosis is poorly visualized (arrows). Since while he was straining, it was not possible to obtain good X-rays during voiding, because the images were blurred. The urethra did open wider than seen here. There are surgical clips above the arrows. (F) Uroflow obtained prior to the urodynamic study show a very different pattern than that seen during the study. VOID: 13/333/0. This flow looks more like he was voiding with a detrusor contraction than by abdominal straining. He says "I always have to push a bit to start, then the urine comes out easily," without the need to strain.

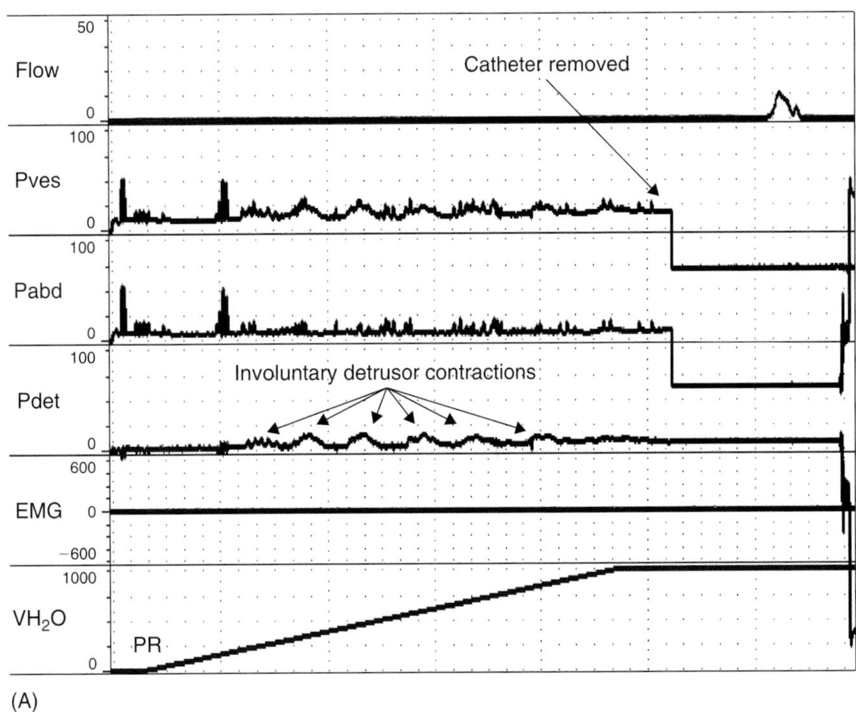

(A)

Fig. 18.5 Bilateral vesicoureteral reflux (VUR) and asymptomatic detrusor overactivity in an 87-year-old man 6 months status post partial cystectomy and augmentation cystoplasty for transitional cell carcinoma of the bladder (P2,N0,M0). (A) Urodynamic study: There are multiple low magnitude involuntary detrusor contractions during bladder filling that do not result in incontinence. FSF = 750 ml, 1st urge = 950 ml, and severe urge = 1001 ml, but he was unable to void with the catheter in place. After removal of the catheter, he had a normal uroflow without abdominal straining, but left a residual urine of 850 ml. Subsequently, in the privacy of the bathroom, he voided to completion.

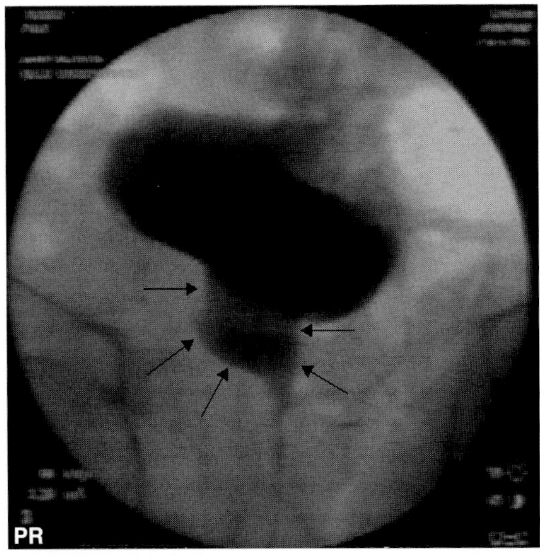

(B)

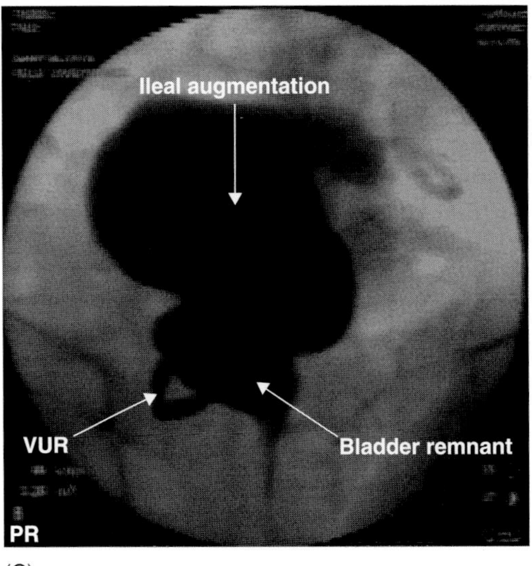

(C)

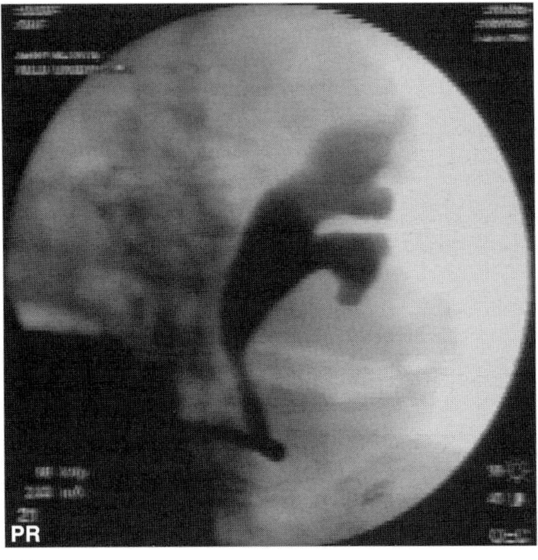

(D)

Fig. 18.5 (continued) (B) X-ray exposed during bladder filling at a volume of 100 ml shows what, at first glance, might be misconstrued as a reasonably normal bladder with a transurethral resection of the prostate (TURP) defect (arrows). (C) With further filling it becomes apparent that what appeared to be a wide open prostatic urethra is actually the bladder remnant and just above this is the augmented portion of the bladder. There is also right Vesicoureteral reflex. (D) During later filling there is grade 3 bilateral vesicoureteral reflux (only the left side is pictured here).

Index